WITHDRAWN

D0392374

ES

STUDIES OF NEUROTRANSMITTERS AT THE SYNAPTIC LEVEL

Advances in Biochemical Psychopharmacology

Volume 6

Advances in Biochemical Psychopharmacology

Series Editors

Erminio Costa, M.D.

Chief, Laboratory of Preclinical Pharmacology
National Institute of Mental Health
Washington, D.C., U.S.A.

Paul Greengard, Ph.D.

Professor of Pharmacology
Yale University School of Medicine
New Haven, Conn., U.S.A.

STUDIES OF NEUROTRANSMITTERS AT THE SYNAPTIC LEVEL

Advances in Biochemical Psychopharmacology
Volume 6

EDITORS

E. Costa, M.D.
Chief, Laboratory of Preclinical
Pharmacology
National Institute of Mental Health
Washington, D.C., U.S.A.

L. L. Iversen, M.D.
Department of Pharmacology
Cambridge University
Cambridge, England

R. Paoletti, M.D.
Professor and Director,
Institute of Pharmacology and Pharmacognosy
University of Milan
Milan, Italy

Raven Press • New York • 1972

© 1972 by Raven Press Books, Ltd. All rights re-
served. This book is protected by copyright. No part
of it may be duplicated or reproduced in any manner
without written permission from the publisher. Made
in the United States of America.

International Standard Book Number 911216–20–0
Library of Congress Catalog Card Number 73–84113

Preface

During the past few years there has been rapid development in neurochemistry, particularly as it relates to neurotransmitters. The contributions described in this volume indicate the level of sophistication that this area of research has attained. The breadth and ingenuity of experimental approaches to the study of the life history of neurotransmitters is impressive. Electron microscopy, histochemistry, cell biology, pharmacology, enzymology, and chemistry have each made special contributions. The use of such a variety of disciplines has proven to be a powerful stimulus for rapid advances in our understanding of the biochemistry and pharmacology of neurotransmitters.

The neuron contains highly branched nerve terminals with specific pre- and postsynaptic uptake and receptor mechanisms. The nerve terminals also contain storage vesicles and enzymes that synthesize and metabolize transmitter substances. These enzymes have a different subcellular localization and are under many controls. In addition, the central nervous system has a varied regional composition of transmitters, cell bodies, nerve terminals, and enzymes. All of this makes the chemistry of the nervous system different from any other organ. Thus, many of the papers described in this volume deal with the regional chemistry at the synaptic level. Some also give a glimpse of the future of this area, the disposition of possible new neurotransmitters, and the physical isolation of postsynaptic receptors.

Julius Axelrod
Washington, D.C.

v

Contents

vii

Advances in Biochemical Psychopharmacology, Vol. 6
Raven Press, New York © 1972

Application of Cytochemical Techniques to the Study of Suspected Transmitter Substances in the Nervous System

Tomas Hökfelt and Åke Ljungdahl

Karolinska Institutet, Stockholm, Sweden

An increasing number of substances are suspected of acting as neurotransmitters in the mammalian central nervous system (see e.g. Hebb, 1970). In order to establish their transmitter nature, several criteria must be fulfilled (Florey, 1960; McLennan, 1963; Werman, 1966), one of which is the demonstration—preferably both at the light- and electron-microscopic levels—of the occurrence of the substance within the neuron from which it is suspected of being released upon the arrival of nerve impulses. This has so far been possible only for a group of biogenic monoamines including dopamine (DA), noradrenaline (NA), and 5-hydroxytryptamine (5-HT), thanks to the development and application of various techniques (for references see Bloom, 1972; Hökfelt and Ljungdahl, 1972) such as the Falck-Hillarp formaldehyde fluorescence method (Falck, Hillarp, Thieme, and Torp, 1962).

In this chapter, some aspects of the intraneuronal localization of the monoamines and their storage sites will be discussed and, against this background, some recent autoradiographic results on the cellular and fine structural localization of several suspected amino acid neurotransmitters will be presented. For a more systematic presentation of the topic, we refer the reader to two recent articles (Bloom, 1972; Hökfelt and Ljungdahl, 1972).

GENERAL ASPECTS ON APPLICATION OF TECHNIQUES

The ideal way to study histochemically the localization of suspected neurotransmitters is to involve the substance itself in a specific, chemical reaction *in situ*, i.e., at the "physiological" storage site in the tissue, resulting in a product visible in a microscope. This principle of a *direct* visualization of the neurotransmitter has been achieved with the Falck-Hillarp method, where the amines react with formaldehyde vapors to form a fluorescent compound (Falck et al., 1962; Corrodi and Jonsson, 1967; Falck and Moore, 1972). In all probability, the ultrastructural demonstration of an electron-dense core (precipitate) within synaptic vesicles in monoamine neurons after various fixation methods (OsO_4, a combined glutaraldehyde-OsO_4 sequence, or $KMnO_4$) may represent similarly direct techniques for electron-microscopic studies (for discussion see Bloom, 1970, 1972; Hökfelt, 1970, 1971). Also in autoradiographic studies of suspected neurotransmitters (see, e.g., Wolfe, Potter, Richardson, and Axelrod, 1962; Aghajanian and Bloom, 1966; Descarries and Droz, 1970) the transmitter substance itself is traced. Future developments of new direct techniques may involve immunological principles — immunohistochemistry — since it has recently been possible to make antibodies to a small molecule such as histamine (Davies and Meade, 1970), one of the suspect neurotransmitters.

A different approach is based on attempts to visualize substances closely related to the suspected transmitter such as the enzymes involved in transmitter metabolism. This *indirect* tracing of transmitters may be exampified by the precipitation techniques for acetylcholine esterase (Koelle and Friedenwald, 1949) or choline acetyltransferase (Burt, 1970; Kása, Mann, and Hebb, 1970) for tracing neurons releasing acetylcholine (ACh) at the synapse. Immunohistochemical methods have also been introduced recently, but so far only for enzymes involved in catecholamine (CA) synthesis (Geffen, Livett, and Rush, 1969; Fuxe, Goldstein, Hökfelt, and Joh, 1970a, 1971; Goldstein, Fuxe, Hökfelt, and Joh, 1971; Hartman and Udenfriend, 1970). Enzymes involved in ACh and γ-aminobutyric acid (GABA) metabolism have also been traced autoradiographically using labeled enzyme inhibitors such as diisopropyl fluorophosphate (Ostrowski and Barnard, 1961), hemicholinium, and thiosemicarbazide (Knyihár and Csillik, 1970).

BIOGENIC MONOAMINES (DA, NA, AND 5-HT)

Methodology

The wealth of information available on the localization of DA, NA, and 5-HT both in nervous and non-nervous tissues stems from a variety of light- and electron-microscopic techniques (see Pearse, 1960). However, a more systematic mapping of the occurrence of monoamines in nervous tissues started out with the introduction of the Falck-Hillarp fluorescence method—based on the formation of fluorescent isoquinolines (from DA and NA) or carbolines (from 5-HT) after paraformaldehyde treatment (see Corrodi and Jonsson, 1967)—leading to a profound knowledge of the distribution of monoamine neurons both in the peripheral and central nervous systems (see Fuxe, Hökfelt, Jonsson, and Ungerstedt, 1970*b;* Falck and Moore, 1972).

The fluorescence histochemical results have provided a valuable basis for attempts to extend the knowledge of localization of monoamines to the ultrastructural level. Such attempts to visualize a substance in the electron microscope are basically dependent on the possibility of involving the amine in a reaction with a heavy metal that will result in an electron-dense precipitate. Fortunately, test-tube experiments have revealed that DA, NA, and 5-HT all react with almost all routine fixatives for electron microscopy to form precipitates (see Table 1). As to one-step fixation procedures with

TABLE 1. *Reaction between various fixatives and amines in test-tube experiments*

Amine	Fixative				
	$OsO_4{}^a$	$KMnO_4{}^b$	PF^c	$Glut.^d$	$Glut. + OsO_4{}^d$ or $K_2Cr_2O_7$
Noradrenaline	+	++	0	+	+
Dopamine	+	++	0	+	+
Adrenaline	+	++	0	0	+
5-Hydroxytryptamine	+	++	0	+	+
L-DOPA	+	++			
Metaraminol	0	+			
β-Phenylethylamine		0			

(From Hökfelt, 1971.)
The formation of a precipitate is indicated by a plus.
[a] Van Orden et al., 1966.
[b] Hökfelt and Jonsson, 1968.
[c] Hopsu and Mäkinen, 1966.
[d] Wood and Barrnett, 1964; Coupland et al., 1964.

metallic oxidants such as OsO_4 and $KMnO_4$, a redox reaction seems to take place, where the amines reduce the fixatives mainly to osmium dioxide and manganese dioxide, respectively. The hydroxyl groups of the amine molecules, mainly the phenolic ones, seem to be responsible for this reaction since NA (with two phenolic OH groups) gives a strong reaction, metaraminol (with one phenolic OH group) gives only a weak reaction, and β-phenylethylamine (with no OH group) gives no reaction when mixed in test tubes with $KMnO_4$ (see Fig. 1). Precipitates are also obtained in test tubes with a

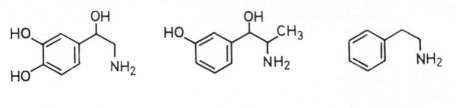

Noradrenaline   Metaraminol   β-Phenylethylamine

FIG. 1. Molecular structures of three monoamine analogs: noradrenaline (with two phenolic hydroxyl groups), metaraminol (with one hydroxyl group) and β-phenylethylamine (with no hydroxyl group). See text and Table 1.

glutaraldehyde-OsO₄ sequence. In the first step, glutaraldehyde probably reacts with the amine group (see, e.g., Tramezzani, Chiocchio, and Wassermann, 1964; Coupland, Pyper, and Hopwood, 1964; Wood and Barrnett, 1964) leaving the OH groups free for a subsequent reaction with OsO₄ as discussed above.

The first evidence from experiments on intact tissues that neuronal monoamines may react with the fixative and give rise to an electron-dense precipitate was obtained already in 1961, when De Robertis and Pellegrino de Iraldi (1961a, b) and Lever and Esterhuizen (1961) described a special type of synaptic vesicles containing an electron-dense precipitate (dense-core or granular vesicles) in probable adrenergic neurons. In subsequent studies on various tissues and species, these findings could sometimes be confirmed, sometimes not. Since then, owing to the introduction of new fixation procedures and pharmacological manipulations (some important advances are listed in Table 2), general agreement now exists that the so-called small granular or dense-core vesicles (see below) are monoamine storage sites (Fig. 2).

Although many pharmacological and experimental results favor the view that the dense core of the small granular vesicles reflects the amine content, there is some doubt about the validity of this correlation, at least for KMnO₄-fixed tissues (see, e.g., Bloom, 1972). This is mainly due to a lack of correlation between the presence of the electron-dense core and the retention of the amine as revealed in experiments with labeled NA (Devine and Laverty, 1968; Hökfelt and Jonsson, 1968). Thus, KMnO₄ fixation gives a high yield of dense-core vesicles (and few empty or agranular vesicles) but a low retention of the amine, whereas a combined fixation with glutaraldehyde and OsO₄ often gives few dense-core vesicles (and many empty vesicles) but a high retention of the amines (Table 3). This has re-

TABLE 2. *Fixation procedures for the demonstration of small granular vesicles in monoamine neurons*

Fixative	Tissue	Reference
A. Metallic oxidants		
1. OsO_4	Pancreas	Lever and Esterhuizen (1961)
	Pineal	De Robertis and Pellegrino de Iraldi (1961a)
	Vas deferens	Richardson (1962)
	Iris	Richardson (1964)
	Intestine	Grillo and Palay (1962)
2. $KMnO_4$	PNS, CNS	Richardson (1966)
		Hökfelt (1968)
B. Aldehyde + metallic oxidants		
1. Glut. ald.-OsO_4	Vas deferens	Bloom and Barrnett (1966); Van Orden et al. (1966)
	Pineal	Machado (1967)
2. Glut. ald.-$K_2Cr_2O_7$	CNS	Wood (1966)
(-OsO_4)	Pineal	Jaim-Etcheverry and Zieher (1968)
	Iris	Tranzer and Thoenen (1968)
3. Glut. ald. + formald. -$K_2Cr_2O_7$(-OsO_4)	Vas deferens	Tranzer and Snipes (1968)
4. Acrylic ald. -$K_2Cr_2O_7$(-OsO_4)	Heart	Woods (1969)
5. Formald.-glut. ald. -$K_2Cr_2O_7$(-OsO_4)	CNS	Wood (1967)
	Pineal (5-HT)	Jaim-Etcheverry and Zieher (1968)
C. Pharmacological tools increasing amine levels		
1. Endogenous, e.g., MAO inhibition		
2. Exogenous		
a) "True" transmitter, e.g., NA		Tranzer and Thoenen (1967b)
		Hökfelt (1968)
b) "False" transmitter, α-methyl-NA		Bondareff (1966)
		Hökfelt (1967, 1968)
5-OH-DA		Tranzer and Thoenen (1967a)

(From Hökfelt, 1971.)

sulted in difficulties with autoradiographic studies on $KMnO_4$-fixed tissues (Taxi, 1968; Bloom, 1970, 1972; Descarries and Droz, 1970).

The specificity of $KMnO_4$ fixation has been discussed previously (Hökfelt and Jonsson, 1968; Hökfelt, 1970, 1971), but the following points may be summarized.

(1) As seen in Table 3, all the amine is not lost but about 50% remains in the tissue, and autoradiographic studies in our laboratory have indeed shown that marked accumulations of grains can be seen, e.g., over nerve

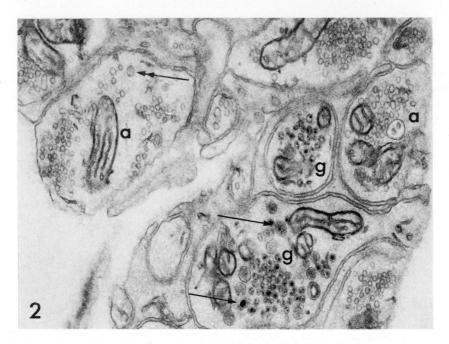

FIG. 2. Electron micrograph of guinea pig iris. A number of varicosities (nerve endings, axonal enlargements) are seen. Two (g), probably adrenergic ones, contain granular vesicles (mainly small ones) with a few of the large type (arrows). The other varicosities (a) contain only agranular vesicles—also, the large ones have an empty interior (double/arrow). They probably belong to cholinergic nerves. $KMnO_4$ fixation. Magnification × 35,000.

TABLE 3. *Fate of ^3H-NA during fixation and dehydration procedure*

	3% $KMnO_4$ (30 min)	5% Glut. (90 min)	5% Glut. (30 min)	1% OsO_4 (90 min)	5% Glut. (30 min) +1% OsO_4 (60 min)
Fixative 1	18[a]	26	15	26	13
Ringer (10 min)	14	10	11	4	9
Fixative 11	—	—	—	—	9
Ringer (10 min)	—	—	—	—	2
Ethanol (45 min)	2	7	4	1	0
Propyleneoxide (30 min)	0	0	0	0	0
Tissue	53	57	70	65	71
Total	87	100	100	96	104

(From Hökfelt and Jonsson, 1968.)

[a] The figures represent the percentage of radioactivity found in solutions and tissue as compared to the total amount of ^3H-NA present in control irides not fixed and processed.

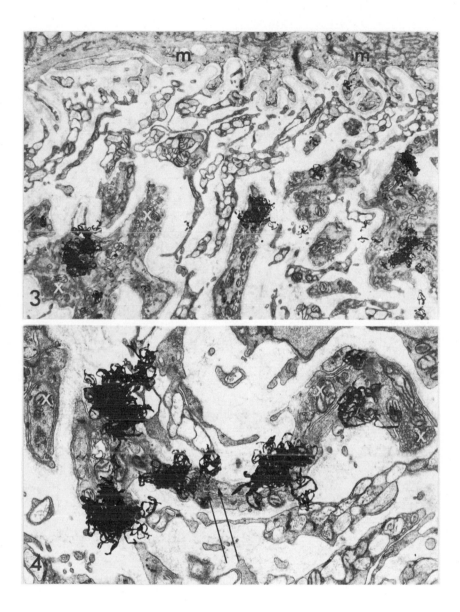

FIGS. 3 and 4. Electron-microscopic autoradiographs of rat iris, incubated with ³H-noradrenaline (10^{-6} M). A number of nerves are seen covered by strong accumulations of grains. The grains almost completely cover the varicosities but granular vesicles can be seen at arrows in Fig. 4. Nerve endings with agranular vesicles (x), however, lack activity. Muscle cells (m) of the dilator muscle plate are seen at the top of Fig. 3. KMnO₄ fixation. Magnifications × 10,000 and 20,000, respectively.

endings in the rat iris after incubation with ^{3}H-NA (10^{-6} M) and $KMnO_4$ fixation (Figs. 3 and 4).

(2) A low retention of amine after fixation does not imply a lack of correlation between precipitate and amine levels. Thus, after the initial redox reaction, the oxidized amine may not be chemically bound within the precipitate and may thus partially be washed out. It is, therefore, possible to state only that the dense core reflects the amine content *at the moment of fixation*, which is sufficient for most studies, with the exception, of course, of autoradiography.

(3) The specificity of the $KMnO_4$ fixation can be seriously questioned since $KMnO_4$ reacts with innumerable substances. Therefore, the correlation between precipitate and amines is not based on a specificity of the reaction between these two substances but rather on the fact that the vesicles contain the amines in extremely high concentrations, as the following calculation shows. The amount of NA in one varicosity of the adrenergic axon terminals in the rat iris dilator muscle has been calculated to be about 5×10^{-3} pg (Dahlström, Häggendal, and Hökfelt, 1966) and the number of vesicles in one varicosity to be roughly 500 (Hökfelt, 1969; see Fig. 5). The radius of one vesicle is about 250 Å of which the membrane constitutes 70 Å; i.e., the radius of the vesicle "cavity" is about 180 Å. If, hypothetically, all the NA is stored within the vesicles [i.e., if none is localized in the extravesicular space and none within the membrane (which in fact makes up about 65% of the total vesicle volume)], the NA concentration in the vesicle is about 2.4 M (Fig. 6)!

(4) In addition to these general considerations, there are a number of more specific experiments favoring the view that the dense core indeed reflects the amine levels in the vesicle. Thus, most pharmacological and experimental (electrical stimulation, denervation) results (summarized, e.g., in Hökfelt, 1968, 1970; Bloom, 1970, 1972) are in agreement with this view

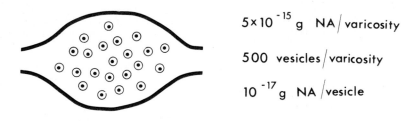

5×10^{-15} g NA/varicosity

500 vesicles/varicosity

10^{-17} g NA/vesicle

FIG. 5. Schematic illustration of an adrenergic varicosity in rat iris dilator muscle with granular vesicles (more than 95% are of the small type; see Hökfelt, 1969). The amount of NA in one vesicle can be calculated to about 10^{-17} g (see text).

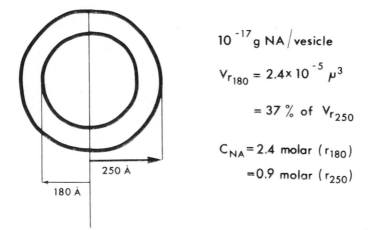

$$10^{-17} \, g \, NA / vesicle$$

$$V_{r_{180}} = 2.4 \times 10^{-5} \, \mu^3$$

$$= 37 \% \text{ of } V_{r_{250}}$$

$$C_{NA} = 2.4 \text{ molar } (r_{180})$$

$$= 0.9 \text{ molar } (r_{250})$$

FIG. 6. Schematic illustration of a small granular vesicle with a diameter of about 500 Å and a membrane thickness of about 70 Å. The concentration of NA in the vesicle can be calculated to lie between 2.4 M (if all NA is in the interior cavity of the vesicle) and 0.9 M (if all NA is equally distributed over the whole vesicle, i.e., also within the membrane) (see text).

although some results have been interpreted to represent discrepancies (see Bloom, 1972; Goldstein and Bloom, 1970).

(5) It may, finally, be added that the term "granular vesicle" may soon give rise to serious confusion. Any successful attempt to visualize in the electron microscope a suspected transmitter substance in a synaptic vesicle will result in a "granular vesicle." Thus, the zinc-iodide-OsO$_4$ technique as used by Akert and colleagues (Akert and Sandri, 1968, 1970) results in electron-dense precipitates in *all* types of small synaptic vesicles and they do probably not reflect the transmitter content (Pellegrino de Iraldi and Gueudet, 1968; Matus, 1970). Furthermore, fixation with OsO$_4$ at +60°C reveals electron-dense precipitates in small vesicles in certain boutons, e.g., in the paraventricular nucleus. These precipitates also occur after reserpine treatment (Bloom and Aghajanian, 1968b) and may thus not be related to amine stores.

Although the concentrations of the amines within the vesicles are high, the absolute amount is, of course, very small, demonstrating the high sensitivity of the fixation technique required to visualize amine stores at the ultrastructural level. With the KMnO$_4$ technique, we observe dense cores in nerves in the iris dilator muscle of rats treated with a catecholamine synthesis inhibitor which lowers amine levels to about 20% of normal. With 5×10^{-3} pg NA present in one normal varicosity and 500 vesicles in this varicosity (see above), the amount detectable with $KMnO_4$ fixation would thus be about 2×10^{-6} pg (Fig. 5). A similar calculation for the sensitivity of the Falck-Hillarp technique gives a figure of 5×10^{-4} pg (Jonsson, 1971).

Small and Large Granular Vesicles

Grillo and Palay (1962) were the first to demonstrate that there seemed to be at least two populations of granular vesicles in the same neuron, distinguished by their size: small granular vesicles with a diameter of about 500 Å and large granular vesicles with a diameter of about 1,000 Å (see Fig. 2). Subsequent studies have justified this classification, and there is now evidence that they differ not only in size but also in chemical composition and function. Some interesting aspects of this topic may be summarized as follows.

Both small and large granular vesicles are present in monoamine neurons, where both types in all probability contain an amine as revealed with the bichromate technique (Wood, 1966; Tranzer and Thoenen, 1968) and $KMnO_4$ (see Fig. 2) (Hökfelt, 1968, 1969), and both types are also able to take up exogenous amines (Tranzer and Thoenen, 1967; Hökfelt, 1968).

However, whereas the small granular vesicles seem to occur exclusively in monoamine neurons, large granular vesicles can in addition be demonstrated also in non-monoamine neurons provided that glutaraldehyde-OsO_4 fixation is used (see, e.g., Coupland, 1965; Fuxe, Hökfelt, and Nilsson, 1965; Fuxe, Hökfelt, Nilsson, and Reinius, 1966; Clementi, Mantegazza, and Botturi, 1966). With $KMnO_4$ fixation, on the other hand, the large vesicles in the monoamine neurons (identified by their content also of small granular vesicles) often have a dense core, whereas in non-monoamine neurons (characterized by small, empty, agranular vesicles) the large vesicles are devoid of a dense core (see Fig. 2) (Hökfelt, 1968, 1969).

Both types of granular vesicles are present in all parts of the neuron although the proportions may vary (Figs. 8–10) (see also below). Thus, the proportion of the large type seems to be higher in the axons than in the varicosities of the axon terminals (Geffen and Ostberg, 1969; Hökfelt, 1969).

It was possible from histochemical experiments alone to propose the hypothesis that the two types of vesicles have a different chemical composition, as shown in Table 4. Recent studies on isolated vesicles from the axons of splenic nerve have, in fact, provided strong evidence that the large granular vesicles contain high amounts of DA-β-hydroxylase and chromogranin A, but comparatively low amounts of NA, whereas the small granular vesicles in all probability contain these substances in reverse proportions

TABLE 4. *Small and large vesicles in monoamine and non-monoamine neurons as revealed after various fixation and/or impregnation procedures*

Procedure	Vesicles in mono-amine neurons		Vesicles in certain non-monoamine neurons	
	Small	Large	Small	Large
Glutaraldehyde-OsO$_4$	(+)[a]	+[b]	−	+
Zinc-iodide-OsO$_4$ (Akert and Sandri, 1968)	+	−	+	−
Bismuth-iodide (Pfenninger et al., 1969)	−	+	−	+
E-PTA[c] (Bloom and Aghajanian, 1968c)	−	+	−	+
KMnO$_4$ (Hökfelt, 1968, 1969)	+	+	+	−

(From Hökfelt, 1970.)

The presence or the absence of an electron-dense precipitate ("dense core") within the two types of vesicles have been recorded as "+" and "−," respectively.

[a] Only in certain peripheral adrenergic neurons and never in central adrenergic neurons.

[b] It should be pointed out that the degree of the density of the large vesicles may vary considerably (see Bloom and Aghajanian, 1968a). Thus, the present division into two groups ("+" or "−") only gives a schematic picture.

[c] E − PTA = ethanolic phosphotungstic acid.

(De Potter, Smith, and De Schaepdryver, 1970; Lagercrantz, 1971; Klein and Thureson-Klein, 1971; see also Geffen and Livett, 1971).

The functional role of the two types of vesicles has been the subject of much discussion. From the large numbers of small granular vesicles in the varicosities and their localization close to the synaptic cleft, it seemed reasonable to associate them rather than the large ones with the release process (see, e.g., Hökfelt, 1968). Evidence for a preferential release from small granular vesicles has indeed recently been obtained in stimulation experiments in combination with subcellular analysis (Fillenz and Howe, 1971). Recently, Geffen and Ostberg (1969) have proposed that the large granular vesicles are produced in the cell body, transported down along the axons and transformed into the small type (see also Smith, De Potter, Moerman, and De Schaepdryver, 1970; Geffen and Livett, 1971). Although this represents a very interesting and attractive hypothesis, we would like to emphasize that Geffen and Ostberg (1969) have based their study solely on OsO$_4$ fixation which *does not* reveal small granular vesicles in the cell body. The presence of small granular vesicles in the cell body as shown with KMnO$_4$ fixation would therefore imply either that a transformation from large to small granular vesicles occurs also in the cell body or that two types of vesicles of different origin are present. It has recently been proposed that the small vesicles may be formed locally in the nerve endings from the axonal endoplasmic reticulum (Machado and Machado, 1971), a hypothesis which may gain some support from studies on adrenergic nerves during the recovery phase after reserpine treatment showing elongated vesicles and tubules containing electron-dense precipitates (Hökfelt, *in preparation*).

Intraneuronal Distribution of Amines

Not only could the monoamine neuron systems be mapped with the Falck-Hillarp fluorescence method, but it was also possible to obtain a rough estimate of the intraneuronal amine levels, revealing a characteristic uneven distribution with low to medium concentrations in the cell body, low in the axons, and high in the terminal axonal enlargements (varicosities, nerve endings) (see Dahlström, 1966) (Fig. 7a–c). When comparing peripheral and central NA neurons, it was found that whereas in the central cell bodies the fluorescence was mainly localized perinuclearly (roughly corresponding to the Golgi apparatus), the fluorescence in the peripheral NA cell bodies was often most intense in the peripheral parts of the cytoplasm (see Fig. 7a).

At the ultrastructural level, the distribution of granular vesicles closely parallels the distribution of fluorescence provided that the KMnO₄ fixation technique is used (Figs. 8–11) (Hökfelt, 1969; Taxi, Gautron, and L'-Hermité, 1969; Van Orden, Burke, Geyer, and Lodoen, 1970; Hökfelt and Van Orden, 1972). Thus, large amounts of small granular vesicles localized in clusters mainly in the peripheral parts of the cell body (Fig. 8) were observed in addition to the few large granular vesicles seen also after, e.g., glutaraldehyde-OsO₄ fixation. It should, however, be emphasized that both Taxi (1965) and Grillo (1966) were able to demonstrate distinct but sparse small granular vesicles in ganglion cell bodies with plain OsO₄ fixation. In other studies, doubt has been expressed about the existence of small granular vesicles in cell bodies. For example, Geffen and Ostberg (1969) performed a quantitative study on the distribution of granular vesicles which

---

FIG. 7. Fluorescence micrographs from the various parts of an adrenergic neuron — cell bodies in the superior cervical ganglion (*a*), axons in the sciatic nerve trunk (*b*), and axon terminals in the iris dilator muscle (*c*) (all tissues from rat). In Fig. 7a, a number of cell bodies are seen. Note the strongly fluorescent dots in the periphery of the cell bodies (arrow heads), in all probability localized in the cytoplasm and probably corresponding to clusters of granular vesicles seen in Fig. 8. Sometimes a thin zone of fluorescence can be seen in the perinulear cytoplasm probably corresponding to the Golgi apparatus (arrows). In Fig. 7b, axons with a varying fluorescence intensity are seen. Note small fluorescent dots probably corresponding to small clusters of granular vesicles sometimes seen in electron micrographs (see Fig. 10). Fig. 7c shows the typical adrenergic ground plexus with

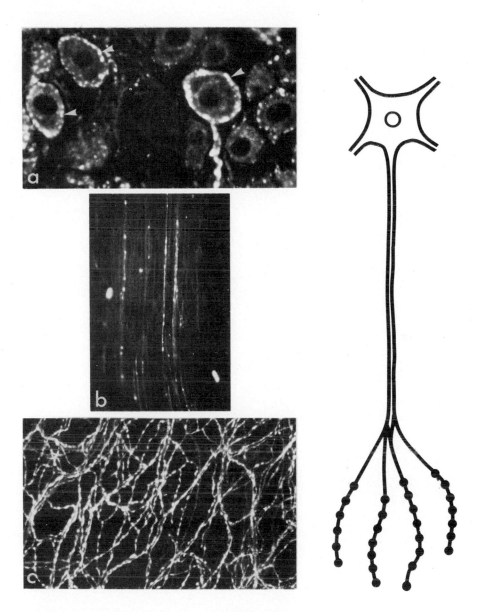

several axon terminals often running in parallell in the same strand. The highest fluorescence intensity is seen in the varicosities which contain large numbers of granular vesicles (see Figs. 2 and 11). Fluorescence method of Falck and Hillarp. Magnifications × 2,900, 400, and 400, respectively. [These excellent micrographs were kindly provided by Dr. L. S. van Orden (from van Orden et al., 1970, with permission of the publisher) (Fig. 7a), Dr. L. Olson (Fig. 7b), and Dr. T. Malmfors (Fig. 7c).]

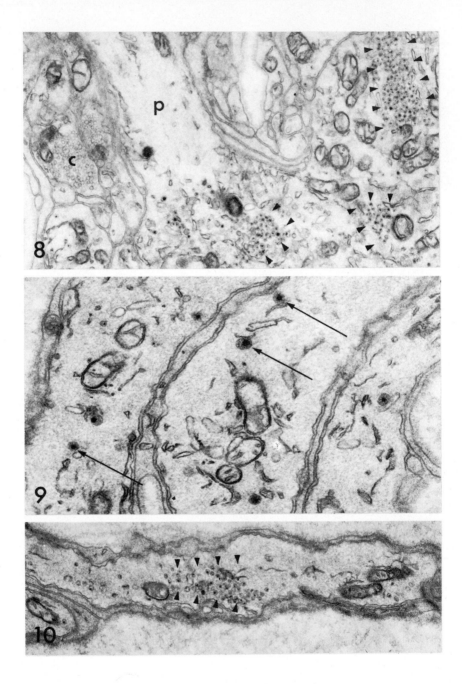

revealed only granular vesicles of the large type in the cell body and in the axon, whereas in the terminal axonal enlargements granular vesicles of both types were seen. In an autoradiographic study on the uptake of exogenous amine in central CA neurons, Descarries and Droz (1970) concluded that amines in the cell body are not vesicle bound but are bound to a macromolecular complex not visible in the microscope. Some recent excellent results published by Van Orden et al. (1970), however, add further weight to the view that amines are vesicle bound even in the cell body. They succeeded in obtaining fluorescence micrographs showing that the fluo-

←
FIG. 8. Electron micrograph of part of a cell body in rat superior cervical ganglion. The peripheral part of the cytoplasm is seen containing clusters of almost exclusively small granular vesicles (arrow heads). Note lack of vesicles in a cell process (p) and the agranular vesicles in the probable cholinergic nerve endings (c). KMnO₄ fixation. Magnification × 20,000. From Hökfelt (1969) with permission of the publisher.

←
FIGS. 9 and 10. Electron micrographs of axons of the internal carotid nerve trunk of rat. In the three axons of Fig. 9, only scattered granular vesicles (arrows), mostly of the large type, are seen, whereas a cluster of small granular vesicles is seen in the axon of Fig. 10. KMnO₄ fixation. Magnifications × 35,000 and 21,000, respectively. Fig. 9 from Hökfelt and Dahlström (1971) with permission of the publisher.

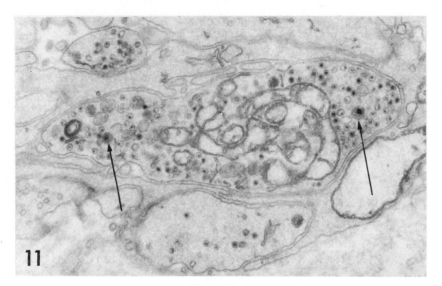

FIG. 11. Electron micrograph of human submandibular gland. Some varicosities containing small and large (arrows) granular vesicles are seen. Note absence of a dense core in many large vesicles. KMnO₄ fixation. Magnification × 30,000. From Norberg et al. (1969) with permission of the publisher.

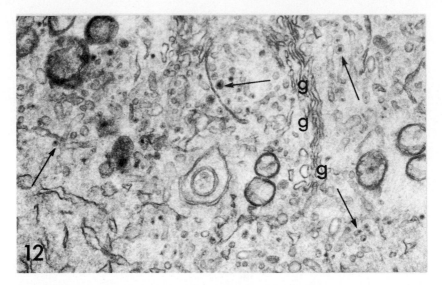

FIG. 12. Electron micrograph of rat lumbar sympathetic ganglion treated with local application of Vinblastine. Many granular vesicles are seen in the neighborhood of the Golgi apparatus. KMnO$_4$ fixation. Magnification × 35,000. From Hökfelt and Dahlström (1971) with permission of the publisher.

rescence in the peripheral parts of the cytoplasm is in fact distributed in a dot-like manner (see Fig. 7a), probably corresponding to accumulations of vesicles as seen in the electron microscope (see Fig. 8), thus confirming early results by Eränkö and Härkönen (1963) often considered as artefacts. Furthermore, recent studies with local application of colchicine and vinblastine, two mitotic inhibitors on sympathetic ganglia have revealed an accumulation of granular vesicles in the cell body, especially in the neighborhood of the Golgi apparatus (Fig. 12) (Hökfelt and Dahlström, 1971). We interpret these findings to indicate that the transport of granular vesicles produced in the Golgi apparatus or its neighborhood is inhibited by the mitotic inhibitors, similar to the inhibition of transport of NA seen after local constrictions or after local application of colchicine on the axons of adrenergic nerves (Dahlström, 1966, 1968).

SUSPECTED AMINO ACID NEUROTRANSMITTERS

Methodology

For the suspected amino acid neurotransmitters GABA, glycine, and glutamate, no histochemical methods exist, to our knowledge, by which they can be directly visualized in the light or electron microscope. Thus, so far little *morphological* data are available as to their localization in the nervous system. Although some enzymes involved in GABA metabolism have been traced histochemically (van Gelder, 1965) and autoradiographically (Csillik and Knyihár, 1970; Knyihár and Csillik, 1970), the present view on the distribution, e.g., of GABA, is based mainly on biochemical (Hirsch and Robins, 1962; Kuriyama, Haber, Siskens, and Roberts, 1966; Fonnum, Storm-Mathisen, and Walberg, 1970; Obata, Otsuka, and Tanaka, 1970) and neurophysiological work (Obata, Ito, Ochi, and Sato, 1967; Krnjević and Schwartz, 1967; Curtis, Hösli, Johnston, and Johnston, 1968; Obata and Takeda, 1969; Iversen, Mitchell, and Srinivasan, 1971). The same is true for glycine (Curtis and Watkins, 1960; Krnjević and Phillis, 1963; Aprison and Werman, 1965; Curtis, Hösli, Johnston and Johnston, 1967; Davidoff, Graham, Shank, Werman, and Aprison, 1967; Werman, Davidoff, and Aprison, 1968).

Considering the monoamine neurons as models, one possibility for localizing hypothetical GABA, glycine, or glutamate "neurons" would be to use autoradiography, as has been extensively done with NA and 5-HT (see, e.g., Wolfe et al., 1962; Aghajanian and Bloom, 1966; Descarries and Droz, 1970). This technique is based on the existence of a specific and efficient uptake mechanism localized at the nerve cell membrane, by which the monoamine neurons can take up and strongly concentrate exogenous amines, a process which in all probability is of considerable physiological importance as an inactivation mechanism for the transmitter after its action at the receptor site (see Iversen, 1967).

Recent studies (Iversen and Neal, 1968) have focused attention on the fact that various amino acids are taken up and concentrated in nervous tissue (see, e.g., Kandera, Levi, and Lajtha, 1968; Battistin, Grynbaum, and Lajtha, 1969), offering a promising basis to perform autoradiography and to obtain information on the uptake and distribution pattern of exogenous amino acids. Since GABA does not easily pass the blood-brain barrier — as elegantly demonstrated by whole-body autoradiography (Hespe, Roberts, and Prins, 1970) — the isotope must either be administered *in vitro* by incubating thin brain slices in a physiological buffer solution containing the labeled amino acid or by intraventricular or intracerebral injections.

We have so far mainly used the *in vitro* technique, although this approach has a number of drawbacks which make the interpretation of the results obtained difficult. The main problems associated with the *in vitro* technique include poor morphology due to a partial destruction of neuronal cell bodies and swelling of glial components and extracellular space (see, e.g., Gerschenfeld, Wald, Zadunaisky, and De Robertis, 1959; Pappius,

Klatzo, and Elliott, 1962; Cohen and Hartman, 1964; Thorack, Dufty, and Haynes, 1965; Elliott, 1970; Harvey and McIlwain, 1970; Pappius, 1970). This swelling may be prevented in part by adding substances of high molecular weight such as dextran (Pharmacia, Sweden) to the incubation medium (see, e.g., Hökfelt, 1968). The damage of neuronal cell bodies and possibly their uptake capacity during the slicing (cutting) procedure and/or incubation procedure may lead to erroneous negative results. The poor morphology makes it difficult to identify at the light-microscopic level the structures accumulating the isotope, for example, to establish whether neurons or glia are responsible for the uptake patterns. Furthermore, comparisons with earlier published work based, e.g., on perfusion fixed tissue are often extremely difficult to perform.

Apart from these specific problems concerning the *in vitro* technique, general "autoradiographic problems" such as dislocation and loss of the isotopes during preparation procedures must also be considered. We have determined the loss of ³H-GABA during fixation (glutaraldehyde) and dehydration procedure to be about 40% (*unpublished data;* see also Faeder and Salpeter, 1970). In an attempt to estimate the effect of such losses, we have used freeze-dried and plastic-embedded tissue in addition to glutaraldehyde (often followed by postfixation in OsO_4)-fixed tissue also, a procedure which seems to prevent loss and diffusion of at least the monoamines (see Hökfelt, 1965; Hökfelt and Ljungdahl, 1971a). Furthermore, the emulsion was applied in a dry form with a special loop technique (Caro and van Tubergen, 1962; Miller, Stone, and Prescott, 1964; Nagata and Nawa, 1966). Another important point concerns the identity of the radioactivity. In studies performed under similar experimental conditions to those used in the present study, Iversen and Neal (1968) and Neal (1971) demonstrated that the radioactivity present in slices after incubation almost exclusively represents unchanged GABA and glycine, respectively.

It may, furthermore, be added that the presence of the neurotransmitters in the incubation medium may influence the membrane properties, e.g., the membrane potential, which in turn may affect the uptake mechanisms.

GABA

The uptake studies have mainly been performed on slices either from normal rats or from rats pretreated with amino-oxyacetic acid (AOAA, 25 mg/kg, i.v.), which is known to inhibit GABA breakdown (Wallach, 1961). The slices were incubated with ³H-GABA (specific activity 2 C/ mmole, New England Nuclear Corp., Boston, Mass.; 4×10^{-6} M) in a

Tyrode buffer solution for 30 or 45 min. Light-microscopic autoradiography revealed characteristic, specific grain distribution patterns for the various brain regions studied. In addition to a general diffuse activity found over the tissue sections, the following main findings may be summarized (see also Hökfelt and Ljungdahl, 1970, 1971a, 1972).

In the *cerebellar cortex* of the rat, grains are found (1) over small cell bodies and over fiber-like or dot-like structures in the molecular layer (Fig. 13), (2) occasionally over cell bodies in the molecular layer close to the Purkinje cell layer, (3) surrounding the basal part of the Purkinje cell bodies (Fig. 21), (4) over dot-like structures and occasionally over large cell bodies in the granular layer (Fig. 14), (5) over small cell bodies in the white matter, (6) over cells lying around the blood vessels, and (7) over the meninges.

In the *cerebral cortex*, high concentrations of grains are seen (1) more or less distinctly dot-like over the whole cortex but with the highest intensity over layer I [small, distinct, dot-like structures are sometimes seen in the close vicinity of small pyramidal cell bodies (Figs. 15 and 16)], (2) over cell bodies in the outer layers (Fig. 15), and (3) over small cell bodies in all other cortical layers (Fig. 15).

Owing to the technical deficiencies mentioned above, it has so far been difficult to identify with certainty the morphological correlates of the grain accumulations, i.e., whether neurons or glia take up GABA. In the cerebellar cortex, preliminary electron-microscopic autoradiography has provided evidence that the small labeled cell bodies in the molecular layer probably correspond to stellate cells, and the dot-like accumulations in the granular layer may correspond to accumulations found over Golgi cell nerve endings. It is tempting to speculate that the accumulations of silver grains over the large cell bodies in the granular layer could correspond to Golgi cell bodies. It may, furthermore, be speculated that the accumulations close to the basal parts of the Purkinje cell bodies may represent nerve endings of basket cells. This is also indicated by the close morphological correlation between the autoradiographic uptake pattern and the silver impregnation picture seen in Fig. 17. Figure 17*b* is considered to show the nerve endings of basket cells terminating on the Purkinje cell (initial axon segment and neighboring cell body).

The lack of activity over Purkinje cell bodies, which from convincing biochemical and neurophysiological studies (for references, see above) represent "GABA-neurons," may seem disappointing. It is, therefore, of some interest to discuss possible explanations for this unexpected negative result, especially since this is a common problem in interpreting autoradiographic pictures. Although the important objection must be considered that

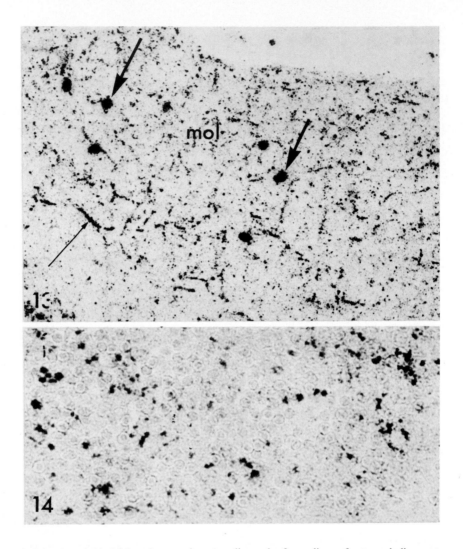

FIGS. 13 and 14. Light-microscopic autoradiographs from slices of rat cerebellar cortex incubated with ³H-GABA (Fig. 14 from AOAA-pretreated rat). Accumulations of grains are seen over cell bodies (large arrows) in the molecular layer (mol) (Fig. 14) and dot-like and fiber-like accumulations are seen both in the molecular layer (thin arrows, Fig. 14) and the granular layer (Fig. 13). Magnifications × 400 and 700, respectively.

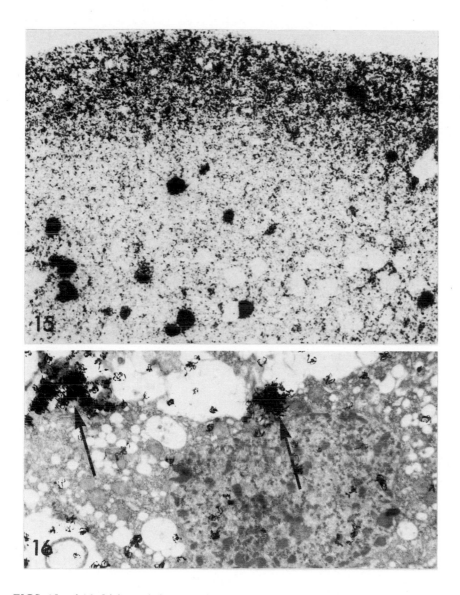

FIGS. 15 and 16. Light- and electron-microscopic autoradiographs of slices of rat cerebral cortex incubated with ^{3}H-GABA (AOAA pretreatment). At the light-microscopic level (Fig. 15), strong accumulations are seen over cell bodies mainly in layer II and over the whole of layer I. At the ultrastructural level (Fig. 16), strong accumulations can be seen over boutons (arrows) in contact with a pyramidal cell. Note deficiencies in morphology due to experimental procedure. Magnifications × 380 and 7,000, respectively. Fig. 15 from Hökfelt and Ljungdahl (1971a) with permission of the publisher.

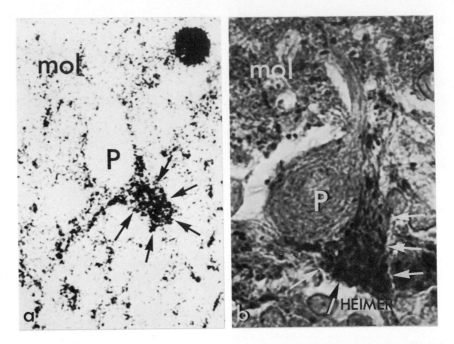

FIG. 17. Light-microscopic autoradiograph (*a*) and micrograph from silver impregnated section (*b*), both from the cerebellar cortex. Fig. 17*a* shows the grain distribution after incubation of a cerebellar slice with ^{3}H-GABA (AOAA pretreatment). Note the close correlation in localization between grain distribution basal to the Purkinje cell body (P) (arrows) in Fig. 17*a* and the precipitates in Fig. 17*b*, probably representing the axon terminals of basket cells, at the corresponding sites close to the Purkinje cells (P). mol = molecular layer. Magnifications × 800 and 1,400, respectively. Fig. 17*b* was kindly supplied by Dr. L. Heimer (Department of Psychology, Massachusetts Institute of Technology, Cambridge, Mass.). The silver impregnation method used is described in Heimer (1967), second modification, page 106.

those neurons which in the present study take up and accumulate GABA do not represent neurons releasing GABA at the synapse, our work and the following discussion are based on the hypothesis that "GABA" and mono-amine neurons share the capacity of taking up exogenous transmitter. Apart from the possibility that Purkinje cells do not represent "GABA neurons," a number of explanations exist for our negative finding.

(1) There are deficiencies in the autoradiographic technique as discussed above.

(2) Damage of the Purkinje cells due to the slicing and/or incubation procedure may result in a damaged uptake mechanism. The large size of

these neurons may render them especially sensitive. However, preliminary studies from intracerebellar injections indicate that after this route of administration the Purkinje cell bodies also fail to accumulate ³H-GABA.

(3) Different types of neurons may have an uptake mechanism of varying efficiency. Furthermore, differences in the surface-to-volume ratio or differences in metabolic processes may also play a role. We have in fact observed intriguing differences in the ability of monoamine cell bodies to take up and accumulate exogenous amines. Thus, whereas DA cell bodies in the arcuate nucleus and substantia nigra accumulate exogenous NA strongly *in vitro*, this does not seem to be the case with NA cell bodies in the locus coeruleus to the same extent (*unpublished data*).

(4) The strong accumulations in surrounding glial (and neuronal?) elements observed may prevent access of the isotope to the Purkinje cell bodies. This would be in agreement with the dense accumulations of label over Schwann cells, but not axons, in the lobster nerve-muscle preparation incubated with ³H-GABA (Orkand and Kravitz, 1971).

In the cerebral cortex, we have identified small neurons, which may represent basket cells, over which grain accumulations were seen. Furthermore, intense accumulations were seen over nerve endings in close contact with small pyramidal cell bodies (Fig. 16). Strong evidence for an intra-neuronal localization of GABA in brain cortex has also been obtained recently in an elegant autoradiographic study by Bloom and Iversen (1971). They were able to demonstrate that ³H-GABA was predominantly taken up into neuronal elements (nerve endings) after incubation both of a nerve ending particle fraction and of cortical slices. The same percentage (about 30%) of the nerve endings seemed to accumulate GABA in both types of experiments, favoring the view that GABA is taken up into a specific neuron population. Also in the rabbit retina, autoradiographic evidence has been obtained for an accumulation of ³H-GABA (and ³H-glycine) in neurons (Ehinger, 1970; Ehinger and Falck, 1971).

There is no doubt, however, that an uptake of ³H-GABA also occurs into glial elements, especially after the inhibition of GABA breakdown by AOAA. Thus, the small labeled cell bodies in the white matter and those closely surrounding the Purkinje cell bodies in all probability represent glial cells (oligodendroglia and Bergmann glia, respectively). This is in agreement with recent studies on a lobster nerve-muscle preparation showing accumulation of ³H-GABA over Schwann cells (Orkand and Kravitz, 1971), indicating that glial uptake may represent an important inactivation mechanism. A similar mechanism seems to operate for glutamate in an insect nerve-muscle preparation (Faeder and Salpeter, 1970).

Glycine

So far we have mainly studied the uptake pattern of glycine in spinal cord slices (see Hökfelt and Ljungdahl, 1971b), which accumulate exogenous glycine by an active, energy-dependent uptake mechanism (Neal, 1971). Transverse slices were incubated with ^{3}H-glycine (specific activity 4.67 C/mmole; New England Nuclear Corp., Boston, Mass.; 2×10^{-7} to 5×10^{-6} M) in a Tyrode buffer solution for 30 or 45 min.

The results indicate at the light-microscopic level an uptake mainly in the gray matter (Fig. 18). Apart from a diffuse activity (intensity is dependent on the distance from the surface of the slice), strong accumulations can be seen over dot- and fiber-like structures and also over small cell bodies (Figs. 18 and 19). Electron-microscopic autoradiography shows that grains are mainly localized over boutons (Fig. 20). According to a preliminary calculation, 50% of the boutons in the anterior horn seem to accumulate the isotope. In addition, certain thin myelinated axons also exhibit intense activity (Fig. 20). These myelinated axons are mostly of a fine caliber and run mainly perpendicular to the long axis of the spinal cord. No obvious accumulations are seen in the vast majority of myelinated axons, either in the columns or in the dorsal roots. A distinct activity can, however, be seen over the Schwann cell bodies. Oligodendroglial cell bodies and their processes also exhibit a strong activity (Fig. 20).

Glycine has been suggested as an inhibitory transmitter in the spinal cord, localized to interneurons (see Aprison, Davidoff, and Werman, 1970). It is an interesting hypothesis that the boutons accumulating glycine may belong to a specific type of neuron which could correspond to these spinal inhibitory interneurons. However, uptake seems to occur also into glial elements which may also represent an important inactivation mechanism, as discussed for GABA (see above).

→

FIGS. 18 and 19. Light-microscopic autoradiographs of rat spinal cord slices incubated with ^{3}H-glycine. The highest activity is found over the grey matter (gm), where many dot-like and fiber-like accumulations are seen. Often dot-like accumulations (arrows) are seen close to the cell bodies of motoneurons (m). Magnifications × 160 and 400, respectively.

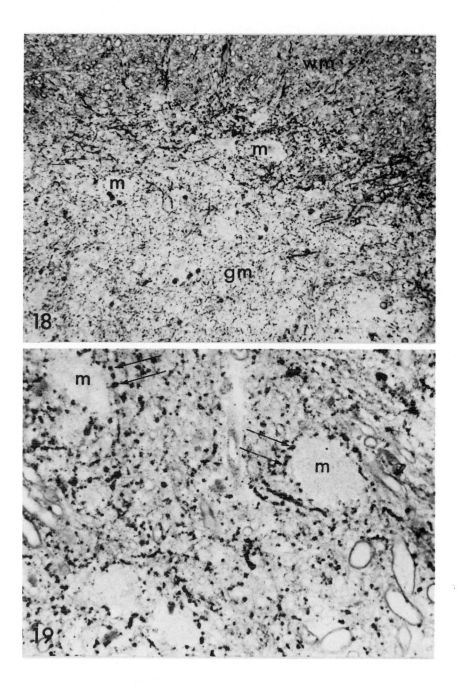

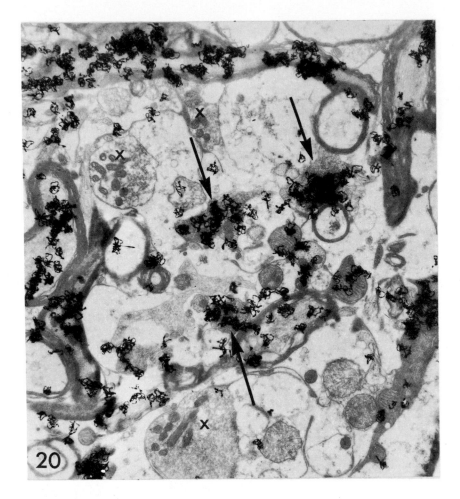

FIG. 20. Electron-microscopic autoradiograph of rat spinal cord slice incubated with
³H-glycine. Grain accumulations are seen over boutons (arrows), thin myelinated axons,
and processes of oligodendrogial cells. Note absence of grains over three boutons (x).
Magnification × 10,000.

Comparison Between Uptake of GABA, Glycine, Glutamate, and NA

To study the specificity of the uptake of GABA and glycine, we have
compared their uptake patterns in rat cerebellar cortex slices with those
of glutamate (specific activity 27 C/mmole; New England Nuclear Corp.,

Boston, Mass.; 2×10^{-7} to 2×10^{-6} M), which is suggested to be an excitatory transmitter in brain cortex (Krnjevic and Phillis, 1963), and NA (specific activity 8.67 C/mmole; New England Nuclear Corp., Boston, Mass.; 10^{-6} M). Some representative autoradiographs from this comparison are shown in Figs. 21–23.

Similarities in the uptake patterns were observed for the accumulation of activity over small glial cell bodies both in the Purkinje cell layer (Bergmann glia and Fañana cells) and in the white matter, which were both seen after incubation with ^{3}H-GABA in combination with AOAA, ^{3}H-glycine, or ^{3}H-glutamate, but not with NA. Thin processes radiating from the glial cells around the Purkinje cell bodies could be seen distinctly, especially after incubation with ^{3}H-glycine and ^{3}H-glutamate. Furthermore, after incubation both with ^{3}H-GABA and ^{3}H-glycine, accumulations of activity were seen over large cell bodies and over small dot-like structures in the granular layer.

Specific uptake patterns, unique to only one of the group of transmitters were seen as follows. (1) Small cell bodies in the molecular layer exhibited increased activity after incubation with ^{3}H-GABA. (2) Strong accumulation of grains surrounding the basal part of the Purkinje cells were seen after incubation with ^{3}H-GABA. (3) Accumulation over small cell bodies in the granular layer was seen after incubation with ^{3}H-glycine. (4) The uptake pattern of ^{3}H-NA was completely different from those of the amino acids. The diffuse activity was very low, and accumulations of grains were seen only over small dot-like structures in all cortical layers (see also Bloom, Hoffer, and Siggins, 1971), closely corresponding to the distribution of NA fibers seen in the fluorescence microscope (Hökfelt and Fuxe, 1969).

In conclusion, the uptake and accumulation of ^{3}H-GABA, ^{3}H-glycine, and ^{3}H-glutamate into what are probably glial cell elements seems to occur into the same type of cells, indicating a lack of specificity in this uptake mechanism. Uptake into what are probably neuronal structures, however, seems to be more specific, since clear differences exist between the patterns observed for ^{3}H-GABA and ^{3}H-glycine. The uptake of ^{3}H-glutamate in cerebellar slices seems to occur almost exclusively in glial cells.

GENERAL CONCLUSIONS

Sensitive histochemical methods are available for visualising both at the light- and electron-microscopic levels NA, DA, and 5-HT, three monoamines suspected of acting as neurotransmitters or modulators. Thus, the neuron systems containing these substances can be mapped and the intra-

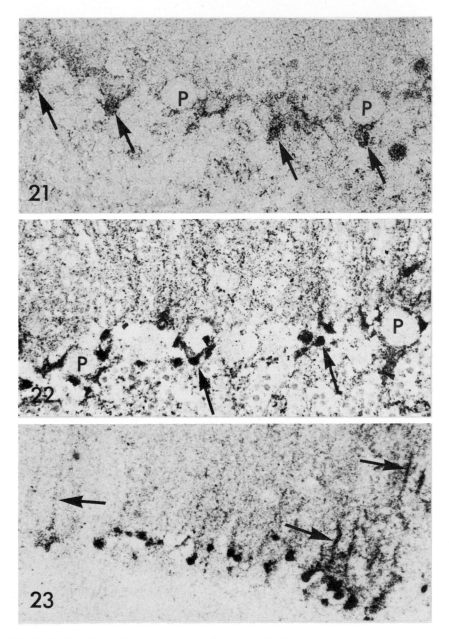

FIGS. 21–23. Light-microscopic autoradiographs of slices of rat cerebellar cortex incubated with ^{3}H-GABA (AOAA pretreatment), ^{3}H-glycine, and ^{3}H-glutamate, respectively. All micrographs from the Purkinje cell (P) layer. After incubation with ^{3}H-GABA (Fig.

neuronal transmitter distribution can be determined. NA, DA, and 5-HT are present not only in the axon terminals, where they may be released upon arrival of nerve impulses, but also in the cell body and the axons. Evidence from $KMnO_4$-fixed tissues indicates that the NA in all parts of the neuron is bound in very high concentrations (about 1 M) to special storage vesicles, of which two types seem to exist, small and large granular vesicles. The bulk of transmitter, at least in the varicosities and the cell body, is present in the small type, which is predominant in these parts (more than 95% of the vesicles in the varicosities are of the small type) whereas the large type, which is more frequent in the axons, may contain enzymes such as DA-β-hydroxylase and only relatively small amounts of amines.

For other suspected neurotransmitters such as the amino acids GABA, glycine, and glutamate, no similar histochemical methods are available at present. To obtain some information, in spite of this, about their possible localization in the nervous system, we have performed autoradiographic studies, incubating thin slices from various brain regions in buffer solutions containing ^{3}H-GABA, ^{3}H-glycine, and ^{3}H-glutamate. Specific distribution patterns were observed for these amino acids, suggesting an uptake and accumulation both in neuronal and glial elements. Further studies are necessary to determine whether the neuronal uptake takes place into neurons utilizing these substances as transmitters. The accumulation of amino acids in glial elements suggests that, in contrast to the monoamine systems, glial uptake may function as an important inactivation mechanism for suspected amino acid neurotransmitters.

ACKNOWLEDGMENT

This work has been supported by grants from the Swedish Medical Research Council (B72–14x–2887–03B and B72–14P–3262–02B) and by grants from Therese and Johan Anderssons Minne, Ollie and Elof Ericssons Stiftelse, and Magnus Bergvalls Stiftelse.

---

21), accumulations are found predominantly surrounding the basal part of the Purkinje cell bodies (arrows) (*cf.* Fig. 17 *a* and *b*). After incubation with ^{3}H-glycine (Fig. 22), accumulations are mainly seen over small cell bodies (arrows), probably of glial origin (Bergmann glia, Fañana cells), surrounding the Purkinje cells (P). Note activity basal to the Purkinje cell body (P) to the right. After ^{3}H-glutamate incubation (Fig. 23), small cell bodies surrounding Purkinje cells accumulate the isotope. Note the accumulation in processes (arrows) radiating through the molecular layer. These processes probably belong to Bergmann glia. Magnification × 370 for all figures.

REFERENCES

Aghajanian, G. K., and Bloom, F. E. (1966): Electron-microscopic autoradiography of rat hypothalamus after intraventricular H^3-norepinephrine. *Science*, 153:308–310.

Akert, K., and Sandri, C. (1968): An electron-microscopic study of zinc iodide-osmium impregnation of neurons. I. Staining of synaptic vesicles at cholinergic junctions. *Brain Research*, 7:286–295.

Akert, K., and Sandri, C. (1970): Identification of the active synaptic region by means of histochemical and freeze-etching techniques. In: *Excitatory Synaptic Mechanisms*, edited by P. Anderson and J. K. S. Jansen. Oslo University Press, Oslo.

Aprison, M. H., Davidoff, R. A., and Werman, R. (1970): Glycine: Its metabolic and possible transmitter roles in nervous tissue. In: *Handbook of Neurochemistry*, edited by A. Lajtha. Plenum Press, New York-London.

Aprison, M. H., and Werman, R. (1965): The distribution of glycine in cat spinal cord and roots. *Life Sciences*, 4:2075–2083.

Battistin, L., Grynbaum, A., and Lajtha, A. (1969): Distribution and uptake of amino acids in various regions of the cat brain in vitro. *Journal of Neurochemistry*, 16:1459–1468.

Bloom, F. E. (1970): The fine structural localization of biogenic monoamines in nervous tissue. International Review of Neurobiology, 13:22–67.

Bloom, F. E. (1972): Localization of neurotransmitters by electron microscopy. In: *Proceedings of the Association for Research in Nervous and Mental Diseases*, Conference on Neurotransmitters, December 4 and 5, 1970, New York City. Williams and Wilkins. Baltimore.

Bloom, F. E., and Aghajanian, G. K. (1968a): An electron microscopic analysis of large granular synaptic vesicles of the brain in relation to monoamine content. *Journal of Pharmacology and Experimental Therapeutics*, 159:261–273.

Bloom, F. E., and Aghajanian, G. K. (1968b): An osmiophilic substance in brain synaptic vesicles not related to catecholamine content. *Experientia*, 24:1225–1227.

Bloom, F. E., and Aghajanian, G. K. (1968c): Fine structural and cytochemical analysis of the staining of synaptic junctions with phosphotungstic acid. *Journal of Ultrastructure Research*, 22:361–375.

Bloom, F. E., and Barrnett, J. (1966): Fine structural localization of noradrenaline in vesicles of autonomic nerve endings. *Nature*, 210:599–601.

Bloom, F. E., Hoffer, B. J., and Siggins, G. R. (1971): Studies on norepinephrine-containing afferents to purkinje cells of rat cerebellum. I. Localization of the fibers and their synapses. *Brain Research*, 25:501–521.

Bloom, F. E., and Iversen, L. L. (1971): Localizing ^{3}H-GABA in nerve terminals of rat cerebral cortex by electron microscopic autoradiography. *Nature*, 229:628–630.

Bondareff, W. (1966): Localization of α-methylnorepinephrine in sympathetic nerve fibers of the pineal body. *Experimental Neurology*, 16:131–135.

Burt, A. M. (1970): A histochemical procedure for the localization of choline acetyltransferase activity. *Journal of Histochemistry and Cytochemistry*, 18:408–415.

Caro, L., and Van Tubergen, R. P. (1962): High resolution autoradiography. I. Methods. *Journal of Cell Biology*, 15:173–188.

Clementi, F., Mantegazza, P., and Botturi, M. (1966): A pharmacologic and morphologic study on the nature of the dense-core granules present in the presynaptic endings of sympathetic ganglia. *International Journal of Neuropharmacology*, 5:281–285.

Cohen, M. M., and Hartman, J. F. (1964): Biochemical and ultrastructural correlates of cerebral cortex slices metabolizing *in vitro*. In: *Morphological and Biochemical Correlates of Neural Activity*, edited by M. M. Cohen and R. S. Synder. Harper & Row, New York.

Corrodi, H., and Jonsson, G. (1967): The formaldehyde fluorescence method for the histochemical demonstration of biogenic amines. *Journal of Histochemistry and Cytochemistry*, 15:65–68.

Coupland, R. E. (1965): Electron microscopic observations on the structure of the rat adrenal medulla. II. Normal innervation. *Journal of Anatomy*, 99:255–272.

Coupland, R. E., Pyper, A. S., and Hopwood, D. (1964): A method for differentiating between noradrenaline- and adrenaline-storing cells in the light and electron microscope. *Nature*, 201:1240–1242.

Csillík, B., and Knyihár, E. (1970): Distribution of ^{14}C-thiosemicarbazide in the rat brain: an attempt to localize sites of γ-aminobutyric acid production. *Nature*, 225:562–563.

Curtis, D. R., and Watkins, J. C. (1960): The excitation and depression of spinal neurones by structurally related amino acids. *Journal of Neurochemistry*, 6:117–141.

Curtis, D. R., Hösli, L., Johnston, C. A. R., and Johnston, I. H. (1967): Glycine and spinal inhibition. *Brain Research*, 5:112–114.

Dahlström, A. (1966): The intraneuronal distribution of noradrenaline and the transport and life-span of amine storage granules in the sympathetic adrenergic neurons. M. D. Thesis, Stockholm.

Dahlström, A. (1968): Effect of colchicine on transport of amine storage granules in sympathetic nerves of rat. *European Journal of Pharmacology*, 5:111–116.

Dahlström, A., Häggendal, J., and Hökfelt, T. (1966): The noradrenaline content of the varicosities of sympathetic adrenergic nerve terminals in the rat. *Acta Physiologica Scandinavica*, 67:289–294.

Davidoff, R. A., Graham, L. T., Jr., Shank, R. P., Werman, R., and Aprison, M. H. (1967): Changes in amino acid concentrations associated with loss of spinal interneurons. *Journal of Neurochemistry*, 14:1025–1031.

Davies, T. R. A., and Meade, K. M. (1970): Biologically active antibodies to histamine. *Nature*, 226:360.

De Robertis, E., and Pellegrino De Iraldi, A. (1961a): Plurivesicular secretory processes and nerve endings in the pineal gland. *Journal of Biophysical and Biochemical Cytology*, 10:361–372.

De Robertis, E., and Pellegrino De Iraldi, A. (1961b): A plurivesicular component in adrenergic nerve endings. *Anatomical Record*, 139:299.

Descarries, L., and Droz, B. (1970): Intraneural distribution of exogenous norepinephrine in the central nervous system of the rat. *Journal of Cell Biology*, 44:385–399.

Devine, C. E., and Laverty, R. (1968): Fixation for electron microscopy and the retention of ^{3}H-noradrenaline by tissues. *Experientia*, 24:1156–1157.

Ehinger, B. (1970): Autoradiographic identification of rabbit retinal neurons that take up GABA. *Experientia*, 26:1063.

Ehinger, B., and Falck, B. (1972): Autoradiography of some suspected neurotransmitter substances: GABA, glycine, glutamic acid, histamine, dopamine, and L-DOPA. *Brain Research*, 33:157–172.

Elliott, K. A. C. (1970): The use of brain slices. In: *Handbook of Neurochemistry*, edited by A. Lajtha. Plenum Press, New York.

Eränkö, O., and Härkönen, M. (1963): Histochemical demonstration of fluoregenic amines in the cytoplasm of sympathetic ganglion cells of the rat. *Acta Physiologica Scandinavica*, 58:285–286.

Faeder, I. R., and Salpeter, M. M. (1970): Glutamate uptake by a stimulated insect nerve muscle preparation. *Journal of Cell Biology*, 46:300–307.

Falck, B., Hillarp, N.-Å., Thieme, G., and Torp, A. (1962): Fluorescence of catecholamines and related compounds condensed with formaldehyde. *Journal of Histochemistry and Cytochemistry*, 10:348–354.

Falck, B., and Moore, R. Y. (1972): *Fluorescence Histochemistry of Biogenic Amines*. Academic Press, New York.

Fillenz, M., and Howe, P. R. C. (1971): The contribution of small and large vesicles to noradrenaline release. *Journal of Physiology*, 212:42P–43P.

Florey, E. (1960): Physiological evidence for naturally occurring inhibitory substances. In: *Inhibition in the Nervous System and γ-Aminobutyric Acid*, edited by E. Roberts, C. F. Baxter, A. van Harreveld, C. A. G. Wiersma, W. R. Adey, and K. F. Killam, Pergamon Press, London.

Fonnum, F., Storm-Mathisen, J., and Walberg, F. (1970): Glutamate decarboxylase in inhibitory neurons. A study of the enzyme in Purkinje cell axons and boutons in the cat. *Brain Research*, 20:259–276.

Fuxe, K., Goldstein, M., Hökfelt, T., and Joh, T. H. (1970a): Immunohistochemical localization of dopamine-β-hydroxylase in the peripheral and central nervous system. *Research Communications in Chemical Pathology and Pharmacology*, 1:627–636.

Fuxe, K., Goldstein, M., Hökfelt, T., and Joh, T. H. (1971): Cellular localization of dopamine-β-hydroxylase and phenylethanolamine-N-methyl transferase as revealed by immunohistochemistry. In: *Histochemistry of Nervous Transmission*, edited by O. Eränkö. Elsevier, Amsterdam.

Fuxe, K., Hökfelt, T., Jonsson, G., and Ungerstedt, U. (1970b): Fluorescence microscopy in neuroanatomy. In: *Contemporary Research Methods in Neuroanatomy*, edited by W. J. H. Nauta and S. O. E. Ebbesson, Springer-Verlag, Berlin.

Fuxe, K., Hökfelt, T., and Nilsson, O. (1965): A fluorescence and electron-microscopic study on certain brain region rich in monoamine terminals. *American Journal of Anatomy*, 117: 33–45.

Fuxe, K., Hökfelt, T., Nilsson, O., and Reinius, S. (1966): A fluorescence and electron microscopic study on central monoamine nerve cells. *Anatomical Record*, 155:33–40.

Geffen, L. B., and Livett, B. G. (1971): Synaptic vesicles in sympathetic neurons. *Physiological Reviews*, 51:98–157.

Geffen, L. B., Livett, B. G., and Rush, R. A. (1969): Immunohistochemical localization of protein components of catecholamine storage vesicles. *Journal of Physiology*, 204:593–605.

Geffen, L. B., and Ostberg, A. (1969): Distribution of granular vesicles in normal and constricted sympathetic neurones. *Journal of Physiology*, 204:583–592.

Gerschenfeld, H. M., Wald, F., Zadunaisky, J. A., and De Robertis, E. (1959): Function of astroglia in the water ion metabolism of the central nervous system. *Neurology*, 9:421–425.

Goldstein, M. L., and Bloom, F. E. (1970): Depletion of granular synaptic vesicles with *in vitro* n-ethylmaleimide. *Pharmacologist*, 12:248.

Goldstein, M., Fuxe, K., Hökfelt, T., and Joh, T. H. (1971): Immunohistochemical studies on phenyl-ethanolamine-N-methyltransferase, DOPA-decarboxylase and dopamine-β-hydroxylase. *Experientia*, 27:951–952.

Grillo, M. (1966): Electron microscopy of sympathetic tissue. *Pharmacological Reviews*, 18:387–399.

Grillo, M., and Palay, S. L. (1962): Granule-containing vesicles in the autonomic nervous system. In: *Electron Microscopy*, edited by S. S. Breese, Jr. Academic Press, New York.

Hartman, B. K., and Udenfriend, S. (1970): Immunofluorescent localization of dopamine-β-hydroxylase in tissues. *Molecular Pharmacology*, 6:85–94.

Harvey, J. A., and McIlwain, H. (1970): Electrical phenomena and isolated tissues from the brain. In: *Handbook of Neurochemistry*, edited by A. Lajtha, Plenum Press, New York.

Hebb, C. (1970): CNS at the cellular level: Identity of transmitter agents. *Annual Review of Physiology*, 32:165–192.

Heimer, L. (1967): Silver impregnation of terminal degeneration in some forebrain fiber systems: A comparative evaluation of current methods. *Brain Research*, 5:86–108.

Hespe, W. Roberts, E., and Prins, H. (1969): Autoradiographic investigation of the distribution of (^{14}C) GABA in tissues of normal and amino-oxyacetic acid-treated mice. *Brain Research*, 14:663–671.

Hirsch, H. E., and Robins, E. (1962): Distribution of γ-aminobutyric acid in the layers of the cerebral and cerebellar cortex. Implications for its physiological role. *Journal of Neurochemistry*, 9:63–70.

Hökfelt, T. (1965): A modification of the histochemical fluorescence method for the demonstration of catecholamines and 5-hydroxytryptamine, using Araldite as embedding medium. *Journal of Histochemistry and Cytochemistry*, 13:518–519.

Hökfelt, T. (1967): The possible ultrastructural identification of tubero-infundibular dopamine containing nerve endings in the median eminence of the rat. *Brain Research*, 5:121–123.

Hökfelt, T. (1968): *In vitro* studies on central and peripheral monoamine neurons at the ultra-structural level. *Zeitschrift für Zellforschung*, 91:1–74.

Hökfelt, T. (1969): Distribution of noradrenaline storing particles in peripheral adrenergic neurons as revealed by electron microscopy. *Acta Physiologica Scandinavica*, 76:427–440.

Hökfelt, T. (1970): Electron microscopic studies on peripheral and central monoamine neu-rons. In: *Aspects of Neuroendocrinology*, edited by W. Bargman and B. Scharrer. Springer-Verlag, Berlin.

Hökfelt, T. (1971): Ultrastructural localization of intraneuronal monoamines. Some aspects on methodology. In: *Histochemistry of Nervous Transmission*, edited by O. Eränkö. Else-vier, Amsterdam.

Hökfelt, T., and Dahlström, A. (1971): Effects of two mitosis inhibitors (Colchicine and Vinblastine) on the distribution and axonal transport of noradrenaline storage particles, studied by fluorescence and electron microscopy. *Zeitschrift fur Zellforschung* (119:460–482).

Hökfelt, T., and Fuxe, K. (1969): Cerebellar monoamine nerve terminals. A new type of af-ferent fibers to the cortex cerebelli. *Experimental Brain Research*, 9:63–72.

Hökfelt, T., and Jonsson, G. (1968). Studies on reaction and binding of monoamines after fixation and processing for electron microscopy with special reference to fixation with po-tassium permanganate. *Histochemie*, 16:45–67.

Hökfelt, T., and Ljungdahl, Å. (1970): Cellular localization of labeled gamma-aminobutyric acid (^{3}H-GABA) in rat cerebellar cortex: An autoradiographic study. *Brain Research*, 22:391–396.

Hökfelt, T., and Ljungdahl, Å. (1971a): Uptake of ^{3}H-noradrenaline and ^{3}H-gamma-amino-butyric acid in isolated tissues of rat: An autoradiographic and fluorescence microscopic study. In: *Histochemistry of Nervous Transmission*, edited by O. Eränkö.

Hökfelt, T., and Ljungdahl, Å. (1971b): Light and electron microscopic autoradiography on spinal cord slices after incubation with labeled glycine. *Brain Research*, 32:189–194.

Hökfelt, T., and Ljungdahl, Å. (1972): Histochemical determination of neurotransmitter distribution. *Proceedings of the Association for Research in Nervous and Mental Diseases*, Conference on Neurotransmitters, Dec. 4 and 5, 1970, New York City. Williams and Wil-kins, Baltimore.

Hökfelt, T., and Van Orden, L. S. (1972): Ultrastructure of amine-containing neurons. In: *Fluorescence Histochemistry of Biogenic Amines*, edited by B. Falck and R. Y. Moore, Academic Press, New York.

Hopsu, U. K., and Mäkinen, E. O. (1966): Two methods for the demonstration of noradrena-line-containing adrenal medullary cells. *Journal of Histochemistry and Cytochemistry*, 14:434.

Iversen, L. L. (1967): *The Uptake and Storage of Noradrenaline in Sympathetic Nerves*. Cambridge University Press, Cambridge.

Iversen, L. L., Mitchell, J. F., and Srinivasan, V. (1971): The release of γ-aminobutyric acid during inhibition in the cat visual cortex. *Journal of Physiology*, 212:519–534.

Iversen, L. L. and Neal, M. J. (1968): The uptake of (^{3}H) GABA by slices of rat cerebral cor-tex. *Journal of Neurochemistry*, 15:1141–1149.

Jaim-Etcheverry, G., and Zieher, L. M. (1968): Cytochemistry of 5-hydroxytryptamine at the electron microscope level. II. Localization in the autonomic nerves of the rat pineal gland. *Zeitschrift für Zellforschung*, 86:393–400.

Jonsson, G. (1971): Quantitation of fluorescence of biogenic monoamines demonstrated with the formaldehyde fluorescence method. *Progress in Histochemistry and Cytochemistry*, 2:299–334.

Kandera, J., Levi, G., and Lajtha, A. (1968): Control of cerebral metabolite levels. II. Amino acid uptake and levels in various areas of the rat brain. *Archives of Biochemistry and Biophysics,* 126:249–260.

Kása, P., Mann, S. P., and Hebb, C. (1970): Localization of choline acetyltransferase. *Nature,* 226:812–816.

Klein, R. L., and Thureson-Klein, Å. (1971): An electron microscopic study of noradrenaline storage vesicles isolated from bovine splenic nerve trunk. *Journal of Ultrastructure Research (in press).*

Knyihár, E., and Csillik, B. (1970): Localizations of inhibitors of the acetylcholine- and GABA-synthesizing systems in the rat brain. *Experimental Brain Research,* 11:1–16.

Koelle, G. B., and Friedenwald, J. S. (1949): A histochemical method for localizing cholinesterase activity. *Proceedings of the Society for Experimental Biology and Medicine,* 70: 617–622.

Krnjević, K., and Phillis, J. W. (1963): Iontophoretic studies of neurones in the mammalian cerebral cortex. *Journal of Physiology,* 165:274–304.

Krnjević, K., and Schwartz, S. (1967): The action of γ-aminobutyric acid on cortical neurons. *Experimental Brain Research,* 3:320–336.

Kuriyama, K., Haber, B., Siskens, B., and Roberts, E. (1966): The γ-aminobutyric acid system in rabbit cerebellum. *Proceedings of the National Academy of Sciences,* 55:846–852.

Lagercrantz, H. (1971): Isolation and characterization of sympathetic nerve trunk vesicles. *Acta Physiologica Scandinavica,* Suppl. 366.

Lever, J. D., and Esterhuizen, A. C. (1961): Fine structure of the arteriolar nerves in the guinea pig pancreas. *Nature,* 192:566–567.

Machado, A. B. M. (1967): Straight OsO$_4$ versus glutaraldehyde-OsO$_4$ in sequence as fixatives for the granular vesicles in sympathetic axons of the rat pineal body. *Stain Technology,* 42:293–300.

Machado, A. B. M. (1971): Electron microscopy of developing sympathetic fibers in the rat pineal body. The formation of granular vesicles. In: *Histochemistry of Nervous Transmission,* edited by O. Eränkö. Elsevier, Amsterdam.

Matus, A. I. (1970): Ultrastructure of the superior cervical ganglion fixed with zinc iodide and osmium tetroxide. *Brain Research,* 17:195–204.

McLennan, H. (1963): *Synaptic Transmission.* W. B. Saunders Company, Philadelphia.

Miller, O. L., Jr., Stone, G. E., and Prescott, D. M. (1964): Autoradiography of soluble materials. *Journal of Cell Biology,* 23:654–658.

Nagata, T., and Nawa, T. (1966): A modification of dry-mounting technique for radioautography of water-soluble compounds. *Histochemie,* 7:370–371.

Neal, M. J. (1971): The uptake of (^{14}C)-glycine by slices of mammalian spinal cord. *Journal of Physiology,* 215:103–118.

Norberg, K.-A., Hökfelt, T., and Eneroth, C.-M. (1969): The autonomic innervation of human submandibular and parotid glands. *Journal of Neuro-Visceral Relations,* 31:280–290.

Obata, K., Ito, M., Ochi, R., and Sato, N. (1967): Pharmacological properties of the postsynaptic inhibition by Purkinje cell axons and the action of γ-aminobutyric acid on Deiters neurones. *Experimental Brain Research,* 4:43–57.

Obata, K., Otsuka, M., and Tanaka, Y. (1970): Determination of gamma-aminobutyric acid in single nerve cells of cat central nervous system. *Journal of Neurochemistry,* 17:697–698.

Obata, K., and Takeda, K. (1969): Release of γ-aminobutyric acid into the fourth ventricle induced by stimulation of the cat's cerebellum. *Journal of Neurochemistry,* 16:1043–1047.

Orkand, P. M., and Kravitz, E. A. (1971): Localization of the sites of γ-aminobutyric acid (GABA) uptake in lobster nerve-muscle preparations. *Journal of Cell Biology,* 49:75–89.

Ostrowski, K., and Barnard, E. A. (1961): Application of isotopically labelled specific inhibitors as a method in enzyme histochemistry. *Experimental Cell Research,* 25:456–468.

Pappius, H. M. (1970): Water spaces. In: *Handbook of Neurochemistry,* edited by A. Lajtha, Plenum Press, New York.

Pappius, H. M., Klatzo, I., and Elliot, K. A. C. (1962): Further studies on swelling of brain slices. *Canadian Journal of Biochemistry and Physiology,* 40:885–898.

Pearse, A. G. E. (1960): *Histochemistry, Theoretical and Applied*. Churchill, London.
Pellegrino de Iraldi, A., and Guedet, R. (1968): Action of reserpine on the osmium tetroxide zinc iodide reactive site of synaptic vesicles in the pineal nerves of the rat. *Zeitschrift für Zellforschung*, 91:178–185.
Pfenninger, K., Sandri, C., Akert, K., and Eugster, C. H. (1969): Contribution to the problem of structural organization of the presynaptic area. *Brain Research*, 12:10–18.
De Potter, W. P., Smith, A. D., and De Schaepdryver, A. F. (1970): Subcellular fractionation of splenic nerve: ATP, chromogranin A and dopamine-β-hydroxylase in noradrenergic vesicles. *Tissue and Cell*, 2:529–546.
Richardson, K. C. (1962): The fine structure of autonomic nerve endings in smooth muscle of the rat vas deferens. *Journal of Anatomy*, 96:427–442.
Richardson, K. C. (1964): The fine structure of the albino rabbit iris with special reference to the identification of adrenergic and cholinergic nerves and nerve endings in its intrinsic muscles. *American Journal of Anatomy*, 114:173–206.
Richardson, K. C. (1966): Electron microscopic identification of autonomic nerve endings. *Nature*, 210:756.
Smith, A. D., de Potter, W. P., Moerman, E. J., and de Schaepdryver, A. F. (1970): Release of dopamine-β-hydroxylase and chromogranin A upon stimulation of the splenic nerve. *Tissue and Cell*, 2:547–568.
Taxi, J. (1965): Contribution a l'étude des connexions des neurons moteurs du système nerveux autonome. *Annales des Sciences Naturelles, Zoologie*, (Paris), 7:413–674.
Taxi, J. (1968): Sur la fixation et la signification du contenu dense des vésicules des fibres adrénergiques étudiées du microscope électronique. *Comptes Rendus de l'Académie Bulgare des Sciences*, 21:1229–1231.
Taxi, J., Gautron, J., and L'Hermite, P. (1969): Données ultrastructurales sue une éventuelle modulation adrénergique de l'activité du ganglion cervical superieur du rat. *Comptes Rendus Hebdomadaires des Séances de l'Academie des Sciences* (Paris), 269:1281–1284.
Thorack, R. M., Dufty, M. L., and Haynes, J. M. (1965). The effect of anisotonic media upon cellular ultrastructure in fresh and fixed rat brain. *Zeitschrift für Zellforschung*, 66:690–700.
Tranzer, J. P., and Snipes, R. L. (1968): Fine structural localization of noradrenaline in sympathetic nerve terminals: a critical study of the influence of fixation. In: *Proceedings of the 4th European Regional Conference on Electron Microscopy*, edited by D. S. Bocciarelli. Tipografia Poliglotta Vaticana, Roma.
Tranzer, J. P., and Thoenen, H. (1967a): Electronmicroscopic localization of 5-hydroxydopamine (3,4,5-trihydroxyphenylethylamine), a new false sympathetic transmitter. *Experientia*, 23:743.
Tranzer, J. P., and Thoenen, H. (1967b): Significance of empty vesicles in postganglionic sympathetic nerve terminals. *Experientia*, 23:123–124.
Tranzer, J. P., and Thoenen, H. (1968): Various types of amine-storing vesicles in peripheral adrenergic nerve terminals. *Experientia*, 209:484–486.
Tramezzani, J. H., Chiocchio, S., and Wassermann, G. F. (1964)· A technique for light and electron microscopic identification of adrenalin- and noradrenalin-storing cells. *Journal of Histochemistry and Cytochemistry*, 12:890–899.
Van Gelder, N. M. (1965): The histochemical demonstration of γ-aminobutyric acid metabolism by reduction of a tetrazolium salt. *Journal of Neurochemistry*, 12:231–237.
Van Orden, L. S., Bloom, F. E., Barrnett, R. J., and Giarman, N. J. (1966): Histochemical and functional relationships of catecholamines in adrenergic nerve endings. I. Participation of granular vesicles. *Journal of Pharmacology and Experimental Therapeutics*, 154:185–199.
Van Orden, L. S., III, Burke, J. P., Geyer, M., and Lodoen, F. V. (1970): Localization of depletion-sensitive and depletion-resistant norepinephrine storage sites in autonomic ganglia. *Journal of Pharmacology and Experimental Therapeutics*, 174:56–71.
Wallach, D. P. (1961): Studies on the GABA pathway. The inhibition of γ-aminobutyric acid-α-ketoglutaric acid transaminase *in vitro* and *in vivo* by U7524 (amino-oxyacetic acid). *Biochemical Pharmacology*, 5:323–331.

Werman, R. (1966): A review—Criteria for identification of a central nervous system transmitter. *Comparative Biochemistry and Physiology*, 18:745–766.

Werman, R., Davidoff, R. A., and Aprison, M. H. (1968): Inhibitory action of glycine on spinal neurons in the cat. *Journal of Neurophysiology*, 31:81–95.

Wolfe, D. E., Potter, L. T., Richardson, K. C., and Axelrod, J. (1962): Localizing tritiated norepinephrine in sympathetic axons by electron microscope autoradiography. *Science*, 138:440–442.

Wood, J. G. (1966): Electron microscopic localization of amines in central nervous tissue. *Nature*, 209:1131–1133.

Wood, J. G. (1967): Cytochemical localization of 5-hydroxytryptamine (5-HT) in the central nervous system (CNS). *Anatomical Record*, 157:343.

Wood, J. G., and Barrnett, R. J. (1964): Histochemical demonstration of norepinephrine at a fine structural level. *Journal of Histochemistry and Cytochemistry*, 12:197–209.

Woods, R. I. (1969): Acrylic aldehyde in sodium dichromate as a fixative for identifying catecholamine storage sites with the electron microscope. *Journal of Physiology*, 35–36P.

Advances in Biochemical Psychopharmacology, Vol. 6
Raven Press, New York © 1972

Gas Chromatography — Mass Fragmentography: A New Approach to the Estimation of Amines and Amine Turnover

F. Cattabeni, S. H. Koslow, and E. Costa

*Laboratory of Preclinical Pharmacology, National Institute of Mental Health,
Saint Elizabeths Hospital, Washington, D.C. 20032*

INTRODUCTION

Dynamics of Catecholamine Pools in Neurons

Currently, the function of synapses that store catecholamines is studied by relating *in vivo* measurements of turnover rates of norepinephrine (NE) and dopamine (DA) to changes of neuronal activity associated with a defined behavioral pattern or drug action. To assess the validity of the conclusions drawn from such studies, we shall consider the neuron as a specialized secretory cell. This cell not only secretes the chemical mediator of nerve impulses but also enzymes (Hartman and Udenfriend, 1970; Smith, De Potter, Moerman, and DeSchaepdryver, 1970) and other proteins (De-Potter, DeSchaepdryver, Moerman, and Smith, 1969; Smith, 1971a) whose functional role is not yet understood.

The specialization involved in this secretory function derives from the extreme elongation of axons and the occurrence of the secretion in axon terminals where the rate of protein synthesis is limited (Droz, 1969). This sluggishness of protein synthesis in nerve terminals as compared to cell bodies (Barondes, 1969) creates a problem because in the nerve terminals the secretion proceeds at a fast rate and there is a great disproportionality between the volume of cell bodies and that of the axons emanating from them. To overcome these difficulties, the particles that store the trans-

37

mitter (synaptic vesicles) are transported from their site of formation (cell body) to the axon terminals by a unique system of axonal flow.

At the axon terminals, the process that brings about the transmitter release must overcome the obstacle created by the two membrane barriers (cellular and vesicular). This obstacle is obviated by the process of exocytosis, an ingenious mechanism which regulates the quantal release of transmitters (Fillenz, 1971). The high concentration of transmitter in the vesicles allows for the rapid shift in the transmitter concentrations at the extracellular receptor sites. We are just beginning to learn how to relate morphology of synaptic vesicles to the case history of their participation in neuronal secretion, and this information must now be considered to build simple biochemical models of neuronal function.

Catecholamines are synthesized in every part of the axon, including its terminal portion (Costa and Neff, 1966) where exocytosis takes place. In contrast, the proteins associated with storage and formation of catecholamines are synthesized in the cell body and packaged into vesicular particles before being transported by specialized mechanisms to the terminal portions of axons (Grillo, 1966; Lentz, 1969). Beams and Kessel (1968) have marshalled circumstantial evidence supporting the view that the packaging of proteins into a particle occurs in the Golgi apparatus or in a closely related structure. It is presently believed that the vesicle, during its life span in the axon, undergoes important morphological and biochemical changes. Several authors have discussed the diverse appearances of vesicles present in cell bodies and axons from that of vesicles in terminal axons (Grillo, 1966; Geffen and Ostberg, 1969). Large dense-cored vesicles prevail in cell bodies whereas small granular vesicles are the abundant subcellular particles in axon terminals (Grillo, 1966). Although both types of vesicles store NE, chromogranin A, and dopamine-β-hydroxylase (DBH), there are some differences in the relative abundance of these compounds (DePotter, Smith, and DeSchaepdryver, 1970). These differences should be kept in mind because they have potential implications in interpreting turnover-rate measurements of transmitters. The NE in small granular vesicles is more readily released by reserpine than is the NE of dense-cored vesicles (Taxi, 1971); the NE uptake by the large dense-cored vesicles is influenced by monoamine oxidase to a greater extent than is the NE uptake by small granular vesicles (Taxi, 1971); the ratio of DBH to NE is higher in large dense-cored vesicles than in small granular vesicles (DePotter, 1971). The large dense-cored vesicles can be found also in cholinergic axons (Taxi, 1961), and it is possible that this vesicle carries secretory and enzymatic proteins in both cholinergic and adrenergic axons (DeIraldi and DeRobertis, 1968). In adrenergic terminals, the small granular vesicles probably originate locally (Geffen and Ostberg, 1969) from the large dense-cored vesicles. Indirectly, the latter hypothesis questions whether the NE stored in the large dense-cored vesicles is ever released extracellularly by nerve impulses. Although this question cannot yet be answered positively, it is pertinent to note that exocytosis has now been demonstrated for large dense-cored vesicles of the adrenal medulla (Grynszpan-Winograd, 1971). It is probable that extracellular release of NE by exocytosis is the first step of the process that generates small granular vesicles from large dense-cored vesicles (Smith, 1971b).

Pools of Catecholamines and Turnover-Rate Measurements

It is presently believed that after exocytosis the membrane fragments of the large dense-cored vesicles reorganize into smaller granular vesicles which still contain DBH and chromogranin A (Smith, 1971a). The ratio between DBH and NE is greater in axons which contain mostly large dense-cored vesicles than in terminals which store small granular vesicles or in the perfusate of a sympathetically innervated tissue (Smith, 1970). We can, therefore, assume that the process which controls NE turnover rate in the small granular vesicles may differ from those in the large dense-cored vesicles because in the former DBH could be a rate-limiting enzyme. These considerations may imply that in terminal axons there are pools of NE with different turnover rates, which depend on the amount of DBH present. Recent studies (Weinshilboum, Johnson, Thoa, Axelrod, and Kopin, 1971), however, have shown no difference between the ratio of DBH and NE in the perfusate and in the sympathetically stimulated vas deferens when the ratio in the tissue was determined between the soluble DBH and the NE. This finding suggests that part of the DBH is membrane bound and that, if the functional enzyme were that bound to the vesicle membrane, then different concentrations of DBH in various types of granules may not necessarily mean differences in NE turnover rates.

Kopin, Breese, Krause, and Weise (1968) reported that newly synthesized NE is preferentially released upon stimulation of the splenic nerve. They assumed that the newly synthesized NE is incorporated in a small NE pool which turns over rapidly, and which would supply the transmitter to be released by nerve impulses. No good reason was ever given to explain why newly synthesized NE is preferentially released. The neuronal model they envisioned is identical to one previously considered by us to explain the biphasic decline of ^{3}H-NE taken up by rat heart tissue following the intravenous administration of DL-^{3}H-NE (Montanari, Costa, Beaven, and

Brodie, 1963). We have discarded this model for its inherent inconsistency, when we found that after administering tracer doses of L-^{3}H-NE, the specific activity of heart NE declined exponentially in a monophasic manner (Costa, Boullin, Hammer, Vogel, and Brodie, 1966). Before the report by Kopin et al. (1968), we also presented evidence that nerve impulses do not release NE from the total store but from a limited pool (Boullin, Costa, and Brodie, 1966). However, we would like to emphasize that in those experiments, as in the experiments reported by Kopin et al. (1968), either the perfusing fluid contained phenoxybenzamine or the frequency of nerve impulses was unphysiologically high. To defend the model with one compartment open at both ends (Neff, Ngai, Wang, and Costa, 1969), we could recall that by perfusing at constant rates with labeled tyrosine (Neff et al., 1969) or with pulse injections of the labeled amino acid (Neff, Spano, Groppetti, Wang, and Costa, 1971), we could calculate the same apparent rate of catecholamine turnover. In these experiments, the fractional rate constant was calculated from the specific activities of precursor and product at various times selected either during the first 25 min immediately after the labeling or between 40 and 240 min after labeling (Table 1). An unsurmountable difficulty in any attempt to calculate absolute synthesis rates of tissue catecholamines is represented by the impossibility of measuring the specific radioactivity of the precursor pool of tyrosine. To overcome this problem, we have entertained the view that O_2 may be the precursor of choice. The source of O_2 for enzymes such as tyrosine hydroxylase is molecular oxygen. This rapidly equilibrating homogeneous oxygen pool is regulated by the diffusion coefficient for O_2 in which the driving gradient is assumed to be concentration difference (Forster, 1964). In a man of 70 kg, who has a rate of O_2 consumption of 300 ml/min, the total O_2 store can be calculated to be 1,546 ml (Rehn, 1964), thus providing a precursor pool with a very rapid turnover.

TABLE 1. *Turnover rates of dopamine in striatum of rats calculated from the specific activity of the precursor and the product at various times after pulse injections of ^{3}H-L-tyrosine*

Method	k (per hr)	nmoles/ g/hr	Reference
Pulse labeling with 3,5^{3}H-tyrosine (k calculated from 40 min to 240 min after label)	0.34	21[a]	Neff et al. (1971)
Pulse labeling with 3,5^{3}H-tyrosine (k calculated from 10 min to 25 min after label)	0.34	22[a]	Costa et al. (1971)

[a] Calculated for a dopamine steady state of 65 nmoles/g.

Use of ^{18}O to Label Catecholamine Pools

It is now well established that the hydroxylation of tyrosine depends on the function of specific hydroxylase belonging to the general group of mixed-function oxygenases (Mason, 1957). This hydroxylase reaction requires both oxygen and an external electron donor, the pteridine cofactor. The requirement for oxygen is specific. In those systems where the reaction has been studied with ^{18}O, it has been shown that the hydroxyl oxygen atom is derived from molecular oxygen. Thus, hydroxylase reactions should be distinguished from hydration reactions where the hydroxyl oxygen is derived from water (Kaufman, 1962). While the intermediary metabolism of various small rapidly turning over molecules is characterized by oxidation via dehydrogenation, the oxidation by addition of molecular oxygen prevails in oxidation of stable organic molecules. The general equation for this reaction as it applies to tyrosine hydroxylase is

$$T_H + D_{H_2} + O_2 \xrightarrow{\text{tyrosine hydroxylase}} T_{OH} + D + H_2O$$

where T_H is the tyrosine, T_{OH} is 3,4-dihydroxyphenylalanine, and D_{H_2} is pteridine cofactor functioning as a hydrogen donor. The molecular oxygen (O_2) that participates in this reaction comes directly from the air. If a stable isotope of oxygen (^{18}O) is introduced in the body by the inspired air, one can attempt to estimate turnover rates of catecholamines by measuring the temporal changes in the abundance of the ^{18}O in the tissue molecular oxygen content and that in the synaptic stores of catecholamines. However, to measure incorporation of ^{18}O into the catecholamine pathway, it is necessary to develop a completely new technology for catecholamine assay based on mass fragmentography (Sweeley, Elliott, and Ryhage, 1966; Hammar, Holmstedt, Lindgren, and Tham, 1969).

In the following sections we shall report the general principles of mass fragmentography and the development of a quantitative mass fragmentographic assay of tissue catecholamines which is the necessary first step to develop turnover-rate measurements with ^{18}O labeling. Since at this time the technique of using ^{18}O to measure turnover rates of catecholamines is still in the developmental stage, we have tried to document the reliability and sensitivity of quantitative mass fragmentography by identifying and measuring small catecholamine pools in various tissues (i.e., locus coeruleus) and characterizing possible functional and morphological differences in the catecholamine pools of the superior cervical ganglion.

BACKGROUND INFORMATION FOR MASS FRAGMENTOGRAPHY OF TISSUE CATECHOLAMINES

We advise the reader interested in a detailed description of mass fragmentography to consult the review published by Hammar et al. (1969). Here we simply summarize some basic principles involved in our adaptation of mass fragmentography to assay tissue concentrations of catecholamines.

Gas Chromatography

In gas chromatographic analysis of primary amines, it is necessary to transform these amines into derivatives with greater volatility and lower polarity than those of the parent compound. A technique has been described by Anggard and Sedvall (1969) to form acylated volatile derivatives of catecholamine metabolites following reaction with pentafluoropropionic anhydride (PFPA). We have adapted this derivative formation to tissue catecholamine analysis. As we shall describe later, we found by mass spectrometry that four pentafluoropropionyl (PFP) groups are added to NE and three PFP groups are introduced into DA.

Gas Chromatography–Mass Spectrometry

The great advantage of connecting a gas chromatograph (GC) (Fig. 1, No. 1) to a mass spectrometer (MS) is given by the superior fractionation capacity of the GC and the analytical specificity of the MS. The GC is connected to the MS by a molecular separator (Fig. 1, No. 2). This molecular separator allows 50% of the molecules, heavier than helium, to enter the ion source, while removing 99% of the carrier gas from the system (Ryhage, 1967). In this way, the carrier gas does not interfere with the mass spectral analysis. Leaving the separator, the molecules enter the ionization chamber (Fig. 1, No. 3) where they are subjected to electron bombardment, resulting in their ionization and fragmentation. The positively charged ions are then accelerated by an electric field. To gain entrance to the flight tube, the ion beam passes through a hole in a total ion current electrode (Fig. 1, No. 4). In this way, 10% of the total ions leaving the ion source are collected by the electrode and the intensity of this current is amplified and recorded on a strip chart (Fig. 1, A). In the flight tube,

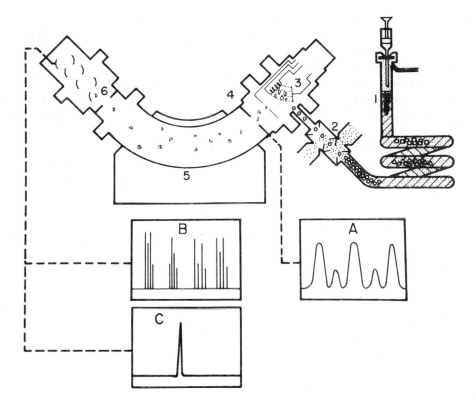

FIG. 1. Schematic drawing of LKB 9000 GC-MS. See text for full description. For normal mass spectroscopy, when the peak of a compound is measured on the total ion current monitor (*A*) the magnetic field is varied and the mass spectrum recorded on the UV recorder (*B*); for mass fragmentography, the magnetic field is held constant at a specific *m/e* during the entire elution of a compound from the GC, and the total ion density of this fragment recorded on the UV recorder (*C*). 1, Gas chromatograph; 2, molecular separator; 3, ionization chamber; 4, total ion current electrode; 5, magnetic field; 6, specific ion (*m/e*) detector.

the ions are subjected to a magnetic field (Fig. 1, No. 5) which deflects them according to their mass to charge ratio[1] (*m/e*). Equation (1) expresses the relationship between the factors involved in mass spectrometry:

$$m/e = \frac{H^2 r^2}{2V} \tag{1}$$

[1] Since in most cases, there is only a single positive charge, the *m/e* is usually equivalent to the mass number of the fragment.

where r is the radius of the curvature of the path of the ions which is constant, H is the strength of the magnetic field, and V is the accelerating voltage. To obtain the mass spectrum of a compund, H^2 is increased, resulting in the successive impingment of ions with an increasing m/e upon the first dynode of the electron multiplier (Fig. 1, No. 6). The resulting secondary electrons are further amplified (10^7) by the remaining dynodes of the electron multiplier, subjected to DC amplification, and the electrical signal recorded on a UV recorder (Fig. 1, B).

To record the mass spectrum of a compound, 10^{-6} to 10^{-7} mole must be used. At the maximum intensity of the total ion current, as recorded on the strip chart (Fig. 1, A), the magnetic field is continually varied, thereby allowing for the measurement and recording (Fig. 1, B) of the fragmentation pattern of the compound. This fragmentation is then expressed in terms of the most abundant fragment (base peak) (Fig. 2).

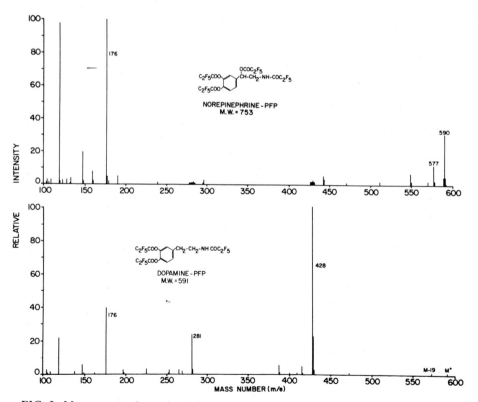

FIG. 2. Mass spectra of norepinephrine, dopamine pentafluoropropionyl derivatives (PFP). For mass spectrometric conditions, see text.

Mass Fragmentography

Equation (1) shows that when H^2 and V are kept constant, only ions with a given m/e will be detected. By keeping the magnetic field constant, the sensitivity of detection is increased so that as little as 10^{-14} to 10^{-15} mole can be detected. This is possible because the ion density of the specific fragment is continually monitored (Fig. 1, No. 6) and recorded (Fig. 1, C) during the entire time the compound is eluted from the GC. The compound is thus identified by its GC retention time and its specific fragmentation at this time. Greater specificity is obtained by simultaneously monitoring two or more fragments (multiple-ion detection). The relative abundance of these fragments to each other is then compared to the relative abundance of these fragments as determined from a normal mass spectrum (see above Section). On the LKB 9000 GC-MS, this may be done by keeping constant the magnetic field and increasing the accelerating voltage [V, Eq. (1)]. However, there are limitations: (1) only three fragments can be simultaneously measured; and (2) the m/e of the three fragments must be within a 10% range of each other. It is obvious from the mass spectra of the NE and DA derivatives (Fig. 2) that multiple-ion detection is not possible since there are no other abundant fragments (m/e) within a 10% range of the base peak, and we must use the base peak to obtain maximal sensitivity. We have therefore increased the specificity of the assay for different tissues by measuring the density of different characteristic fragments in separate analysis, using the internal standards to correct for variations between individual runs (Koslow, Cattabeni, and Costa, 1972).

Routinely we focus only on the base peaks of the endogenous amines and the closest most abundant peaks (m/e) of the internal standards (Table 2). To do this, the magnetic field is set to the specific m/e value prior to the

TABLE 2. *Gas chromatography (GC) retention time and mass spectrometric specifications for mass fragmentographic analysis of pentafluoropropionyl (PFP) derivities of norepinephrine, dopamine, and their internal standards*

PFP-amine derivative	GC retention time (min)	m/e of assayed fragment	Min focused on m/e of fragment to be assayed
α-Methylnorepinephrine[a]	2.08	190 (100)[b]	0–2.5
Norepinephrine	2.83	176 (100)	2.5–3.6
α-Methyldopamine[a]	4.36	442 (33)	3.6–5.1
Dopamine	5.83	428 (100)	5.1–7.0

[a] Internal standard.
[b] In parentheses the relative abundance of fragments (100-base peak).

compounds' elution from the GC. The magnetic field is then held constant during the entire elution of the compound thereby recording the ion density of a specific fragment (m/e) (Table 2). The magnetic field is then altered to record the specific fragment of the next compound eluted from the GC column. In this manner, structural specificity is derived from the m/e value of the fragment recorded when the compound is eluted from the GC at an exact retention time.

ANALYSIS OF TISSUE CATECHOLAMINES

Selection of the Internal Standard

To correct for losses in the preparation of the samples and to relate ion density generated by a specific fragment to the concentration of the compound present in the tissue specimen, it is necessary to immediately add an appropriate internal standard to the tissue homogenate. A compound qualifies as an internal standard for quantitative mass fragmentographic analysis of a catecholamine if it meets the following requirements. (1) The rates of the forward and backward reactions of the standard with the acylating reagent must be identical to that of the catecholamine considered. (2) The derivatives of the standards must have GC retention times similar to the catecholamines. (3) The fragmentation pattern and the percent of the total ion current represented by the base peak of the standard must be similar to that of the catecholamine. (4) When using an LKB 9000, the m/e value of the base peak of the catecholamine and the standard must be within 10% in order to be monitored simultaneously by alternating the accelerating voltage. However, requirement (4) is not essential if the retention time of the internal standard and that of the catecholamine are sufficiently different to allow time for the refocusing of the instrument to their respective m/e values. As a result of the search for appropriate internal standards for the assay of tissue catecholamine content by mass fragmentography, we found that α-methylnorepinephrine (α-MNE) and α-methyldopamine (α-MDA) are appropriate internal standards for NE and DA, respectively.

Reaction Condition

In the formation of derivatives for quantitative anlaysis, it is required that the time necessary for the reaction to reach completion applies to a wide concentration range of the catecholamines. We have shown by GC–mass fragmentography that when NE, DA, α-MNE, and α-MDA in concentrations of 0.5 to 200 pmoles react with PFPA (100 μl of PFPA in 20 μl ethylacetate) at 60°C, the acylation of catecholamines reaches a steady state in 30 min. The yield of the reaction was estimated fluorimetrically after concentrations of NE and DA between 300 and 1,000 pmoles and concentrations of α-MNE and α-MDA 10-fold greater were reacted with PFPA at 60°C for 30 min. At the end of the reaction, the acylated derivatives were extracted into benzene and the unreacted amines detected fluorimetrically. These tests revealed that 90 to 100% of the catecholamines and their internal standards were acylated by PFPA. The acylated amines are stable for at least 24 hr if maintained with an excess of PFPA and the other products of the reaction. The acylated derivatives are unstable as soon as the other reactants and PFPA are removed. However, we have ascertained that the rate constant for the backward reaction is equal for both catecholamines and their respective internal standards.

Mass Spectra of the PFP Derivatives of Catecholamines α-MDA and α-MNE

The gas chromatographic conditions are: 12-ft glass column (i.d. 2 mm) packed with OV 17, 3% on Gas Chrom Q (100–120 mesh); flash heater, 280°C; column oven, 180°C; helium flow, 20 ml/min. The mass spectrometric conditions are: molecular separator, 240°C; ion source, 290°C; electron energy, 80 eV, trap current 60 μamp; and electron multiplier 3.7 kV. Mass spectral analysis of NE-PFP and DA-PFP (Fig. 2) revealed that these compounds have their most abundant fragment at m/e 176 and m/e 428, respectively. Their internal standards show the same type of fragmentation pattern. α-MNE and α-MDA both have their most abundant fragments at m/e 190, and α-MDA has a second intense fragment at m/e 442. A complete explanation of the fragmentation pattern of these four compounds is found elsewhere (Koslow et al., 1972).

Linearity of the Reaction

To test the linearity of the reaction, we kept the concentrations of the internal standards (α-MNE, α-MDA) constant (20 pmoles) and varied the amount of NE and DA (0.5 to 200 pmoles). In practice, an exact amount of catecholamines and their internal standard dissolved in 0.1 M formic acid and 50 mM ascorbic acid are placed into a 0.3-ml screw-cap reaction vial. The solutions are dried under a jet of nitrogen, and to each vial 100 μl of PFPA and 20 μl of ethylacetate are added. The vials are capped

(Teflon-lined caps) and incubated at 60°C for 30 min. Immediately before analysis, the excess PFPA is evaporated and the residue dissolved in 10 μl of ethylacetate. Usually we inject 2 μl and at the retention times listed (Table 2) we record the ion density generated by the fragments corresponding to the base peaks. Plotting the ion-density ratio between NE and its internal standard on the ordinate and the absolute amine concentrations on the abscissa, a linear relationship is obtained (Fig. 3). Similar linearity is obtained for DA and α-MDA.

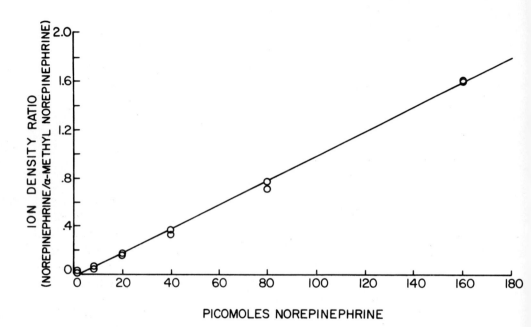

FIG. 3. Using the procedure described in the text, a linear relationship is obtained for standard NE with its α-methyl analog as internal standard.

Assay Procedure

Tissue samples (usually a few mg or less) were homogenized in a constant volume of a 50 mM solution of ascorbic acid in 0.1 M formic acid. An aliquot of the homogenate is used for protein assay (Lowry, Rosebrough, Farr, and Randall, 1951) and the remainder centrifuged at 4°C for 15 min at 1.2×10^4 g. A small volume of this supernatant is added to vials containing the two internal standards (20 pmoles) and processed as described above.

The concentrations of NE and DA found in a constant aliquot of various dilutions of a superior cervical ganglion homogenate are graphically displayed in Fig. 4. These data show that the analysis is linear over a wide range of tissue concentrations, supporting the reliability of our quantitative assay. Figure 5 depicts a typical mass fragmentogram obtained by analyzing a volume of homogenate equivalent to $1/60$ of a rat superior cervical ganglion (approximately 15 μg of tissue).

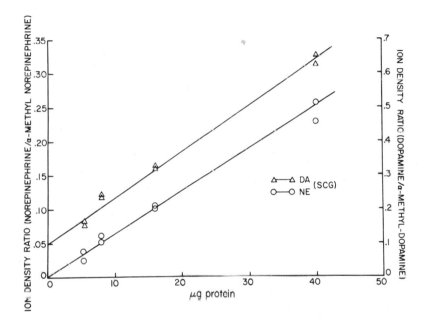

FIG. 4. A linear relationship is obtained when analyzing the endogenous levels of NE and DA using different quantities of a homogenate of one superior cervical ganglion (SCG) of the rat.

COMPARING THE SENSITIVITY OF MASS FRAGMENTOGRAPHY TO OTHER METHODS USED TO ASSAY TISSUE CATECHOLAMINES

We have determined in two separate assays the NE and DA concentrations in various rat tissues by the spectrophotofluorometric and the mass fragmentographic method (Table 3). The results obtained with the two methods show reasonable agreement. The high DA value obtained for the

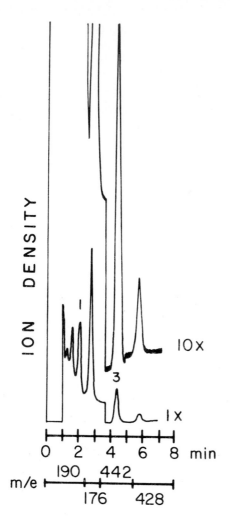

FIG. 5. Mass fragmentogram obtained from analysis of $\frac{1}{60}$ of a homogenate of a rat superior cervical ganglion. Internal standards (peaks 1 and 3) were added to the sample before processing. The peak between 1 and 3 and the one immediately after 3 correspond to the peaks for NE and DA, respectively (Table 1).

striatum with the mass fragmentography method may be explained by the fact that only the center most portion of the caudate nucleus was analyzed; whereas the spectrophotofluorometric analysis was performed on the entire striatum. By showing the data of Table 3, we do not intend to emphasize that mass fragmentography is more sensitive than fluorometric methods; we are showing these data simply to document that the values obtained with the two methods are similar. In fact, it is possible to develop gas chromatographic methods based on this acylation reaction which may meas-

TABLE 3. *Assay of tissue norepinephrine (NE) and dopamine (DA) content mass fragmentography compared with spectrophotofluorometry*

Tissue	Mass fragmentography			Spectroflurometry[a]		
	NE	DA	Wet wt. (mg)	NE	DA	Wet wt. (mg)
Cerebellum	1.1 ± 0.26[b] (4)	0.21 ± 0.04 (5)	250	1.1 ± 0.13 (4)	0.29 ± 0.031 (12)	750
Superior cervical ganglion	78 ± 6.1 (7)	13 ± 1.7 (7)	1.4	[c]	[c]	1.3
Striatum	2.0 ± 0.07 (3)	83 ± 5.1 (3)	27	[c]	54 ± 8.2 (4)	50
Salivary gland	7.3 ± 0.38 (4)	0.092 ± 0.016 (4)	250	5.3 ± 0.32 (4)	[c]	330

[a] Spectrophotofluorometric assay was carried out according to the procedure described by Neff et al. (1966).

[b] Catecholamine concentrations are given as the mean ± SE, nmole/g wet weight of tissue. Number of rats in parentheses.

[c] This amine could not be detected by processing the total amount of tissue sampled. Brain was dissected as described in Costa et al. (1971).

ure as little as 3 to 5 pmoles of catecholamines using electron capture detectors (Karoum, Cattabenni, Costa, Ruthvan, and Sandler, 1972). However, the sensitivity of the fragmentographic method is probably at least 20-fold greater (0.06 to 0.1 pmole). Where the greater sensitivity of our method is more evident is in the measurement of DA which can be performed simultaneously with that of NE without any additional manipulation.

The specificity of the fluorometric method rests on the chemical separation of the compounds. Unless one combines ion-exchange chromatography and adsorption onto Al_2O_3, one cannot be absolutely sure that he is measuring the amines rather than the acidic metabolites or the amino acid precursors. This danger is particularly evident when dealing with biological fluids or with tissues of animals receiving either amino acid precursors or drugs which block decarboxylation or the efflux of the acidic metabolites of catechols. The specificity of mass spectrometry depends on the separation of the compounds before reaching the ion source and of the structural recognition of ion detection at specific m/e values.

We would like to emphasize that, by using high-resolution instruments, one cannot achieve equal specificity because high resolution cannot compensate for gas chromatographic separation. In this case, a high-resolution instrument may help to recognize the chemical composition of the fragment but this recognition does not indicate whether a given fragment originates from the same compound unless at the time of the analysis only one compound reaches the ion source. Quantitative measurement of amine content in brain with a high-resolution mass spectrometer using the direct-inlet probe rather than gas chromatography for the introduction of the sample have been reported by Majer and Boulton (1970). The values given in that paper and in other communications by the same authors are at variance with values reported by other authors (Gunne and Jonsson, 1965). A reason for this discrepancy might be the fact that Majer and Boulton (1970) attempted quantitative analysis by introducing an impure sample into the instrument with the heated direct-inlet system; with this procedure several compounds may vaporize simultaneously. Other obvious sources for error are unsymmetrical peaks (envelope) and the lack of an internal standard. These essentials cannot be overlooked when quantitative analysis is the object of a study. The use of the direct inlet cannot be compared with mass fragmentography where the derivatization of the compound, recognition of ions by fragmentography, and retention time on the gas chromatograph give three extra dimensions of accuracy that make the assay very specific.

To summarize, (a) derivatization, (b) retention time, (c) presence of suitable internal standards, (d) measurement of ion density at a given m/e value, and (e) measurement of ratios of two characteristic fragments contribute to making mass fragmentography a powerful qualitative and quantitative tool for neurochemical analysis.

CHARACTERIZING TISSUE DOPAMINE STORES ASSOCIATED WITH SYNAPTIC FUNCTION

The data reported in Table 3 show that DA is present in various tissues; its concentrations are very low in the cerebellum and salivary gland as compared to its levels in the superior cervical ganglion and striatum. Histochemical and biochemical evidence (Dahlström and Fuxe, 1964; Fuxe and Andén, 1966; Fuxe and Hökfelt, 1966, and 1967) suggests that fluorescent fibers in the striatum contain dopamine. More controversial are the attempts made to explain the origin of the DA in sympathetic ganglia. The superior cervical sympathetic ganglion of the rat has three distinct neuronal populations: the noradrenergic sympathetic neurons, a few cholinergic neurons, and the small intensely fluorescent (S1F) cells. It was initially suggested that these S1F cells contain serotonin (Eranko and Harkonen, 1965), but later studies strongly indicate that these cells contain a catecholamine (Norberg, Ritzen, and Ungerstedt, 1966). Comparatively high concentrations of DA have been identified in sympathetic ganglia (Bjorklund, Cegrell, Falck, Ritzen, and Rosengreen, 1970), and we have confirmed this for the superior cervical ganglion of the rat with mass fragmentography (Table 3). It is thus possible that the S1F cells contain dopamine, although proof of this would require the dissection of S1F cells and the measurement of their NE and DA content.

This naturally brings up the question whether the mass fragmentographic method is sufficiently sensitive to assay the catecholamine concentrations in single cells. Fuxe and Andén (1966) have estimated that a cell body in the substantia nigra contains between 5 to 20 femtomoles (10^{-15} mole) of dopamine in a volume ranging between 10^4 and 2×10^4 μ^3, to a final concentration of 60 to 200 μg/g wet weight. Since the fluorescent intensity of S1F cells is higher than that of cells in the substantia nigra, S1F cells may contain a greater concentration of DA. The sensitivity limit of the method we have just described is 30 to 60 femtomoles. We have occasionally succeeded in detecting catecholamine peaks from the analysis of single isolated neurons from the rat superior cervical ganglion. We have, however, failed to perform such measurements on single cells reproducibly.

Since we cannot yet take the direct approach of determining the molecular nature of the transmitter stored in S1F cells, we have attempted to answer this question indirectly by using pharmacological agents. Norberg, Ritzen, and Ungerstedt (1966) and Van Orden, Burke, Geyer, and Loeden (1970) have shown by histofluorometry that the catecholamine stored in S1F cells is resistant to depletion by high doses of reserpine. The experiments reported in Table 4 show that ganglionic DA is more resistant than NE to depletion by reserpine. In fact, when compared to control values, 0.1 mg/kg of reserpine i.v. depletes NE by 82% and does not significantly alter the DA concentration. A reserpine dose of 0.5 mg/kg depletes NE by 92% and DA by only 55%. These results suggest that the reserpine-resistant amine stores of the S1F cells contain DA rather than NE as suggested by Van Orden et al. (1970). The catecholamine which modulates synaptic transmission in sympathetic ganglia (Costa, Revzin, Kuntzman, Spector, and Brodie, 1961; Eccles and Libet, 1961) may be DA. This amine applied locally hyperpolarizes the membrane of ganglion cells without changing its conductance to various ions (Libet and Tosaka, 1969, 1970). The reserpine-resistant DA store is, however, insufficient evidence to implicate this store in synaptic transmission.

What does resistance to reserpine depletion indicate? The adrenal medulla is another tissue where catecholamine stores are resistant to the depletion elicited by reserpine. It may be important that S1F cells in ganglia and chromaffin cells in adrenals both contain large dense-cored vesicles and

TABLE 4. *Reserpine depletion of norepinephrine (NE) and dopamine (DA) in the superior cervical ganglion of rats*

Reserpine (mg/kg i.v.)	NE	DA	NE	DA
	(pmoles/mg protein) (mean ± SE)		(% depletion)	
0	940 ± 96 (12)	100 ± 13 (11)	0	0
0.1	170 ± 12[a] (3)	76 ± 2.3 (3)	81.6	25.1
0.5	73 ± 10[a] (9)	46 ± 7.0[a] (9)	92.2	54.9
5.0	67 ± 8.5[a] (3)	18 ± 3.9[a] (3)	93.8	72
10.0	59 (2)	21 (2)	94.7	79.4

Animals were sacrificed 2 hr after reserpine. Number of animals in parentheses.
[a] $p < 0.05$ when compared to mean of ganglia from untreated rats.

have short processes (Williams and Palay, 1969). If these characteristics are related to reserpine resistance, then one might think that the depletion of catecholamines by reserpine can be evidenced more promptly if the cells are transporting synaptic vesicles over elongated cellular processes. This view is supported by the finding that the time course of the reserpine depletion is shorter-lasting in the cell body than in the nerve terminals (Dahlström, Fuxe, and Hillarp, 1965). Considering the dynamic aspects of the renewal of granules in S1F cells and adrenal cells, and that of synaptic vesicles in axon terminals, we might propose that the percentage of the storage granules replaced per unit of time is high in the chromaffin and S1F cells and comparatively low in the axon terminals. The view that it is easy to deplete amines by reserpine in the sites where the replacement of granules occurs at a slow rate is supported by a report of Andén and Lundborg (1970) which shows that recovery of catecholamines after reserpine depends on axonal transport of granules.

    We explored whether diethyldithiocarbamate (DDC) could be used as a tool to exclude the possibility that DA plays a role only as a precursor of NE. This drug inhibits DBH (Goldstein, Anagnoste, Lauber, and Mc-Kereghan, 1964); hence, it should change the NE and DA concentrations in opposite directions if the cell secretes NE and the DA is the precursor of NE. If DA and NE are in different cells, and if only a part of the DA present in the tissue serves as the NE precursor, DDC should decrease NE but the increase of DA would be relatively insignificant. DDC was administered (200 mg/kg, iv.) to rats to determine whether DA in superior cervical ganglia is an end product or is related to catecholamine biosynthesis (Table 5). A dose of DDC which decreases NE concentrations in ganglion or in the cerebellum by more than 50% fails to increase the DA concentration in the ganglion, but it increases by 20-fold or more the concentration of DA in the cerebellum. In the same rats, the changes in the NE and DA content of the salivary gland, although not statistically significant, do suggest that here DA is a precursor for NE synthesis. Obviously, rates of NE turnover and the half-life of the drug must be considered in interpreting these data.

Can we then conclude that DA has a synaptic action in those tissues where there is no change in its concentration after injections of high doses of DDC? From inspection of Table 5, this conclusion could be accepted provisionally if it were not for the results of the experiments with locus coeruleus, which presumably does not contain dopaminergic nerves, but does not respond to DDC. As a tentative explanation for such discrepancies, we would like to suggest that in the locus coeruleus, which contains cell bodies of noradrenergic neurons, DA may not change after DDC because the recently synthesized granules may contain DBH in excess.

TABLE 5. *Norepinephrine (NE) and dopamine (DA) concentrations[a] in tissues of rats receiving saline or diethyldithiocarbamate (DDC) intravenously[b]*

Tissue	Control		DDC	
	NE	DA	NE	DA
Superior cervical ganglion	100 ± 8.6 (7)	18 ± 2.3 (7)	44 ± 2^c (5)	17 ± 1.8 (5)
Locus coeruleus	20 ± 1.6 (6)	3.2 ± 0.25 (6)	16 ± 1.3 (5)	$3.7 + 0.6$ (5)
Cerebellum	270 ± 66 (4)	53 ± 10 (5)	67 ± 8.2^c (4)	170 ± 21^c (4)
Salivary gland	1.800 ± 94 (4)	23 ± 3.9 (4)	$1,300 \pm 250$ (3)	55 ± 12 (3)
Striatum	54 ± 2 (3)	$2,200 \pm 140$ (3)	39 ± 0.58^c (3)	$2,200 + 48$ (3)

[a] Mean $\pm$ SE, pmoles/total tissue sampled.

[b] 200 mg/kg was injected 2 hr before killing the rats. Number of rats in parentheses. The weight for the locus coeruleus (about 0.1 mg) cannot be accurately given since invariable slight excess of surrounding tissue was included to ensure complete dissection of this nucleus. For weights of other tissues sampled, see Table 3.

[c] Significantly different from control values ($p < 0.05$).

SUMMARY

One of the problems encountered in estimating catecholamine turnover after injection of radioactive tyrosine is that of measuring the specific activity of the amino acid precursor. We cannot isolate the precursor and, while we measure the specific activity of the amino acid in the tissue, its specific activity may not be uniform in the various functional pools (Neff et al., 1971). Using ^{18}O as precursor, mass fragmentography offers the possibility of measuring the changes with time of the abundance of ^{18}O into the O_2 and the catecholamine pools. Since the O_2 pool of tissue is in rapid flux, the error of the turnover-rate measurements by this method should be negligible.

We have described a mass fragmentographic assay for tissue catecholamines which is readily applicable to the quantitation of catecholamines labeled with heavy isotopes. In addition to this unique capability, this method is also rapid, sensitive, and imparts greater specificity than other available methods (enzymatic and fluorometric). This method also allows for the simultaneous detection of DA with a sensitivity about 100 times greater than that of the most sensitive method presently available.

The problem of identifying whether DA functions as a transmitter in a tissue that contains both NE and DA can be investigated but not solved by the use of DDC. The test of reserpine resistance combined with the study of the action of DDC is not sufficient to give a final answer to the question of whether a tissue containing noradrenergic neurons also contains neurons which "exclusively" store DA. A final answer to this question requires isolation of the neurons and their analysis with mass fragmentography. Mass fragmentography possesses sufficient sensitivity to detect the concentrations of catecholamines in single neurons.

REFERENCES

Andén, N-E., and Lundborg, P. (1970): Recovery of the amine uptake-storage mechanism in nerve granules after reserpine treatment inhibition by axotomy. *Journal of Pharmacy and Pharmacology*, 22:233–235.

Anggard, E., and Sedvall, G. (1969): Gas chromatography of catecholamine metabolites using electron capture detection and mass spectrometry. *Analytical Chemistry*, 41:1250–1256.

Barondes, S. H. (1969): Two sites of synthesis of macromolecules in neurons. In: *Cellular Dynamics of the Neuron*, edited by S. H. Barondes. Academic Press, London, pp. 351–364.

Bjorklund, A., Cegrell, L., Falck, B., Ritzen, M., and Rosengreen, E. (1970): Dopamine containing cells in sympathetic ganglia. *Acta Physiologica Scandinavica*, 78:334–338.

Boullin, D. J., Costa, E., and Brodie, B. B. (1966): Apparent depletion of NE stores after repetitive stimulation of cat colon in presence of phenoxybenzamine. *International Journal of Neurochemistry*, 5:293–298.

Costa, E., Boullin, D. J., Hammer, W., Vogel, W., and Brodie, B. B. (1966): Interactions of drugs with adrenergic neurons. *Pharmacological Reviews*, 18:577–597.

Costa, E., Naimzada, M., and Revuelta, A. (1971): Phenmetrazine, aminorex, and (±) *p*-chloroamphetamine: Their effects on motor activity and turnover rate of brain catecholamines. *British Journal of Pharmacology*, 43:570–580.

Costa, E., and Neff, N. H. (1966): The physiological role of monoamine oxidase (MAO) in monoamine oxidase inhibitors. In: *Monoamine Oxidase Inhibitors: Relationship Between Pharmacological and Clinical Effects*, edited by J. Cheymol and J. R. Boissier. Proceedings of the Third International Pharmacology Meeting, 10:15–32.

Costa, E., Revzin, A. M., Kuntzman, R., Spector, S., and Brodie, B. B. (1961): Role for ganglionic norepinephrine in sympathetic synaptic transmission. *Science*, 133:1822–1823.

Dahlström, A., and Fuxe, K. (1964): Evidence for the existence of monoamine containing neurons in the central nervous system. *Acta Physiologica Scandinavica*, 62: Suppl. 232.

Dahlström, A., Fuxe, K., and Hillarp, N. A. (1965): Site of action of reserpine. *Acta Pharmacologica et Toxicologica*, 22:277–292.

Delraldi, A. P., and DeRobertis, E. (1968): The neurotubular system of the axon and the origin of granulated and nongranulated vesicles in regenerating nerves. *Zietschrift für Zellenforschung und Mikroskopische Anatomie*, 87:330–344.

DePotter, W. P. (1971): Noradrenaline storage particles in splenic nerve. *Philosophical Transactions of the Royal Society of London*, 261:313–317.

DePotter, W. P., DeSchaepdryver, A. F., Moerman, E. J., and Smith, A. D. (1969): Evidence for the release of vesicle proteins together with noradrenaline upon stimulation of the splenic nerves. *Journal of Physiology*, 204:102–104.

DePotter, W. P., Smith, A. D., and DeSchaepdryver, A. F. (1970): Subcellular fractionation of splenic nerve: ATP, chromogranin A and dopamine-β-hydroxylase in noradrenergic vesicles. *Tissue and Cell*, 2:529–546.

Droz, B. (1969): Protein metabolism in nerve cells. *International Review of Cytology*, 25:363–390

Eccles, R. M., and Libet, B. (1961): Origin and blockade of the synaptic responses of curarized sympathetic ganglia. *Journal of Physiology*, 157:484–503.

Eranko, O., and Harkonen, M. (1965): Monoamine-containing small cells in the superior cervical ganglia of the rat and an organ composed of them. *Acta Physiologica Scandinavica*, 63: 511–512.

Fillenz, M. (1971): Fine structure of noradrenaline storage vesicles in nerve terminals of the rat vas deferens. *Philosophical Transactions of the Royal Society of London*, 261:319–339.

Forster, R. E. (1964): Factors affecting the rate of exchange of O_2 between blood and tissues. In: *Oxygen in the Animal Organism*, edited by F. Dickens and E. Neil. Pergamon Press, Oxford, pp. 393–407.

Fuxe, K., and Andén, N-E. (1966): Studies on central monoamine neurons with special reference to the nigro-neostriatal dopamine neuron system. In: *Biochemistry and Pharmacology of the Basal Ganglia*, edited by E. Costa, L. Cote, and M. D. Yahr. Raven Press, New York, pp. 123–129.

Fuxe, K., and Hokfelt, T. (1966): Further evidence for the existence of tubero-infundibular dopamine neurons. *Acta Physiologica Scandinavica*, 66:245–246.

Fuxe, K., and Hokfelt, T. (1967): The influence of central catecholamine neurons on the hormone secretion from the anterior and posterior pituitary. In: *Neurosecretion*, edited by F. Stutinsky, Springer-Verlag; Berlin, pp. 165–177.

Geffen, L. B., and Ostberg, A. (1969): Distribution of granular vesicles in normal and constricted sympathetic neurons. *Journal of Physiology*, 204:583–592.

Goldstein, M., Anagnoste, B., Lauber, E., and McKereghan, M. R. (1964): Inhibition of dopamine-β-hydroxylase by disulfiram. *Life Sciences*, 3:763–767.

Grillo, M. A. (1966): Electron microscopy of sympathetic tissues. *Pharmacological Reviews*, 18:389–399.

Grynszpan-Winograd, O. (1971): Morphological aspects of exocytosis in the adrenal medulla. *Philosophical Transactions of the Royal Society of London*, 261:291–292.

Gunne, L.-M., and Jonsson, J. (1965): On the occurrence of tyramine in the rabbit brain. *Acta Physiologica Scandinavica*, 64:434–438.

Hammar, G. C., Holmstedt, B., Lindgren, J-E., and Tham, R. (1969): The combination of gas chromatography and mass spectrometry in the identification of drugs and metabolites. *Advances in Pharmacology*, 7:53–89.

Hartman, B. K., and Udenfriend, S. (1970): Immunofluorescent localization of dopamine-β-hydroxylase in tissue. *Molecular Pharmacology*, 6:85–94.

Karoum, F., Cattabeni, F., Costa, E., Ruthvan, C. R. J., and Sandler, M. (1972): Gas chromatographic assay of picomole concentrations of biogenic amines. *Analytical Biochemistry (in press)*.

Kaufman, S. (1962): Oxygenases: In: *Aromatic Hydroxylation*, edited by O. Hayaishi. Academic Press, New York, p. 129–180.

Kopin, I. J., Breese, G. R., Krauss, K. R., and Weise, V. K. (1968): Selective release of newly synthesized norepinephrine from the cat spleen during sympathetic nerve stimulation. *Journal of Pharmacology and Experimental Therapeutics*, 161:271–278.

Koslow, S. H., Cattabeni, F., and Costa, E. (1972): Norepinephrine and dopamine: Assay by mass fragmentography in the picomole range. *Science*, 176:177–180.

Lentz, T. L. (1969): Vesicle and granule content of sympathetic ganglion cells during limb regeneration of the newt triturus. *Zietschrift für Zellenforschung und Mikroskopische Anatomie*, 102:447–458.

Libet, B., and Tosaka, T. (1969): Slow inhibitory and excitatory responses in single cells of mammalian sympathetic ganglia. *Journal of Neurophysiology*, 32:43–50.

Libet, B., and Tosaka, T. (1970): Dopamine as a synaptic transmitter and modulator in sympathetic ganglia: A different mode of synaptic action. *Proceedings of the National Academy of Sciences*, 67:667–673.

Lowry, O. H., Rosebrough, N. J., Farr, A. L., and Randall, R. J. (1951): Protein measurement with the folin phenol reagent. *Journal of Biological Chemistry*, 193:265–275.

Majer, J. R., and Boulton, A. A. (1970): Absolute unambiguous, ultramicroanalysis of metabolites present in complex biological extracts. *Nature*, 225:658–660.

Mason, H. S. (1957): Mechanisms of oxygen metabolism. *Advances in Enzymology*, 19:79–233.

Montanari, R., Costa, E., Beaven, M. A., and Brodie, B. B. (1963): Turnover rates of norepinephrine in hearts of intact mice, rats, and guinea pigs using tritiated norepinephrine. *Life Sciences*, 4:232–240.

Neff, N. H., and Costa, E. (1966): The influence of monoamine oxidase inhibition on catecholamine synthesis. *Life Sciences*, 5:951–959.

Neff, N. H., Ngai, S. H., Wang, C. T., and Costa, E. (1969): Calculation of the rate of catecholamine synthesis from the rate of conversion of ^{14}C tyrosine to catecholamines: Effect of adrenal demedullation on synthesis rates. *Molecular Pharmacology*, 5:90–99.

Neff, N. H., Spano, P. F., Groppetti, A., Wang, C. T., and Costa, E. (1971): A simple procedure for calculating the synthesis rate of norepinephrine, dopamine, and serotonin in rat brain. *Journal of Pharmacology and Experimental Therapeutics*, 176:701–710.

Norberg, K. A., Ritzen, M., and Ungerstedt, U. (1966): Histochemical studies on a special catecholamine containing cell type in sympathetic ganglia. *Acta Physiologica Scandinavica*, 67:260–270.

Rehn, H. (1964): Oxygen stores in man. In: *Oxygen in the Animal Organism*, edited by F. Dickens and E. Neil. Pergamon Press, Oxford, pp. 609–618.

Ryhage, R. (1967): Efficiency of molecule separators used in gas chromatograph-mass spectrometer applications. *Arkiv. Kemi*, 26:305–16.

Smith, A. D. (1970): Proteins of vesicles from sympathetic axons: Chemistry, immunoreactivity and release upon stimulation. *Neuroscience Research Program Bulletin*, 8:377–382.

Smith, A. D. (1971a): Secretion of proteins (chromogranin A and dopamine-β-hydroxylase) from a sympathetic neuron. *Philosophical Transactions of the Royal Society of London*, 261:363–370.

Smith, A. D. (1971*b*): Summing up: Some implications of the neuron as a secreting cell. *Philosophical Transactions of the Royal Society of London*, 261:423–437.

Smith, A. D., DePotter, W. P., Moerman, E. J., and DeSchaepdryver, A. F. (1970): Release of dopamine-β-hydroxylase and chromogranin A upon stimulation of the splenic nerve. *Tissue and Cell*, 2:547–568.

Sweeley, C. C., Elliott, W. H., and Ryhage, R. (1966): Mass spectrometric determination of unresolved components in gas chromatographic effluents. *Analytical Chemistry*, 38:1549–1553.

Taxi, J. (1961): Étude de l'ultrastructure des zones synaptiques dans les ganglions sympathetiques de grenouille. *Compte Rendus Hebdomadapires des Seances de l'Academié de Science (Paris) D*, 252:174–176.

Taxi, J. (1971): Ultrastructural data on the cytology and cytochemistry of the autonomic nervous system. *Philosophical Transactions of the Royal Society of London*, 261:311–312.

VanOrden, L. S., III, Burke, J. P., Geyer, M., and Lodoen, F. V. (1970): Localization of depletion-sensitive and depletion resistant norepinephrine storage sites in autonomic ganglia. *Journal of Pharmacology and Experimental Therapeutics*, 174:56–71.

Weinshilboum, R., Johnson, D. G., Thoa, N., Axelrod, J., and Kopin, I. (1971): Proportional release of dopamine-β-hydroxylase (DBH) and norepinephrine (NE) during sympathetic nerve stimulation. *Pharmacologist*, 13:229.

Williams, T. H., and Palay, S. L. (1969): Ultrastructure of the small neurons in the superior cervical ganglion. *Brain Research*, 15:17–34.

Advances in Biochemical Psychopharmacology, Vol. 6
Raven Press, New York © 1972

Application of Enzymatic Cycling to the Measurement of Gamma-Aminobutyric Acid in Single Neurons of the Mammalian Central Nervous System

Masanori Otsuka and Yuhei Miyata

Department of Pharmacology, Faculty of Medicine, Tokyo Medical and Dental University, Bunkyo-ku, Tokyo, Japan

The distributions of neurotransmitters in the nervous system have been extensively studied. Accumulated evidence suggests that both acetylcholine and norepinephrine are specifically concentrated in cholinergic and adrenergic neurons, respectively (Loewi and Hellauer, 1938; MacIntosh, 1941; von Euler, 1956). γ-Aminobutyric acid (GABA), which has recently been shown to be an inhibitory transmitter in the crustacean nervous system (Kravitz, Kuffler, and Potter, 1963; Takeuchi and Takeuchi, 1965; Otsuka, Iversen, Hall, and Kravitz, 1966), is present in a high concentration in inhibitory neurons of the lobster and in a quite low concentration in the excitatory neurons (Kravitz and Potter, 1965; Otsuka, Kravitz, and Potter, 1967).

Whether a similar specific GABA distribution may be found in mammalian CNS is a very interesting problem. There is a good evidence suggesting that GABA functions as an inhibitory transmitter in mammalian CNS (for reviews, see Krnjević, 1970; Curtis and Johnston, 1970; Otsuka, 1972). Mammalian brain contains a large amount of GABA. If this GABA were selectively distributed in certain inhibitory neurons, GABA would serve as a neuronal marker labeling a great number of inhibitory neurons. In order to test this hypothesis, the first step would be to reveal the distribution of GABA in mammalian CNS and correlate it with the relevant physiological and anatomical findings. For this purpose, an ideal solution would be a histochemical method visualizing GABA in tissue sections. In

61

spite of many attempts, however, such a method is not yet available (*cf.* van Gelder, 1968). We have, therefore, adopted direct cytochemical approaches. In this chapter we describe two methods which permit the study of GABA distribution in mammalian CNS at a cellular level.

ANALYSIS OF GABA IN SINGLE ISOLATED NERVE CELLS OF CAT CNS

Determination of GABA

Hirsch and Robins (1962) described an enzymatic method for GABA analysis. This method permits the measurement of GABA in an amount of 5×10^{-12} moles. This sensitivity was enough for the analysis of GABA in single crustacean neurons (Kravitz and Potter, 1965; Otsuka et al., 1967), but it is far from adequate for the single-cell analysis of mammalian CNS, mainly because mammalian central neurons are generally smaller than the crustacean neurons.

In the enzymatic GABA assay of Hirsch and Robins (1962), GABA is converted to succinate by the action of bacterial enzymes (GABA-glutamate transaminase and succinate semialdehyde dehydrogenase) with the formation of an equivalent amount of NADPH, which is then determined fluorometrically. In 1961, Lowry and his collaborators developed a chemical amplification method, which by the use of enzymatic cycling permits an increase of the sensitivity of pyridine nucleotide determination by a factor of several thousand-fold (Lowry, Passonneau, Schulz, and Rock, 1961). We have combined Lowry's cycling method with the enzymatic GABA analysis of Hirsch and Robins. Since the details of our method have already been published (Otsuka, Obata, Miyata and Tanaka, 1971), only an outline will be described.

The first step is the conversion of GABA to succinate with a concomitant reduction of equimolar amounts of $NADP^+$ by the action of the bacterial enzymes [reactions (1) and (2) in Fig. 1]. In order to keep the blank values at a low level, it is important at this stage to reduce the concentration of $NADP^+$ in the reaction mixture (30 μM in our experiments), and also to reduce the volume of the reagent (0.13 μl). In order to prevent evaporation of the reaction mixture, incubation of each sample was carried out in a small space of about 5-μl volume formed by the bottom of a conical microtube and a Parafilm stopper (Fig. 2).

Unreacted $NADP^+$ was destroyed by heating with weak NaOH. To each sample, $NADP^+$ cycling reagent was added and under the action of glu-

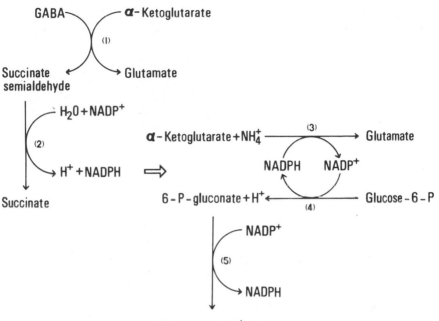

FIG. 1. Principle of micro-determination of GABA by enzymatic cycling. After Scott and Jakoby (1959) and Lowry et al. (1961).

tamate dehydrogenase and glucose-6-P dehydrogenase, $NADP^+$ catalyzed the cycling reactions (3) and (4) of Fig. 1. After 90 min of incubation at 38°C, for every molecule of GABA or NADPH added, 5,000 to 10,000 molecules of 6-P-gluconate were formed. 6-P-Gluconate was then oxidized by the action of 6-P-gluconate dehydrogenase with the formation of an equimolar amount of NADPH [reaction (5) of Fig. 1]. The native fluorescence of the NADPH produced was recorded. Figure 3 shows an example of the standard curve.

Isolation of Nerve-Cell Bodies

Tissue slices were removed from CNS of anesthetized cat. The surface of the slice was stained with 0.1% brilliant blue 6B Locke-solution. This dye is much less satisfactory for visualizing nerve cells than methylene blue or toluidine blue. The latter dyes, however, cannot be used for the present

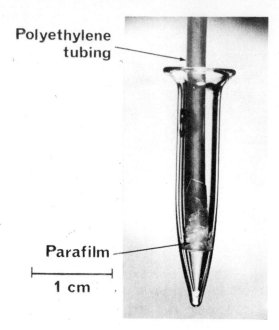

FIG. 2. Microtube containing 0.13 µl of water, and Parafilm stopper.

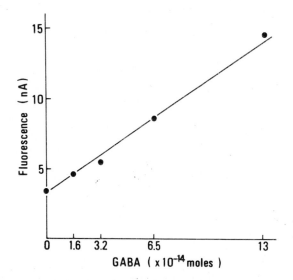

FIG. 3. Standard curve for GABA obtained by the enzymatic cycling method. For details of procedures, see Otsuka et al. (1971). Fluorescence units are galvanometer readings. Each point is the average of duplicate measurements.

purpose because they interfere with the GABA assay. Under a dissecting microscope, a single nerve-cell body was isolated from the surface of the slice by the use of a fine glass needle with a tip diameter of about 1 μm. The isolated nerve cell attached to the tip of a glass needle was soaked in xylene and examined under a compound microscope (Fig. 4A). Xylene was used at this stage because GABA is insoluble in xylene and tissue GABA is not lost

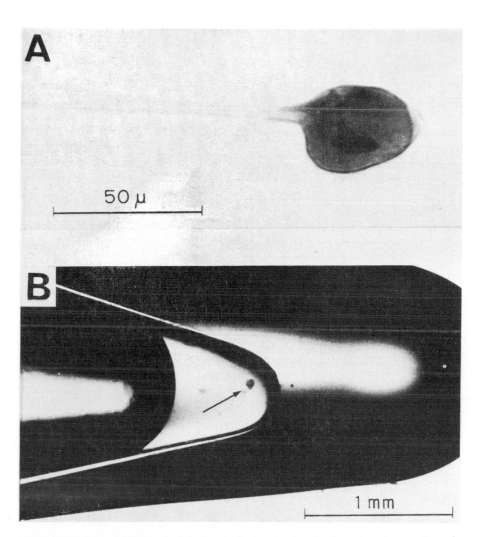

FIG. 4. *A:* A single Deiters cell body attached to the tip of a dissecting glass needle and placed in xylene. *B:* A single Deiters cell (arrow) was transferred into 0.13 μl of 0.1 N HCl at the bottom of a microtube. From Otsuka et al. (1971).

during microscopic observation (Otsuka et al., 1967). If the cell was markedly contaminated by surrounding tissue, it was discarded. The isolated nerve cell was then photographed to estimate its volume, and, after being dried in vacuum, was transferred into 0.1 μl of 0.1 N HCl in the bottom of a 0.1-ml microtube (Fig. 4B). Tubes were kept in a desiccator to remove HCl and water by evaporation.

Analytical Results

Table 1 shows the results obtained on single cell bodies of spinal motoneurons. The GABA content of an isolated spinal motoneuron ranged from 0 to 6.8×10^{-14} moles, and the average GABA concentration was 0.9 mM. Table 2 shows the results of GABA analysis on single Deiters cell bodies isolated from the dorsal part of Deiters nucleus. The average GABA content of an isolated dorsal Deiters cell was more than 10 times higher and the average GABA concentration 7 times higher than the corresponding values of spinal motoneurons.

Isolated nerve-cell preparations analyzed in the present study were very probably contaminated by presynaptic nerve terminals attached to the cell bodies. The high GABA values obtained for dorsal Deiters cells, therefore, may be due to GABA being present at high concentrations in the

TABLE 1. *GABA analysis on single spinal motoneurons isolated from cat spinal cord (L7-S1)*

GABA content (10^{-14} moles)	Volume (10^{-12} liter)	GABA conc. (mM)
0	32.4	0
1.1	38.4	0.3
1.6	16.3	1.0
4.8	33.6	1.4
3.6	24.6	1.5
6.8	50.8	1.3
2.5	36.8	0.7
1.8	19.8	0.9
0.6	26.9	0.2
5.1	35.3	1.4
Mean ± SEM 2.8 ± 0.7	31.5 ± 3.2	0.9 ± 0.2

From Otsuka et al. (1971).

TABLE 2. *GABA analysis on single Deiters cell bodies isolated from the dorsal part of Deiters nucleus*

GABA content (10^{-14} moles)	Volume (10^{-12} liter)	GABA conc. (mM)
45.2	60.6	7.5
16.7	24.4	6.9
45.7	67.8	6.7
63.5	60.8	10.4
7.6	22.2	3.4
70.0	88.0	8.0
15.2	49.6	3.1
20.9	77.1	2.7
46.0	64.7	7.1
31.4	43.0	7.3
Mean ± SEM 36.2 ± 6.7	55.8 ± 6.7	6.3 ± 0.8

From Otsuka et al. (1971).

nerve terminals. It is known that axon terminals of Purkinje neurons originating from cerebellar vermis form inhibitory synapses with dorsal Deiters neurons (Ito, Kawai, and Udo, 1968). Furthermore, there is evidence suggesting that GABA is the transmitter at these inhibitory synapses (Obata, Ito, Ochi, and Sato, 1967; Obata and Takeda, 1969). Based on these considerations, denervation experiments were performed in order to see if GABA is concentrated in the Purkinje axon terminals synapsing with dorsal Deiters cells. As shown in Table 3, the average GABA concentration in isolated dorsal Deiters cells was 6.3 mM in normal cats, and it was reduced to 1.7 mM after the removal of the cerebellar vermis. The GABA concentra-

TABLE 3. *Effect of denervation (removal of cerebellar vermis) on GABA concentration in isolated Deiters cell bodies*

	GABA conc. (mM)	
Cells	Normal cats	Operated cats
Dorsal Deiters	6.3 ± 0.8	1.7 ± 0.7
Ventral Deiters	2.7 ± 0.2	2.7 ± 0.4

Each value represents the mean of 8 to 11 determinations on individual nerve cells ± SEM.
From Otsuka et al. (1971).

tions in ventral Deiters cells of normal cats, on the other hand, showed intermediate values and they were not influenced by the denervation.

Our results on Deiters cells therefore suggest that GABA is concentrated in inhibitory axon terminals of Purkinje neurons originating from the cerebellar vermis and synapsing with dorsal Deiters cells. Since these inhibitory terminals probably occupy only a minor portion of the total volume of our isolated nerve-cell preparation, it is likely that the GABA concentration in the nerve terminals is much higher than 6.3 mM assessed for the average GABA concentration of isolated dorsal Deiters cells of normal cats. It may be noted that our results of GABA analysis on Deiters

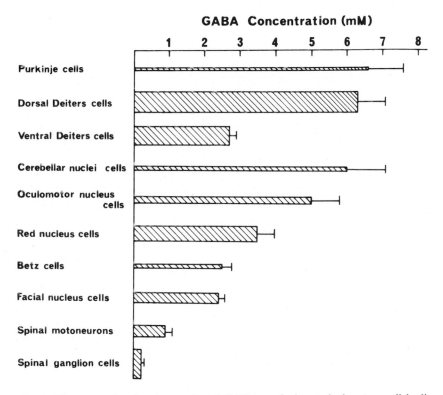

FIG. 5. Histogram showing the results of GABA analysis on single nerve-cell bodies. Length of each bar represents the average GABA concentration in isolated nerve-cell bodies and SEM. Width of each bar is proportional to the average volume of an isolated nerve cell. Large cells were collected from different parts of cat CNS. For each type of neuron, seven to ten determinations were made on individual cell bodies, except spinal ganglion cells, for which analyses were made on pooled cells. After Miyata et al. (1970) and Otsuka et al. (1971).

cells of normal and denervated cats are quite consistent with the recent findings of Fonnum and his collaborators on the GABA synthesizing enzyme glutamate decarboxylase (Fonnum, Storm-Mathisen, and Walberg, 1970; see also Fonnum, this volume).

Figure 5 shows the summarized results of GABA analysis of single nerve-cell bodies of various types in cat CNS. It is to be noted that the GABA concentration of isolated oculomotor neurons was high when compared with spinal and facial motoneurons (Miyata, Obata, Tanaka, and Otsuka, 1970). This fact may be correlated with the findings that inhibitory postsynaptic potentials recorded from oculomotor neurons were blocked by picrotoxin (Ito, Highstein, and Tsuchiya, 1970) and that the iontophoretic application of GABA onto oculomotor neurons produced a depressant effect (Obata and Highstein, 1970).

DISTRIBUTION OF GABA IN THE SPINAL CORD

Although a histochemical staining method for GABA is not yet available, it is possible to reveal GABA distribution in tissue sections at almost cellular resolution by using a direct analytical method with high sensitivity. We will describe our study on the spinal cord.

Cat spinal cord (L5–L7 segments) was frozen in isopentane at about −70°C, and was cut in a cryostat at 150-μm thickness. The tissue section was mounted on a glass slide coated with epoxy resin, kept at room temperature for about 10 min, and photographed in a compound microscope. At this stage it is possible to recognize the rough structure of the spinal cord and large nerve cells (Fig. 6A). The tissue section was transferred to a cold box with a plastic front as described by Aprison and Hancock (1970), and at −25°C was divided into small rectangular blocks at 200 to 500-μm intervals under a binocular microscope with a hand-held broken razor blade (Fig. 6B). The temperature in the cold box was then lowered to −50°C, and each block was taken out and transferred into 5 to 20 μl of 0.1 N HCl in the bottom of a fluorometer tube. Water and HCl were removed by evaporation.

The GABA contents of large blocks (500 × 500 × 150 μm) can be assayed by the usual enzymatic assay (Hirsch and Robins, 1962; Kravitz and Potter, 1965). Small blocks (200 × 200 × 150 μm) were analyzed by a micromethod using enzymatic cycling. The principle of the micromethod is the same as that described in the preceding section, but the procedure was simplified so that 100 samples could be assayed in several hours with a rea-

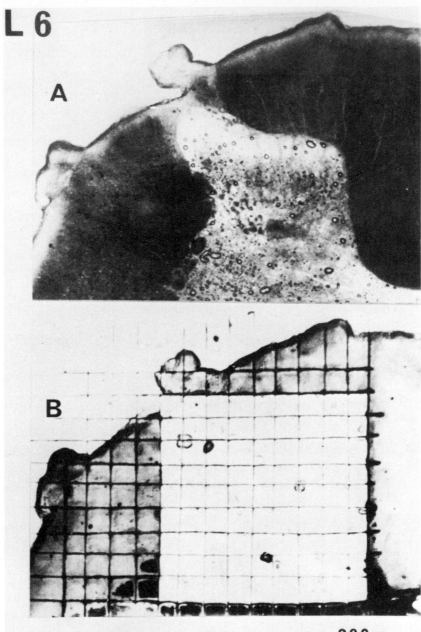

200μ

sonable expense but with a slightly lower sensitivity. Details of the microassay method will be published elsewhere.

Figure 7 shows the results on cat spinal cord. The results are essentially
consistent with the previous analyses of Graham, Shank, Werman, and
Aprison (1967) and Rizzoli (1968), but much more detail has been revealed
in the present study. GABA levels in the dorso-medial region of dorsal
funiculus was very low, about 0.1 mM; those in the motoneuron area were
relatively low, around 0.8 mM. The highest GABA levels (2.2 to 2.6 mM)
were found in an area roughly corresponding to laminae III and IV of

←

FIG. 6. *A:* Photomicrograph of cross-section (150 μm thickness) of cat spinal cord, at
room temperature. Only a dorsal quadrant is shown. *B:* The same section after being
frozen and the samples for GABA analysis had been removed. Traces of razor blade are
seen on epoxy resin coating on slide glass.

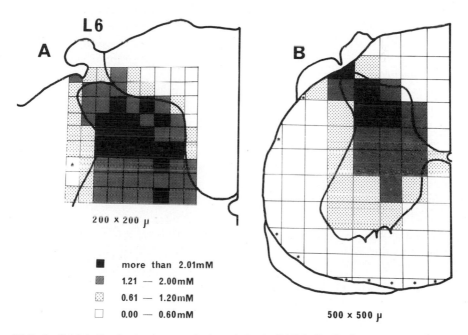

FIG. 7. GABA distribution in cat spinal cord. In *A*, GABA distribution was mapped at
200-μm resolution. The average length of a side of each rectangle is 200 μm. The same tissue
section as shown in Fig. 6 was used. In *B*, GABA distribution was mapped at 500-μm
resolution. A cross-section adjacent to the one shown in Fig. 7*A* was analyzed.

Contours of grey and white matters and spinal roots were traced from photomicro-
graphs. * Assay failed or was not performed.

Rexed. In this connection, it is interesting to note that the origin of the dorsal root potential produced by cutaneous volleys has been located around this area (Eccles, Kostyuk, and Schmidt, 1962; Wall, 1964).

. GENERAL COMMENTS

The present study shows that it is possible, without a histochemical staining method, to reveal GABA distribution in nervous tissues at a cellular level. Studies of GABA distribution in the nervous system have the following advantages over similar studies on other neurotransmitters. (1) The sensitivity of direct chemical analysis of GABA is very high; the lowest detectable amount of GABA is 2×10^{-14} moles by the cycling method. This may be compared with the maximum sensitivity of bioassay for acetylcholine of 6×10^{-15} moles (Cottrell, Powell, and Stanton, 1970). (2) GABA concentrations in nervous tissues are quite high. For example, mouse brain contains about 4 μmoles/g wet weight of GABA (Weinstein, Roberts, and Kakefuda, 1963), whereas it contains only 0.013 μmoles/g of acetylcholine (Takahashi, Nasu, Tamura and Kariya, 1961) and 0.003 μmoles/g of norepinephrine (Smith, 1965). (3) So far, only inhibitory effects of GABA on vertebrate central neurons are known. Therefore, a high GABA content may label a neuron of mammalian CNS as inhibitory.

In the crustacean nervous system, the activity of the GABA synthesizing enzyme glutamate decarboxylase is more than 100 times higher in inhibitory neurons than in excitatory neurons (Hall, Bownds, and Kravitz, 1970). It might, therefore, be thought that glutamate decarboxylase activity may label GABA-releasing neurons. However, a considerable activity of this enzyme was found in cat ventral roots, which consist of cholinergic neurons (Graham and Aprison, 1969).

Although the results presented in this chapter are consistent with the hypothesis that GABA is selectively distributed in certain inhibitory neurons of mammalian CNS (cf. Otsuka et al., 1971), further studies on GABA distribution will be needed in order to prove or disprove this hypothesis. These studies, if the hypothesis turned out to be true, would indicate the location of a great number of inhibitory neurons in the nervous system.

REFERENCES

Aprison, M. H., and Hancock, C. J. (1970): A controlled humidity constant temperature cold box for dissection of small frozen tissue sections. In: *Experiments in Physiology and Biochemistry*, Vol. 3, edited by G. A. Kerkut. Academic Press, New York, pp. 39–48.

Cottrell, G. A., Powell, B., and Stanton, M. (1970): A simple method for measuring a pico-gram of acetylcholine using the clam (*Mya arenaria*) heart. *British Journal of Pharmacology*, 40:866–870.

Curtis, D. R., and Johnston, G. A. R. (1970): Amino acid transmitters. In: *Handbook of Neurochemistry*, Volume IV, edited by A. Lajtha, Plenum Press, New York, pp. 115–134.

Eccles, J. C., Kostyuk, P. G., and Schmidt, R. F. (1962): Central pathways responsible for depolarization of primary afferent fibres. *Journal of Physiology*, 161:237–257.

Fonnum, F. (1972): Application of microchemical analysis and subcellular fractionation techniques to the study of neurotransmitters in discrete areas of mammalian brain. (*This volume*).

Fonnum, F., Storm-Mathisen, J., and Walberg, F. (1970): Glutamate decarboxylase in inhibitory neurons. A study of the enzyme in Purkinje cell axons and boutons in the cat. *Brain Research*, 20:259–275.

Graham, L. T., Jr., and Aprison, M. H. (1969): Distribution of some enzymes associated with the metabolism of glutamate, aspartate, γ-aminobutyrate and glutamine in cat spinal cord. *Journal of Neurochemistry*, 16:559–566.

Graham, L. T., Jr., Shank, R. P., Werman, R., and Aprison, M. H. (1967): Distribution of some synaptic transmitter suspects in cat spinal cord: glutamic acid, aspartic acid, γ-aminobutyric acid, glycine, and glutamine. *Journal of Neurochemistry*, 14:465–472.

Hall, Z. W., Bownds, M. D., and Kravitz, E. A. (1970): The metabolism of gamma aminobutyric acid in the lobster nervous system. Enzymes in single excitatory and inhibitory axons. *Journal of Cell Biology*, 46:290–299.

Hirsch, H. E., and Robins, E. (1962): Distribution of γ-aminobutyric acid in the layers of the cerebral and cerebellar cortex. Implications for its physiological role. *Journal of Neurochemistry*, 9:63–70.

Ito, M., Highstein, S. M., and Tsuchiya, T. (1970): The postsynaptic inhibition of rabbit oculomotor neurones by secondary vestibular impulses and its blockage by picrotoxin. *Brain Research*, 17:520–523.

Ito, M. Kawai, N., and Udo, M. (1968): The origin of cerebellar-induced inhibition of Deiters neurones. III. Localization of the inhibitory zone. *Experimental Brain Research*, 4:310–320.

Kravitz, E. A., Kuffler, S. W., and Potter, D. D. (1963): Gamma-aminobutyric acid and other blocking compounds in *Crustacea*. III. Their relative concentrations in separated motor and inhibitory axons. *Journal of Neurophysiology*, 26:739–751.

Kravitz, E. A., and Potter, D. D. (1965): A further study of the distribution of γ-aminobutyric acid between excitatory and inhibitory axons of the lobster. *Journal of Neurochemistry*, 12:323–328.

Krnjević, K. (1970): Glutamate and γ aminobutyric acid in brain. *Nature*, 228:119–124.

Loewi, O., and Hellauer, H. (1938): Über das Acetylcholin in peripheren Nerven. *Pflügers Archiv für die Gesamte Physiologie des Menschen und der Tiere*, 240:769–775.

Lowry, O. H., Passonneau, J. V., Schulz, D. W., and Rock, M. K. (1961): The measurement of pyridine nucleotides by enzymatic cycling. *Journal of Biological Chemistry*, 236:2746–2755.

MacIntosh, F. C. (1941): The distribution of acetylcholine in the peripheral and the central nervous system. *Journal of Physiology*, 99:436–442.

Miyata, Y., Obata, K., Tanaka, Y., and Otsuka, M. (1970): Determination of γ-aminobutyric acid in isolated nerve cells of the brain stem of the cat. *Journal of the Physiological Society of Japan*, 32:377–378.

Obata, K., and Highstein, S. M. (1970): Blocking by picrotoxin of both vestibular inhibition and GABA action on rabbit oculomotor neurones. *Brain Research*, 18:538–541.

Obata, K., Ito, M., Ochi, R., and Sato, N. (1967): Pharmacological properties of the postsynaptic inhibition by Purkinje cell axons and the action of γ-aminobutyric acid on Deiters neurones. *Experimental Brain Research*, 4:43–57.

Obata, K., and Takeda, K. (1969): Release of γ-aminobutyric acid into the fourth ventricle induced by stimulation of the cat's cerebellum. *Journal of Neurochemistry*, 16:1043–1047.

Otsuka, M. (1972): γ-Aminobutyric acid in the nervous system. In: *The Structure and Function of Nervous Tissue*, Vol. IV, edited by G. H. Bourne. Academic Press, New York, pp. 249–289.

Otsuka, M., Iversen, L. L., Hall, Z. W., and Kravitz, E. A. (1966): Release of gamma-aminobutyric acid from inhibitory nerves of lobster. *Proceedings of the National Academy of Sciences*, 56:1110–1115.

Otsuka, M., Kravitz, E. A., and Potter, D. D. (1967): Physiological and chemical architecture of a lobster ganglion with particular reference to gamma-aminobutyrate and glutamate. *Journal of Neurophysiology*, 30:725–752.

Otsuka, M., Obata, K., Miyata, Y., and Tanaka, Y. (1971): Measurement of γ-aminobutyric acid in isolated nerve cells of cat central nervous system. *Journal of Neurochemistry*, 18: 287–295.

Rizzoli, A. A. (1968): Distribution of glutamic acid, aspartic acid, γ-aminobutyric acid and glycine in six areas of cat spinal cord before and after transection. *Brain Research*, 11: 11–18.

Scott, E. M., and Jakoby, W. B. (1959): Soluble γ-aminobutyric-glutamic transaminase from *Pseudomonas fluorescens*. *Journal of Biological Chemistry*, 234:932–936.

Smith, C. B. (1965): Effects of *d*-amphetamine upon brain amine content and locomotor activity of mice. *Journal of Pharmacology and Experimental Therapeutics*, 147:96–102.

Takahashi, R., Nasu, T., Tamura, T., and Kariya, T. (1961): Relationship of ammonia and acetylcholine levels to brain excitability. *Journal of Neurochemistry*, 7:103–112.

Takeuchi, A., and Takeuchi, N. (1965): Localized action of gamma-aminobutyric acid on the crayfish muscle. *Journal of Physiology*, 177:225–238.

van Gelder, N. M. (1968): Hydrazinopropionic acid: A new inhibitor of aminobutyrate transaminase and glutamate decarboxylase. *Journal of Neurochemistry*, 15:747–757.

von Euler, U. S. (1956): *Noradrenaline*. Charles C Thomas, Springfield, Ill.

Wall, P. D. (1964): Presynaptic control of impulses at the first central synapse in the cutaneous pathway. *Progress in Brain Research*, Vol. 12, *Physiology of Spinal Neurons*, edited by J. C. Eccles and J. P. Schadé. Elsevier, Amsterdam, pp. 92–118.

Weinstein, H., Roberts, E., and Kakefuda, T. (1963): Studies of sub-cellular distribution of γ-aminobutyric acid and glutamic decarboxylase in mouse brain. *Biochemical Pharmacology*, 12:503–509.

Advances in Biochemical Psychopharmacology, Vol. 6
Raven Press, New York © 1972

Application of Microchemical Analysis and Subcellular Fractionation Techniques to the Study of Neurotransmitters in Discrete Areas of Mammalian Brain

F. Fonnum

Norwegian Defense Research Establishment, Division for Toxicology, 2007-Kjeller, Norway

In brain the identity of the transmitter substance used by a particular type of neuron is in most cases unknown. It is regarded as one of the characteristic features of chemical transmitters that they are specifically localized in the neurons that use them. In our laboratory we have been investigating whether putative transmitters are preferentially synthesized within different types of neurons in the cerebellum, hippocampus, and substantia nigra. In particular we have tried to find out whether glutamate decarboxylase (GAD), the enzyme governing the level of gamma-aminobutyric acid (GABA) within the brain (Baxter, 1970), is concentrated in inhibitory neurons or whether the enzyme is present in all types of neurons. The former would indicate that GABA may be involved in the chemical transmission; the latter would suggest that GABA is merely involved in energy metabolism.

This problem has been approached in three ways: (1) by correlating the distribution of GAD with the distribution of inhibitory neurons; (2) by studying the effect on enzyme activities in axons and terminals following interruption of specific neuronal pathways; and (3) by investigating whether synaptosomes are a hetereogeneous population and whether GAD is distributed differently from other enzymes synthesizing transmitter candidates. In this investigation we have compared the distribution of GAD with choline acetyltransferase (ChAc) and/or 3,4-dihydroxyphenylalanine decarboxylase (DOPA-Dec).

We have chosen to study the distribution of the enzymes synthesizing the transmitters instead of the transmitters themselves. There is excellent correlation between the levels of GAD and ChAc and the levels of GABA and acetylcholine (ACh) in different regions of the brain (Hebb, 1963; Baxter, 1970). It is more difficult to establish such a correlation for DOPA-Dec since this enzyme is involved in the synthesis of noradrenaline, dopamine, and serotonin. High levels of these amines are, however, usually accompanied by a high level of DOPA-Dec (Kuntzman, Shore, Bogdanski, and Brodie, 1961). There are several technical advantages in studying the distribution of enzymes instead of the chemical transmitters. The enzymes are less diffusible and less readily metabolized than the transmitter substances. It is therefore less likely that they should be redistributed in the tissue or that their concentrations should be altered during the preparation of the tissue. Only very small amounts of tissue are required for the determination of enzyme activities, in contrast to the assay of the transmitter substances.

Sensitive radiochemical microassay methods have been developed for each of the three enzymes. GAD was determined by a modification (Fonnum, Storm-Mathisen, and Walberg, 1970) of the method developed by Albers and Brady (1959). ChAc was determined by measuring the conversion of $[1-^{14}C]$acetyl-CoA to $[1-^{14}C]$ACh which was isolated by Kalignost extraction (Fonnum, 1969b). DOPA-Dec was measured by decarboxylation of $[2-^{14}C]$DOPA to $[1-^{14}C]$dopamine in the presence of nialamide, a monoamine oxidase inhibitor. $[1-^{14}C]$Dopamine has, unlike DOPA, a positive charge at pH 6 and may therefore be isolated by Kalignost extraction (Fonnum, 1969a). Kalignost extraction is an example of liquid cation exchange, and further details of this method have been described elsewhere (Fonnum, 1969a). Microdissection was carried out on freeze-dried sections of tissue, and the samples (1 to 10 μg) were weighed on a quartz fiber microbalance (Lowry, 1953). The enzyme activity was determined by the micromethods described above. The substrate solutions contained 0.2% Triton in order to release all enzyme activity. Fractions from density gradients were obtained by tube puncture, and the samples were pipetted directly into the incubation vessel. Occluded ChAc activity was determined by assaying the enzyme in the presence or the absence of Triton.

Extensive morphological and electrophysiological data exist concerning the distribution and function of the inhibitory neurons in cerebellum (Eccles, Ito, and Szentágothai, 1967); this area is, therefore, particularly attractive for studying the distribution of GAD. Some data will also be presented on the distribution of enzymes in substantia nigra, the region in the brain with the highest content of GAD and GABA (Baxter, 1970). Regional differences in the subcellular distribution of ChAc, GAD, and DOPA-Dec will also be discussed.

CEREBELLUM

The cerebellum can be separated into cortex, white matter, and nuclei. The cerebellar cortex contains a narrow layer of Purkinje cells whose axons form inhibitory (Ito, Yoshida, and Obata, 1964; Ito and Yoshida, 1966) synapses in the cerebellar nuclei and the dorsal part of the lateral vestibular nucleus (Jansen and Brodal, 1940; Walberg and Jansen, 1961, 1964). The basket cells in the cerebellum are situated close to the Purkinje cells and form inhibitory synapses on the somata of the latter (Andersen, Eccles, and Voorhoeve, 1963; Hamori and Szentagothai, 1965). The superficial stellate cells are localized in the molecular layer of the cerebellar cortex and form inhibitory synapses on the Purkinje cell dendrites. The Golgi cells form inhibitory synapses on the granular cells. The main afferents to the cerebellum are the climbing fibers and the giant mossy fibers which are both believed to be exitatory (Eccles et al., 1967).

The cerebellar cortex thus contains three inhibitory interneurons and one inhibitory cell sending its axons out of the cortex. It is, therefore, not surprising that several investigators have studied the distribution of GAD and GABA in the different layers of the cerebellar cortex (Albers and Brady, 1959; Hirsch and Robins, 1962; Kuriyama, Roberts, Sisken, and Sano, 1966).

The results (Kuriyama et al., 1966) showed that the Purkinje cell layer in rabbit contained a slightly higher concentration (about 30%) of GABA and GAD than the molecular and granular layers. These results did not distinguish whether the enzyme was situated in the Purkinje cells, in the basket cell terminals, or in both. The high activities of GAD in the other layers could be due to the presence of the enzyme in Purkinje cell dendrites and axons or in the other inhibitory neurons.

To extend these investigations (Fonnum and Storm-Mathisen, *unpublished*), we compared the activities of ChAc and GAD in freeze-dried sections from cortex and from nucleus interpositus. The samples from cortex were taken from the hemisphere slightly rostral to the nuclei and contained the full depth of the gray matter. Particular care was taken to dissect out samples that contained equal amounts of the granular and molecular layers. The results showed that both enzymes were present in high activities in nucleus interpositus (Table 1). The results on ChAc are in agreement with those of Goldberg and McCaman (1967).

When the peduncles were transected to interrupt the afferents to the cerebellum, ChAc showed a marked decrease whereas GAD was unchanged both in cerebellar nuclei and cortex (Table 1). The lesion in the

TABLE 1. *GAD and ChAc in rat cerebellum after transection of the peduncles*

Location	Enzyme	Normal	After lesion	
			4 days	7 days
Cortex	GAD	47 ± 3.6	54.0 ± 2.9	46 ± 2.2
	ChAc	1.8 ± 0.17	0.93 ± 0.01	0.15 ± 0.05
Nucleus interpositus	GAD	150 ± 20	130 ± 13	
	ChAc	15 ± 4.0	3.3 ± 0.3	

The results are expressed in μmoles/hr/g dry wt. Mean values ± SD. Six samples from each animal.

seventh-postoperative-day animals involved only the ventral part of the nuclei and was therefore not assayed. The results demonstrated that ChAc is present in fibers afferent to the cerebellum, whereas GAD is localized in cerebellar neurons, i.e., in Purkinje cells, basket cells, Golgi cells, or stellate cells.

   Subcellular fractionation of cerebellar cortex and nuclei with white matter (Table 2) shows that ChAc is predominantly present in a particulate form whereas more GAD is in the supernatant fraction. Furthermore, ChAc from the cerebellar nuclei was recovered in the P_2 fraction whereas ChAc from cortex was mainly recovered in the P_1 fraction. The latter observation is in agreement with the previous work of Israel and Whittaker (1967) suggesting that ChAc in cerebellum is also present in large nerve terminals, presumably those of the mossy fibers. The high proportion of ChAc in the nerve-terminal fraction agrees with the results of the denervation experiments. GAD was isolated in both a particulate and a soluble form from cerebellar cortex thus suggesting that the enzyme was present in both nerve terminals and cell bodies. This excludes the possibility that the enzyme

TABLE 2. *Subcellular distribution of GAD and ChAc in cerebellum*

Enzyme	Rat cortex			Rat nuclei + white matter			Cat n. interpositus	
	P_1	P_2	S_2	P_1	P_2	S_2	P	S
GAD	27	29	44	27	26	47	42	58
ChAc	42	40	18	19	48	33	75	25

The results are expressed as percent of total recovered enzyme activities. Mean values of three experiments.

activity in cortex could be due solely to its presence in the Purkinje cell bodies.

The high concentration of GAD in the cerebellar nuclei required further investigation. A sample of white matter dissected immediately dorsal to the nucleus had only 12% of the GAD activity of the nucleus. The axons of the Purkinje cells in the cerebellar cortex of cat (Fig. 1) terminate in the ipsi-lateral intracerebellar nuclei (nn fastigii, interpositus and lateralis) (Jansen and Brodal, 1958; Walberg and Jansen, 1961). A lesion in the left cerebellar hemisphere of the cat would therefore destroy the Purkinje cells that pro-ject to the left nucleus interpositus. When part of this hemisphere was de-

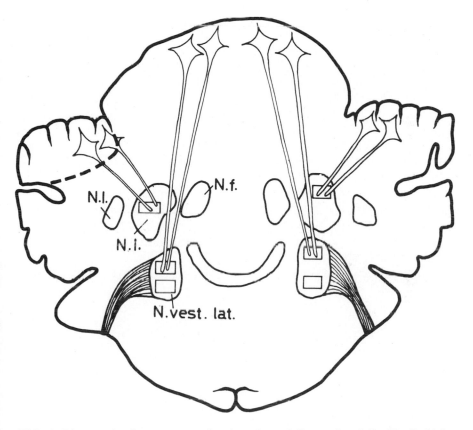

FIG. 1. Diagram showing a cross-section through cerebellum and medulla. The Purkinje cells in the hemisphere terminate in the ipsilateral n. interpositus whereas the Purkinje cells in the vermis, mainly of the anterior lobe, enter the lateral vestibular nucleus from the dorsal aspect and terminate in the dorsal part of the nucleus only.

stroyed, the activity of GAD in the ipsilateral nucleus interpositus was reduced by 50 to 70%. The activity in the contralateral nucleus was, however, unchanged (Table 3; Fonnum et al., 1970). In contrast, the level of ChAc was the same in both nuclei. The level of ChAc in the nucleus interpositus of cats is low when compared to the rat nucleus showing a remarkable species differences between rat and cat cerebella.

The axons of the Purkinje cells of the vermis, mainly of the anterior cerebellar lobe, enter the lateral vestibular nuclei from the dorsal aspect and terminate in the dorsal, not in the ventral part of the nucleus (Fig. 1). When samples were dissected from freeze-dried sections and analyzed for GAD activity (Fonnum et al., 1970), it was shown that the enzyme activity was two to three times higher in the dorsal (Purkinje terminal-rich) than in the ventral part (Table 4). When the Purkinje cells in the vermis were destroyed, the enzyme activity decreased in the dorsal but not in the ventral part. The decrease was related to the extent of the lesion; thus, in animal C_4 where the lesion, by accident, was mainly confined to the right side only, the enzyme activity decreased more markedly on this side.

Also in the lateral vestibular nucleus of the rat we found two to three times higher activities in the dorsal than in the ventral part, and the activity in the dorsal part was reduced by 70% after transection of the peduncles.

The results obtained by comparing the activities of GAD in the dorsal and ventral parts of the lateral vestibular nucleus, the loss of GAD activities in the nucleus interpositus and lateral vestibular nucleus after destruction of the Purkinje cells, and the results from subcellular fractionation suggest that GAD is mainly confined to the Purkinje axon terminals in the intracerebellar nuclei and in the lateral vestibular nucleus. Similar investigations have been carried out on GABA in the lateral vestibular nucleus (Otsuka, Obata, Minyata, and Tanaka, 1971).

Most probably, since our lesions cannot destroy all the Purkinje cells,

TABLE 3. *GAD and ChAc activity in nucleus interpositus in normal and operated cats*

Cat	Enzyme	Activity	
		Right side	Left side
C7 (normal)	GAD	18 ± 5.0	19 ± 3.9
C5 (operated)	GAD	15 ± 1.8	7.3 ± 1.4
C6 (operated)	GAD	14 ± 3.0	4.4 ± 2.1
C5 (operated)	ChAc	1.1 ± 0.2	1.3 ± 0.2

The results are expressed as μmoles/hr/g dry wt. Mean ± SD. From Fonnum et al., (1970).

TABLE 4. *GAD activity in the dorsal and ventral parts of lateral vestibular nucleus in normal and operated cats*

Cat	Side	Activity	
		Dorsal	Ventral
C1 (normal)	R and L	15 ± 3.8 (10)	7.1 ± 2.0 (9)
C6 (normal)	R and L	18 ± 3.8 (9)	6.0 ± 0.9 (9)
C7 (normal)	R and L	15 ± 2.2 (9)	6.2 ± 1.7 (9)
C2 (operated)	L	9.6 ± 2.0 (4)	7.7 ± 1.4 (6)
C2 (operated)	R	6.7 ± 1.6 (6)	6.1 ± 0.9 (7)
C3 (operated)	L	9.8 ± 3.5 (5)	7.0 ± 1.2 (5)
C3 (operated)	R	6.5 ± 2.9 (5)	7.4 ± 1.2 (6)
C4 (operated)	L	11 ± 2.7 (3)	6.4 ± 0.6 (4)
C4 (operated)	R	5.6 ± 1.4 (4)	6.2 ± 0.6 (4)

The results are given as μmoles CO_2/hr/g dry wt. Mean values ± SD. The survival times were 7 days for C2 and 12 days for C3 and C4. No. of samples in parentheses. From Fonnum et al. (1970).

all the GAD activity in these areas is present in the Purkinje axons and terminals. This excludes the possibility that GABA is a general constituent of all neurons, and makes it most likely that GABA is connected with transmission in inhibitory neurons, probably as the inhibitory transmitter.

On a tissue-volume basis, GAD must be highly concentrated in the Purkinje axon terminals. Only about 5% of the area in the lateral vestibular nucleus consists of nerve terminals (Fonnum et al., 1970). After electron-microscopic examination of terminals in this area following a lesion similar to that described in Table 3, we found that 85 out of 507 terminals showed signs of degeneration (50 unclassified structures). These values were obtained by cutting two sections of area 1 mm^2 and 0.8 mm^2 through the dorsal part of the nucleus and selecting at random 50 electron micrographs. The number of degenerating terminals is probably an underestimate, but it indicates that most of the GAD activity may be confined to as little as 0.5 to 1.5% of the total area of the lateral vestibular nucleus (Fonnum and Walberg, *unpublished*).

Electrophysiological, pharmacological, and other biochemical observations support the concept that GABA is the inhibitory transmitter of the Purkinje cells. Both the inhibition by GABA applied electrophoretically and the inhibition produced by stimulation of the Purkinje cells were strychnine resistant (Obata, Ito, Ochi, and Sato, 1967) and blocked by bicuculline (Curtis, Duggan, and Felix, 1970). In addition stimulation of the Purkinje cells leads to a release of GABA into the fourth ventricle (Obata and Takeda, 1969).

SUBSTANTIA NIGRA

Substantia nigra is one of the regions of the brain that contain the highest concentrations of GAD and GABA (Baxter, 1970). The region is morphologically divided into two main parts: pars compacta, a region rich in nerve cells and containing relatively few nerve terminals; and pars reticulata, a region rich in nerve terminals and containing few nerve cells. The only well-defined afferent fibers to substantia nigra are derived from caudate nucleus and putamen (Grofova and Rinvik, 1970).

In our laboratory, we have studied the distribution of GAD, ChAc, AChE, and DOPA-dec in the two parts of cat substantia nigra. The results (Table 5) show that GAD is only slightly more concentrated in pars reticulata than in pars compacta. The results are strikingly different from those with DOPA-dec which is particularly concentrated in pars compacta, probably due to the abundance of DOPA-minergic cells in this region (Dahlström and Fuxe, 1965). In a portion of substantia nigra dissected from fresh tissue, we found 6,000 times higher activity of AChE than of ChAc, compared to a corresponding ratio of 80 in hippocampus (Fonnum, 1970). These results are in agreement with those of Bull, Hebb, and Ratković (1970), who also found an abnormally high ratio between AChE and ChAc for this area of human brain. AChE is therefore an unreliable marker for cholinergic structures in this region.

Destruction of striatum excluding globus pallidus did not result in any substantial loss of GAD, AChE, or ChAc from substantia nigra even 8 months after the lesion.

More than 80% of GAD and less than 20% of lactate dehydrogenase was obtained in a particulate form after homogenization of pars compacta and pars reticulata, and the enzyme is, therefore, mainly confined to nerve terminals.

TABLE 5. *Enzyme activities in substantia nigra*

Location	Activity		
	GAD	DOPA-dec	ChAc
Reticulata	240 ± 39	4.5 ± 0.9	1.8 ± 0.7
Compacta	170 ± 34	$16 \quad \pm 3.9$	3.5 ± 1.8

Activities expressed as μmoles/hr/g dry wt. Mean values $\pm$ SD.

In conclusion, our results on the distribution of GAD in substantia nigra indicate that a higher proportion of the nerve terminals in pars compacta than in pars reticulata must contain GAD. The results are compatible with the view that GAD-containing synapses are particularly concentrated on the soma and proximal dendrites of neurons in the substantia nigra.

SUBCELLULAR FRACTIONATION

When brain tissue is homogenized in isoosmotic sucrose under carefully controlled conditions, ChAc, GAD, and DOPA-Dec are recovered after centrifugation in either a particulate occluded or "soluble" form. According to present views, the particulate form of the enzyme is derived from the detached nerve terminals (synaptosomes) whereas the soluble form is derived from the disruption of cell bodies and probably axons and dendrites (Gray and Whittaker, 1962). By scaling down the homogenizing equipment, it has been possible to study the subcellular distribution of ChAc in small samples of tissue. It was then found (Fonnum, 1970) that 81% of ChAc from ventral root was soluble, 50% from ventral horn, 10 to 15% from caudate nucleus, and 21 to 37% from nucleus interpositus. Such results are in agreement with the above-mentioned concept.

By differential centrifugation according to Gray and Whittaker (1962), the main proportion of enzyme activity was recovered either in the crude synaptosomal fraction (P_2) or in the high-speed supernatant (S_2). The proportion of enzyme activity in S_2 varied with different enzymes and in different regions of the brain (Fig. 2). Thus ChAc was mainly particulate in hippocampus, caudate nucleus, and cortex and mainly soluble in septum. In the three first regions, ChAc was mainly localized in the nerve terminals. Such results are in part supported by denervation experiments, since disruption of the afferents to hippocampus (Lewis, Shute, and Silver, 1967) is accompanied by a large loss of hippocampal ChAc activity. The septum, on the other hand, is believed to contain a high proportion of cholinergic perikarya sending their axons into the hippocampus (Lewis and Shute, 1967).

GAD was recovered in the synaptosome fraction from the above regions. Interestingly GAD and ChAc were distributed similarly in hippocampus, although ChAc is present solely in axons and terminals whereas GAD is probably present in intrinsic neurons (Fonnum and Storm-Mathisen, 1969; Storm-Mathisen and Fonnum, 1971). Such results can only be explained if the basket cells of the hippocampus have short axons and a large number of terminals, or if GAD is highly concentrated in these nerve terminals.

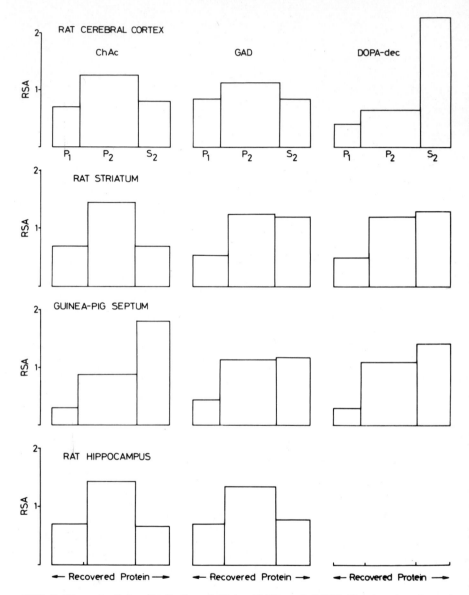

FIG. 2. The subcellular distribution of ChAc, GAD, and DOPA-Dec in rat cortex, rat striatum, guinea pig septum, and rat hippocampus. The results are expressed as RSA (percent enzyme activity/percent protein content of each fraction).

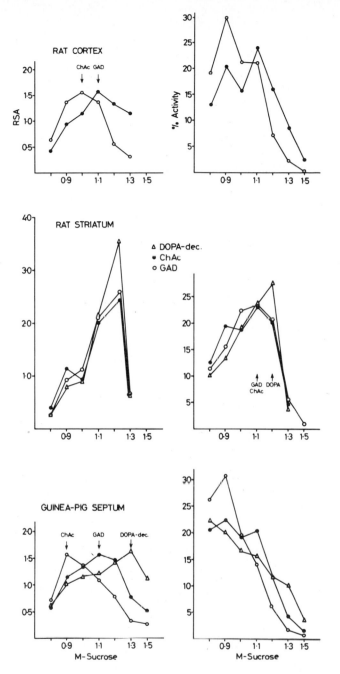

FIG. 3. The distribution of ChAc, GAD, and DOPA-Dec after loading a gradient with the P₂ fraction derived from 250 mg of original wet wt. of tissue and centrifuging for 25 min at 50,000 × g. The results are expressed either as RSA (percent enzyme activity/percent protein of each fraction) or as percent enzyme activity of each fraction.

DOPA-Dec is the most soluble of the three enzymes. The enzyme is less concentrated in nerve terminals than tyrosine-hydroxylase (McGeer, Bagchi, and McGeer, 1965). A large proportion of DOPA-Dec activity in cortical homogenates is recovered in the supernatant fraction, although this region does not contain any aminergic cells (Fuxe and Dahlström, 1964). It may be that the enzyme is also present extraneuronally (e.g., in capillaries), and in areas of low enzyme activity this source may become more important.

When the P_2 fraction was resuspended in 0.32 M sucrose and centrifuged to non-equilibrium on a discontinuous sucrose gradient consisting of equal volumes of 0.8, 0.9, 1.0, 1.1, 1.2, 1.3, and 1.5 M sucrose, the peak of enzyme activities and the specific activity (RSA) relative to protein content varied as shown in Fig. 3. This technique has been developed by Gfeller, Kuhar, and Snyder (1971). Due to the possible binding of ChAc to membranes, the gradient shows the distribution of occluded ChAc activities. The results showed that the peaks of enzyme activity in the gradient varied considerably although considerable overlap occurred. DOPA-Dec was separated from the other enzymes in striatum and septum. GAD sedimented further than ChAc in cerebral cortex and septum. In striatum they were similarly distributed.

In conclusion, ChAc, GAD, and DOPA-Dec showed some regional variation with regard to the proportion of soluble enzyme and with regard to their behavior on density gradient centrifugation. The results are compatible with the view that the synaptosome population is very hetereogeneous.

ACKNOWLEDGMENT

Part of this work was carried out in collaboration with Dr. Jon Storm-Mathisen at the Norwegian Defense Research Establishment and with Dr. Eric Rinvik and Professor Fred Walberg at the Anatomical Institute, University of Oslo.

REFERENCES

Albers, R. W., and Brady, R. O. (1959): The distribution of glutamate decarboxylase in the nervous system of the rhesus monkey. *Journal of Biological Chemistry*, 234:926–928.
Andersen, P., Eccles, J. C., and Voorhoeve, P. E. (1963): Inhibitory synapses on somas of Purkinje cells in the cerebellum. *Nature*, 199:655–656.
Baxter, C. F. (1970): The nature of γ-aminobutyric acid. In: *Handbook of Neurochemistry*, Vol. 3, edited by A. Lajtha. Plenum Press. New York, pp. 289–335.

Bull, G., Hebb, C., and Ratković, D. (1970): Choline acetyltransferase activity of human brain tissue during development and at maturity. *Journal of Neurochemistry*, 17:1505–1515.
Curtis, D. R., Duggan, A. W., and Felix, D. (1970): GABA and inhibition of Deiters' neurones. *Brain Research*, 23:117–120.
Eccles, J. C., Ito, M., and Szentágothai, J. (1967): *The Cerebellum as a Neuronal Machine*. Springer-Verlag, Berlin, 335 pp.
Fonnum, F. (1968): The distribution of glutamate decarboxylase and aspartate transaminase in subcellular fractions of rat and guinea-pig brain. *Biochemical Journal*, 106:401–412.
Fonnum, F. (1969a): Isolation of choline esters from aqueous solutions by extraction with sodium tetraphenylboron in organic solvents. *Biochemical Journal*, 113:291–298.
Fonnum, F. (1969b): Radiochemical micro assays for the determination of choline acetyltransferase and acetylcholinesterase activities. *Biochemical Journal*, 115:465.
Fonnum, F. (1970): Subcellular localization of choline acetyltransferase in brain. In: *Drugs and Cholinergic Mechanisms in the CNS*, edited by E. Heilbronn and A. Winter. Försvarets Forskningsorganisation, Stockholm.
Fonnum, F. and Storm-Mathisen, J. (1969): GABA synthesis in rat hippocampus correlated to the distribution of inhibitory neurones. *Acta Physiologica Scandinavia*, 76:35A–37A.
Fonnum, F., Storm-Mathisen, J., and Walberg, F. (1970): Glutamate decarboxylase in inhibitory neurons. A study of the enzyme in Purkinje cell axons and boutons in the cat. *Brain Research*, 20:259–275.
Fuxe, K. (1964): Evidence for the existence of monoamine neurons in the central nervous system. *Acta Physiologica Scandinavica*, 64, suppl. 247:39–85.
Gfeller, E., Kuhar, M. J., and Snyder, S. H. (1971): Neurotransmittor-specific synaptosomes in rat corpus striatum: Morphorlogical variations. *Proceedings of the National Academy of Sciences*, 68:155–159.
Goldberg, A. M., and McCaman, R. E. (1967): A quantitative microchemical study of choline acetyltransferase and acetylcholinesterase in the cerebellum of several species. *Life Sciences*, 6:1493–1500.
Gray, E. G., and Whittaker, V. P. (1962): The isolation of nerve endings from brain: and electronmicroscopic study of cell fragments derived by homogenization and centrifugation. *Journal of Anatomy*, 96:79–88.
Grofova, I., and Rinvik, E. (1970): An experimental electron microscopic study on the striatal-nigral projection in the cat. *Experimental Brain Research*, 11:249–263.
Hamori, J., and Szentagothai, J. (1965): The Purkinje cell basket; ultrastructure of an inhibitory synapse. *Acta Biologica Academia Science Hungari*, 15:465–479.
Hebb, C. O. (1963): Formation, storage and liberation of acetylcholine. In: *Handbuch der experimentellen Pharmakologie*, vol. 15, edited by G. B. Koelle. Springer-Verlag, Berlin, pp. 55–88.
Hirsch, H. E., and Robins, E. (1962): Distribution of γ-aminobutyric acid in the layers of the cerebral and cerebellar cortex. Implications for its physiological role. *Journal of Neurochemistry*, 9:63–70.
Ito, M., and Yoshida, M. (1966): The origin of cerebellar-induced inhibition of Deiters' neurons I Monosynaptic initiation of the inhibitory postsynaptic potentials. *Experimental Brain Research*, 2:330–349.
Ito, M., Yoshida, M., and Obata, K. (1964): Monosynaptic inhibition of the intracerebellar nuclei induced from the cerebellar cortex. *Experientia*, 20:575–576.
Israel, M., and Whittaker, V. P. (1967): Isolation of giant mossy fibre endings from the cerebella from different species. *Experentia*, 21:325.
Jansen, J., and Brodal, A. (1940): Experimental studies on the intrinsic fibers of the cerebellum. II. Cortico-nuclear projection. *Journal of Comparative Neurology*, 73:267–321.
Jansen, J., and Brodal, A. (1958): *Handbuch der Microscopischen Anatomie des Menshen. IV. Nervensystem*. Das Kleinhirn, Springer-Verlag, Berlin, 323 pp.
Kuntzman, R., Shore, P. A., Bogdanski, D., and Brodie, B. B. (1961): Microanalytical procedures for fluorometric assay of brain DOPA-5HTP decarboxylase, norephinephrine and

serotonin and a detailed mapping of decarboxylase activity in brain. *Journal of Neurochemistry*, 6:226–232.

Kuriyama, J., Haber, B., Sisken, B., and Roberts, E. (1966): The γ-aminobutyric acid system in rabbit cerebellum. *Proceedings of the National Academy of Sciences*, 55:846–852.

Lewis, P. R., Shute, C. C. D., and Silver, A. (1967): Confirmation from choline acetylase analysis of a massive cholinergic innervation to the rat hippocampus. *Journal of Physiology*, 191:215–224.

Lewis, P. R., and Shute, C. C. D. (1967): The cholinergic limbic system: Projections to hippocampal formation, medial cortex, nuclei of the ascending cholinergic reticular system, and the subfornical organ and supra optic crest. *Brain*, 90:521–540.

Lowry, O. H. (1953): The quantitative histochemistry of the brain. *Journal of Histochemistry and Cytochemistry*, 1:420–428.

McGeer, P. L., Bagchi, S. P., and McGeer, E. G. (1965): Subcellular localization of tyrosine hydroxylase in beef caudate nucleus. *Life Sciences*, 4:1859–1867.

Obata, K., Ito, M., Ochi, R., and Sato, N. (1967): Pharmacological properties of the postsynaptic inhibition by Purkinje cell axons and the action of γ-aminobutyric acid on Deiters' neurons. *Experimental Brain Research*, 4:43–57.

Obata, K., and Takeda, K. (1969): Release of γ-aminobutyric acid into the fourth ventricle induced by stimulation of the cat's cerebellum. *Journal of Neurochemistry*, 16:1043–1047.

Otsuka, M., Obata, K., Minyata, Y., and Tanaka, K. (1971): Measurement of γ-aminobutyric acid in isolated nerve cells of cat central nervous system. *Journal of Neurochemistry*, 18:287–296.

Storm-Mathisen, J., and Fonnum, F. (1971): Quantitative histochemistry of glutamate decarboxylase in the rat hippocampal region. *Journal of Neurochemistry*, 18:1105–1111.

Walberg, F., and Jansen, J. (1961): Cerebellar cortico-vestibular fibers in the cat. *Experimental Neurology*, 3:32–52.

Walberg, F., and Jansen, J. (1964): Cerebellar cortico-nuclear progection studied experimentally with silver impregnation methods. *Journal Hirnforschung*, 6:348–354.

Advances in Biochemical Psychopharmacology, Vol. 6
Raven Press, New York © 1972

Sympathetic Reinnervation of the Rat Iris *in vitro*

Irwin J. Kopin, Stephen D. Silberstein, David G. Johnson, Ingeborg Hanbauer, and David M. Jacobowitz

Laboratory of Clinical Science, National Institute of Mental Health, Bethesda, Maryland 20014

It is well known that after complete division of a peripheral nerve, recovery occurs by means of a downgrowth of the nerve fibers from the proximal stump. When sympathetic axons are divided, reinnervation occurs by growth of the axonal fibers from neurons in the sympathetic ganglia. Recently, Olson and Malmfors (1970) showed that rat superior cervical ganglia transplanted into the anterior chamber of the rat eye will reinnervate the iris. Sympathetic ganglia also survive in artificial media and the neurons continue to respond to acetylcholine stimulation for over 1 week after their isolation *in vitro* (Larrabee, 1970). These observations led us to examine the possibility that sympathetic ganglia could establish neuroeffector junctions *in vitro*.

Organ cultures were prepared using rat superior cervical ganglia or rat irides (Silberstein, Johnson, Jacobowitz, and Kopin, 1971*b*). The tissues were cultured separately or with a ganglion overlapping the margins of the iris. After one or more days in culture, the tissues were removed and examined for their ability to take up and store radioactive norepinephrine (Dengler, Michaelson, Spiegel, and Titus, 1962) and for histofluorimetric evidence of catecholamines (Falck and Owman, 1965). Nerve growth factor plays an important role in the development of the sympathetic nervous system (Levi-Montalcini, 1952). The effect of nerve growth factor on equine anti-mouse nerve growth factor serum was assessed, and the actions of drugs known to interact with neurotubular protein (colchicine and vinblastin) or inhibit protein synthesis were also examined.

Sympathetically innervated tissues take up norepinephrine and concentrate the amine in the adrenergic neurons (Dengler et al., 1962). The ability of a tissue to retain norepinephrine appears to be related to the extent of adrenergic innervation (Kopin, Gordon, and Horst, 1965); chronically denervated tissues rapidly lose their ability to concentrate catecholamines (Hertting, Axelrod, Kopin, and Whitby, 1961). As expected from their dense sympathetic innervation (Falck and Owman, 1965), freshly removed irides concentrate norepinephrine when incubated in a physiologic medium containing the labeled catecholamine (Olson and Malmfors, 1970). The ability of cultured irides to take up labeled norepinephrine was used as an index of the extent of sympathetic innervation of the tissue (Silberstein et al., 1971b). After varying intervals of culture with or without contact with superior cervical ganglia, the irides were incubated for 30 min at 37°C in a Krebs-Ringer bicarbonate solution containing ascorbic acid (200 mg/liter) and DL-norepinephrine-7-^{3}H (10^{-7} M, 8.76 C/mmole). After incubation, the tissue was washed with fresh Krebs-Ringer solution for 10 min, and the total radioactivity retained in the iris was assayed by liquid scintillation spectrometry after the tissue had been digested in NCS solubilizer (Amersham/Searle Corporation, Arlington Heights, Ill.).

Uptake of ^{3}H-norepinephrine was almost completely abolished 24 hr after incubation in organ culture whether or not the iris had been kept in contact with a ganglion (Silberstein et al., 1971b). On histofluorimetric examination, the disappearance of the catecholamine-containing nerve fibers suggested that the diminished uptake of the labeled amine was the result of degeneration of the sympathetic nerve endings; this is consistent with the rapid disappearance of norepinephrine, catecholamine uptake, and tyrosine hydroxylase from the rat salivary glands *in vivo* after removal of the superior cervical ganglion (Sedvall and Kopin, 1967).

On the second day in organ culture, irides grown in contact with superior cervical ganglia were found to take up about one-third as much catecholamine as freshly removed irides. The ability to take up ^{3}H-norepinephrine from the medium increased gradually. After 8 days in culture, ^{3}H-norepinephrine uptake was about 20% greater than that found in fresh irides. Irides incubated alone (or separated from superior cervical ganglia) did not recover the ability to take up the amine.

The increase in uptake of ^{3}H-norepinephrine by irides incubated in contact with ganglia correlated well with the degree of reinnervation evident in the reappearance of nerve fibers containing fluorescence characteristic of catecholamines (Silberstein et al., 1971b). After 4 days of culture with ganglia, irides contained a dense network of fluorescent fibers adjacent to the point of contact with the ganglion. The density of innervation was greater than that seen in fresh irides, but the fibers were smooth and did not appear to contain the varicosities which are typical of normal sympathetic nerve endings.

After 8 days in culture, the area of innervation increased, but still did not include the whole iris. At this time, however, varicosities typical of the fluorescent nerve fibers in freshly removed irides appeared along the grown nerve fibers.

The rate and extent of reinnervation was related to nerve growth factor. Nerve growth factor added to the culture medium was required for the degree of reinnervation obtained; when this factor was omitted, less extensive reinnervation occurred. ^{3}H-Norepinephrine uptake, our index of reinnervation, was further diminished when antibody to nerve growth factor had been added to the medium, suggesting that nerve growth factor which is normally present in iris and ganglia (Johnson, Gorden, and Kopin, 1972) plays some role in enhancing axonal regrowth.

When culture medium contains colchicine or vinblastin (5×10^{-7}M), the uptake of ^{3}H-norepinephrine and ^{3}H-metaraminol by irides cultured in contact with ganglia does not increase (Silberstein, Johnson, Hanbauer, and Kopin, 1971a). These drugs, which disrupt neurotubules, do not prevent uptake of these amines in freshly removed irides. It appears, therefore, that neurotubules appear to be essential for the processes of reinnervation.

These observations indicate that the stimulus for reinnervation of sympathetically denervated tissue does not require either nerve impulses or factors which derive from sources other than sympathetic ganglia or target tissue. The rate and extent of reinnervation is influenced by nerve growth factor and requires neurotubular protein.

REFERENCES

Dengler, H. J., Michaelson, I. A., Spiegel, H. E., and Titus, E. (1962): The uptake of labelled norepinephrine by brain and other tissues of the cat. *International Journal of Pharmacology*, 1:23–28.

Falck, B., and Owman, C. (1965): A detailed methodological description of the fluorescence method for the cellular demonstration of biogenic amines. *Acta University Lund*, 7:1–23.

Hertting, G., Axelrod, J., Kopin, I. J., and Whitby, L. G. (1961): Lack of uptake of catecholamines after chronic denervation of sympathetic nerves. *Nature*, 189:66.

Johnson, D. G., Gorden, P., and Kopin, I. J. (1972): A sensitive radioimmunoassay for 7S nerve growth factor antigens in serum and tissues (*in press*).

Kopin, I. J., Gordon, E. K., and Horst, W. D. (1965): Studies of uptake of L-norepinephrine-C^{14}. *Biochemical Pharmacology*, 14:753–759.

Larrabee, M. G. (1970): Metabolism of adult and embryonic sympathetic ganglia. *Federation Proceedings*, 29:1919–1920.

Levi-Montalcini, R. (1952): Effects of mouse tumor transplantation on the nervous system. *Annals of the New York Academy of Sciences*, 55:330–334.

Olson, L., and Malmfors, T. (1970): Growth characteristics of adrenergic nerves in the adult rat. *Acta Physiologica Scandinavica* (Suppl.), 348:1–112.

Sedvall, G., and Kopin, I. J. (1967): Influence of sympathetic denervation and nerve activity of tyrosine hydroxylase in the rat submaxillary gland. *Biochemical Pharmacology,* 16:39–46.

Silberstein, S. D., Johnson, D. G., Hanbauer, I., and Kopin, I. J. (1971a): Sympathetic reinnervation of the rat iris in organ culture. *The Pharmacologist,* 13:203.

Silberstein, S., Johnson, D. G., Jacobowitz, D. M., and Kopin, I. J. (1971b): Sympathetic reinnervation of the rat iris in organ culture. *Proceedings of the National Academy of Sciences,* 68:1121–1124.

Advances in Biochemical Psychopharmacology, Vol. 6
Raven Press, New York © 1972

Disposition and Role of Newly Synthesized Amines in Central Catecholaminergic Neurons

J. Glowinski, M. J. Besson, A. Cheramy, and A. M. Thierry

Groupe NB, Collège de France, 11 place Marcelin Berthelot, Paris 5e, France

The present state of our knowledge and techniques very often leads neurobiologists to choose experimental preparations as simple as possible to study the metabolism of neurotransmitters at the synaptic level. Therefore, it may appear unduly optimistic to perform metabolic studies with a particular transmitter in specific synapses of the brain. Nevertheless, biochemical research on substances involved in neurotransmission, particularly the monoamines, can already be undertaken on discrete structures or localized areas of the brain rich in populations of terminals containing known neurotransmitters. Attempts can also be made to correlate global changes in synaptic quantities of the amines with specific physiological events. Furthermore, since various earlier studies or unexplained data have suggested that amines are not stored homogenously in their respective terminals, progress may also be obtained with new investigations of the characteristics of the various storage forms of these amines. We shall discuss results obtained with three different experimental approaches. They provide more precise information about the complex disposition of catecholamines (CA) in central noradrenergic and dopaminergic neurons; these three lines of research consist of: (1) the estimation of norepinephrine (NE) utilization under conditions of activation of central noradrenergic neurons induced by stress; (2) the estimation of dopamine (DA) release from terminals of the nigro striatal dopaminergic neuronal system; (3) the estimation, with the help of a synthesis inhibitor, of the role of CA in the control of ovulation and self-stimulation. These three types of studies are complementary. They give information about events occurring at the presynaptic level, in the synapse, and indirectly at the receptor sites.

FUNCTIONAL AND STORAGE COMPARTMENTS

Isotopic studies suggest that NE is found in various storage forms in central catecholaminergic neurons (Iversen and Glowinski, 1966a; Glowinski and Iversen, 1966; Thierry, Blanc, and Glowinski, 1971a). In particular, it has been shown that NE previously taken up or synthesized from its precursors in central NE neurons disappears multiphasically from the whole brain or from discrete structures of the rat brain. Two exponential phases of NE decline were observed 10 min after the intracisternal injection of the ^{3}H amine or 80 min after the intracisternal injection of L-3,5-^{3}H-tyrosine, 27 C/mmole (Thierry et al., 1971a). Exogenous D,L-(7-^{3}H)NE (9.7 C/mmole) declines initially very rapidly (half-life = 30 min) and then much more slowly (half-life = 180 min) from the brain stem. This may correspond to two forms of NE utilized at different rates. It appeared interesting to investigate if these two hypothetical forms were affected differently during the physiological activation of central NE neurons. We have shown previously (Thierry, Javoy, Glowinski, and Kety, 1968) that electrical shocks applied to the feet of rats induce an acceleration of the overall turnover of NE in different structures of the rat brain. Therefore, this stress has been used as a tool to explore the characteristics of NE in its different storage forms. When a mild stress of short duration (15 min) was applied to the animals, it had no significant effect on the endogenous levels of NE in the brain stem. This procedure, however, induced in the brain stem a marked decrease in the accumulation of the labeled amine either taken up or synthesized from (2-^{3}H)-DA (6.2 C/mmole) or L-3,5-^{3}H tyrosine (27 C/mmole) after intracisternal injection of D,1-(7^{3}H)NE (9.7 C/mmole) or its precursors. In 15 min, ^{3}H-NE levels were decreased by about 20 to 27% in NE neurons labeled either with D,L-(^{3}H) NE or its ^{3}H precursors (Table 1); this indicates a very rapid acceleration of the ^{3}H-amine utilization. However, the effect of the mild and short-lasting stress was only detected when ^{3}H-NE had been recently taken up or synthesized, during a period in which ^{3}H-NE normally disappears very rapidly. No changes in ^{3}H-NE utilization could be seen when this 15-min stress was applied 2 or 3 hr after the initial labeling of the CA neurons with exogenous NE (Fig. 1) or its precursors. This clearly suggests that ^{3}H-NE newly taken up or newly synthesized behaves similarly and that this form of the amine is preferentially utilized during the activation of NE neurons when compared with ^{3}H-NE stored in tissues for a longer time. Nevertheless, the ^{3}H-amine remaining in the tissues a few hours after its injection or forma-

TABLE 1. *Effect of a 15-min stress on ³H-NE newly taken up or newly synthesized in the brain stem*

		³H-Norepinephrine (nC/g)	
	Exogenous	Synthesized From ³H-Dopamine	Synthesized From ³H-Tyrosine
Control	555 ± 25	53 ± 2	15 ± 1
Stress	450 ± 7[c]	43 ± 2[b]	11 ± 1[a]
% Change from control	−19	−20	−27

Animals received intracisternal injections of 3.1 μC of D,L-(7³H)-NE (9.7 C/mmole) or 10.8 μC of (2 ³H)-DA (6.2 C/mmole) or 23 μC of L-3,5-³H-tyrosine (27 C/mmole). Three groups of rats were submitted to the 15-min stress at 10, 20, and 2 min after ³H-NE, ³H-DA, and ³H-tyrosine administration, respectively. The stress consisted of electric shocks applied to the feet of the animals. The other groups served as respective controls. ³H-NE was estimated in the brain stem. Results are the mean values of groups of eight animals ± SEM.
[a] $p < 0.02$.
[b] $p < 0.01$.
[c] $p < 0.001$ (Thierry, Blanc, and Glowinski, 1971).

tion may be utilized at a faster rate in emergency situations such as those induced by a very severe stress (Fig. 1). As shown previously, a 3-hr stress session, consisting of six periods of electrical shocks lasting for 10 min each alternating with rest periods of 20 min each, markedly increased the utilization of the stored ³H-amine (Fig. 1). In this situation, the endogenous levels of NE decreased slightly (about 15 to 20%); consequently, the specific activity of NE was much lower in tissues of stressed animals than in controls, indicating a marked acceleration of amine turnover (Thierry et al., 1968). Two forms of NE turning over at different rates and exhibiting different sensitivities in their mobilization and utilization under conditions of neuronal activation seem to exist in NE terminals. These results are in agreement with the two compartment models originally proposed by Sedvall and coworkers to explain the intraneuronal distribution of NE in peripheral and central neurons (Sedvall, Weise, and Kopin, 1968). Further convincing evidence in favor of this hypothesis has been obtained recently in our laboratory. NE levels were estimated in the cortex of the rat, a structure rich in NE terminals, at various times after the administration of α-methyl-p-tyrosine (α-MpT) (200 mg/kg i.p.) (Spector, Sjoerdsma, and Udenfriend, 1965) and FLA 63 [bis-(4-methyl-1-homopiperazinyl-thiocarbonyl)disulfide] (40 mg/kg i.p.) (Svensson and Waldeck, 1969; Florvall and Corrodi, 1970), the inhibitors of the first and last step of NE synthesis, respectively. Surprisingly, 5 min after α-MpT was administered, NE levels

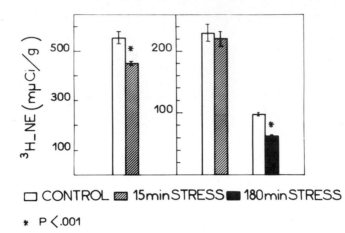

FIG. 1. Effect of stress of short or long duration on ³H-NE newly taken up (*left*) or stored for longer time period (*right*) in the brainstem of the rat. Electrical shocks were applied to the feet of rats for 15 min (short stress), 10 min (left), or 3 hr (right) after the intracisternal injection of D,L-(7³H)NE (3.1 μC, 9.7 C/mmole). In a second experiment animals were stressed for 180 min (long stress: 6 periods of 10 min each of electrical foot shocks alternating with 20 min rest periods) 2 hr after the intracisternal injection of the labeled amine (3.1 μC) (*right*). The animals were killed in all cases at the end of the stress session. ³H-NE was estimated in the brainstem of all animals. Results are the mean ±SEM of groups of eight rats. *$p < 0.01$.

were significantly increased. This initial event was followed by two phases of NE decline, a short-lasting phase (45 min) during which the amine disappeared rapidly (half-life = 45 min), followed by the well-known slower phase during which the amine disappeared with a half-life of 3 hr. The curve of NE disappearance obtained after the administration of FLA 63, a very rapidly acting inhibitor of DA-NE conversion, was quite different. NE levels decreased immediately and very rapidly during the first 5 min; this first period was followed successively by a small rise in the amine levels, which returned almost to the control levels in a few minutes, and by a long-lasting phase of decline which was much more rapid (half-life = 2 hr) than that observed after α-MpT (Thierry, Blanc, and Glowinski, 1971*b*).

The differences between the effects of α-MpT and FLA 63, particularly the faster disappearance of NE observed after FLA 63 already mentioned by other workers (Persson and Waldeck, 1970) may be explained by the persistent formation of NE from stored DA in α-MpT-treated animals (Thierry, Blanc, and Glowinski, 1971*c*). Similar conclusions may be drawn from the earlier results of Goldstein and Nakajima (1967), who also observed a faster disappearance of NE after disulfiram, another dopamine-β-hydroxylase inhibitor, than after α-MpT. The small rise of NE between the two phases of NE decline after FLA 63 is still unexplained but might be attributed to the delivery of NE to cortical nerve terminals by axonal flow. Besides the two new problems just mentioned, it should be pointed out that after both α-MpT (200mg/kg i.p.) and FLA 63 (40 mg/kg i.p.), NE levels did not decline in a simple exponential manner as previously described (Brodie, Costa, Dlabac, Neff, and Smookler, 1966; Iversen and Glowinski, 1966*b;* Costa and Neff, 1970). The decline occurred instead in two main phases, exhibiting different characteristics, and corresponding probably to the two forms of storage already described in the previous experiments. In summary, on the basis of these various and complementary observations, it appears that an appreciable part of newly synthesized or newly taken up NE is localized in NE terminals in a small compartment in which its rate of utilization is very rapid (half-life less than 10 min). Furthermore, the amine localized in this compartment can be rapidly mobilized for release, as suggested by the stress experiments. This "functional compartment" co-exists with a "main storage compartment" much larger in size and containing NE stored in tissues for a longer time, in which the amine is utilized at a much slower rate and is probably released only in emergency situations. The release of the amine from the "main storage compartment" may be observed after depletion of the amine contained in the "functional compartment" or when release of NE from the latter compartment is not compensated for by an acceleration of synthesis.

ROLE OF NEWLY SYNTHESIZED CA IN RELEASE PROCESS

An increased utilization of a transmitter in tissues represents only indirect evidence for enhanced release at the synaptic level. Direct information about the release of newly synthesized CA may be obtained in *in vitro* studies. After incubation of slices of structures rich in NE or DA-containing terminals with L-3,5-^{3}H-tyrosine of high specific activity (27 C/mmole), the synthesis and release of ^{3}H-amines into the incubating medium can be estimated. An increased release of newly synthesized NE has been demonstrated in this way with brain stem slices incubated with desmethylimipramine (DMI), a potent inhibitor of the NE reuptake process (Thierry and Blanc, *unpublished observations*). Changes in the release of labeled DA recently synthesized from its precursor tyrosine in DA-containing terminals of the rat striatum have been observed after treatment with drugs acting on DA neurons, such as amphetamine (Besson, Cheramy, and Glowinski, 1969), apomorphine (Goldstein, Freedman, and Backstrom, 1970), benztropine, and atropine (Goldstein, Fuxe, Battista, Backstrom, and Nakatani, 1970). The indirect activation of DA neurons with thioproperazine (5 mg/kg i.p.), a potent neuroleptic, induced an enhanced release of DA from dopaminergic terminals; the *in vivo* activation of DA neurons by this drug can also be detected *in vitro* (Cheramy, Besson, and Glowinski, 1970). The release of endogenously synthesized CA can also be studied by superfusing continuously with a physiological medium an isolated structure of the brain previously labeled with L-3,5-³H-tyrosine (28 C/mmole) (Besson, Cheramy, Feltz, and Glowinski, 1969). Thus ACh and serotonin, two transmitters normally found in high concentrations in the striatum, were able to induce a marked increase in the release of ³H-DA from this structure in *in vitro* studies, suggesting the existence of interrelations between cholinergic and serotoninergic neurons and the nigro-striatal dopaminergic system. Changes in transmitter release induced pharmacologically are thus detectable *in vitro,* particularly when the release of newly synthesized CA is examined.

However, more direct evidence for the role of newly synthesized amines in events occurring at the synaptic level was obtained in *in vivo* studies. During the last two years, attempts have been made in our laboratory to study the release of DA from dopaminergic terminals of the nigro-striatal system of the cat. Successful results were obtained by superfusing superficial dopaminergic terminals with a cup placed on the ventricular surface of the caudate nucleus; L-3,5-³H-tyrosine (52 C/mmole) was introduced continuously into the cup and the ³H-DA released in the superfusing fluid was collected simultaneously and estimated in successive fractions (Besson, Cheramy, Feltz, and Glowinski, 1971). With this experimental approach, both the spontaneous and pharmacologically-induced release of ³H-dopamine could be easily demonstrated. More recently, an evoked release of the amine in response to electrical stimulation of specific areas of the brain has also been shown (Besson, Cheramy, Gauchy, Glowinski, and Albe-Fessard, *in preparation*). We would like to describe two experiments which were designed to test the hypothesis of a preferential release of newly synthesized ³H-DA. In the first one, the releasing effect of pheniprazine on ³H-DA newly synthesized and ³H-DA stored for a longer time in tissues was examined. The drug, an MAO inhibitor structurally related to amphetamine, was introduced into the cup for a short period during the continuous superfusion of dopaminergic terminals with L-3,5-³H-tyrosine (52 C/mmoles) (continuous labeling), or about 2 hr after a pulse labeling of the tissue with L-3,5-³H-tyrosine (52 C/mmole). In the pulse-labeling experiment, ³H-tyrosine was introduced for 30 min into the cup, and the tissue was then superfused with a physiological medium free of labeled amino acid. In the continuous labeling experiment, the amounts of ³H-DA in the two fractions containing pheniprazine were 4 to 6 times those of the immediately preceding fractions, indicating a very powerful releasing effect of the drug on newly synthesized ^{3}H-DA (Fig. 2). In the acute labeling experiment, the amounts of ^{3}H-DA in the pheniprazine fractions were only 1.5 times greater than those in the fractions preceding drug superfusion.

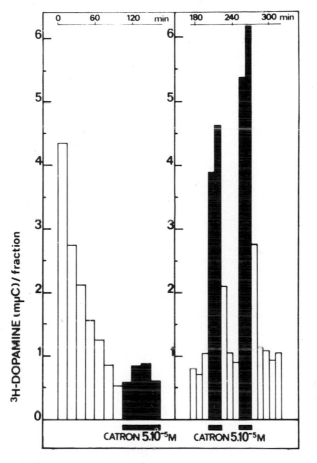

FIG. 2. Effect of pheniprazine (Catron) on the release of ^{3}H-DA newly synthesized or stored for a longer time. The left part of the figure illustrates the effects of Catron application on the release of ^{3}H-DA previously synthesized from L-3,5-^{3}H-tyrosine (27 C/ mmole). DA-containing terminals were pulse labeled during 30 min with ^{3}H-tyrosine (50 µC) and then superfused with a physiological medium, collected in fractions of 15 min each. Pheniprazine was added to the superfusing fluid 105 min after the end of the labeling session. The effect of pheniprazine application on the release of ^{3}H-DA newly synthesized in dopaminergic terminals labeled continuously with ^{3}H-tyrosine (40 µC/ml) is on the right. Superfusates were collected in fractions of 10 min each. ^{3}H-DA was estimated in all collected fractions. Numbers at the top indicate the time (in min) of superfusion. (Figure taken from Besson, Cheramy, Feltz, and Glowinski, 1971).

Thus pheniprazine had only a slight releasing effect on ³H-DA synthesized and stored in tissues for at least 2 hr (Fig. 2). In the second experiment, L-3,5-³H-tyrosine (52 C/mmole) was introduced continuously into the cup and about 2 hr later ³H-DA synthesis was inhibited by injecting α-MpT (100 mg/kg) intravenously. Despite the persistence of large quantities of ³H-DA in the tissue, the spontaneous release of ³H-DA was immediately and markedly decreased after α-MpT injection (Table 2). Moreover, the effects of amphetamine on ³H-DA release during its continuous formation were quite different from those observed after the amine synthesis inhibition. The amounts of ³H-DA released by amphetamine were about 4 times higher than those of the preceding fraction during continuous synthesis, and only 1.6 times higher after inhibition of synthesis (Table 3). These re-

TABLE 2. *Effect of α-MpT on the release of ³H-DA in the cat caudate nucleus*

	No. of fraction after the onset of super-fusion	³H-DA (nC/10 min) released in successively collected fractions
During	9	1.5
continuous ³H-DA	10	1.6
synthesis	11	1.6
Immediately → α-MpT	12	1.0
after α-MpT	13	0.9
injection	14	0.6

The surface of the caudate nucleus of an unanaesthesized cat immobilized with flaxedil was superfused with L-3,5-³H-tyrosine (52 C/mmole) (40 μC/ml) at a rate of 6 ml using a cup. ³H-DA collected continuously was estimated in superfusate fractions of 10 min each during continuous synthesis and immediately after the intravenous injection of α-MpT (100 mg/kg).

TABLE 3. *Effects of amphetamine on ³H-DA newly synthesized or stored for longer time in dopaminergic terminals of the cat caudate nucleus*

	Before	Amphetamine	After
³H-DA released (nC/20 min) during normal synthesis	3	13	7
³H-DA released (nC/20 min) after synthesis inhibition	2	3	2

The surface of the caudate nucleus of an unanaesthesized cat immobilized with flaxedil was superfused with L-3,5-³H-tyrosine (52 C/mmole) (40 μC/ml) as indicated in Table 2. ³H-DA was estimated in superfusate fractions of 20 min each immediately before, during, or just after the addition of amphetamine (10⁻⁶ M) to the superfusing medium in the cup. The experiment was performed during continuous synthesis of ³H-DA from ³H-tyrosine and immediately after the inhibition of ³H-DA synthesis with α-MpT (100 mg/kg i.v.).

sults again suggest that amphetamine released newly synthesized ^{3}H-DA preferentially to ^{3}H-DA stored in tissues for a longer time. As previously shown for central NE terminals, at least two forms of DA storage exhibiting different characteristics are thus present in dopaminergic terminals of the nigro-striatal system. This conclusion is in agreement with earlier studies on DA release performed on the isolated striatum of the rat and *in vivo* on the cat caudate nucleus. ^{3}H-DA levels in successive superfusate fractions decreased in two distinct phases after a pulse labeling of DA terminals with L-3,5-^{3}H-tyrosine (27 C/mmole). A rapid and short-lasting phase (half-life about 15 min) was followed by a long-lasting period during which ^{3}H-DA levels decreased more slowly (half-life = 60 min) in both *in vivo* and *in vitro* experiments. Further evidence for the heterogenous storage of DA in DA terminals was also obtained by studying in detail the effects of α-MpT on DA levels as a function of time in the striatum of the rat (Javoy and Glowinski, 1971). As for cortical NE after FLA 63 administration, striatal DA did not decline in a simple exponential manner after α-MpT injection (200 mg/kg i.p.). Two distinct phases of DA disappearance were observed separated by a short period during which DA levels did not decrease or even increase slightly. Fifteen minutes after α-MpT injection, at the end of the first phase of DA disappearance, DA levels had already significantly decreased by about 25%, indicating a very rapid initial utilization of the amine. This may represent the depletion of the functional compartment of DA in DA terminals. The amine declined much more slowly thereafter; 40 min after α-MpT, its half-life was 2 hr, as previously reported (Costa and Neff, 1966). This second phase of DA disappearance may be attributed to the utilization of DA stored in the main storage compartment.

The two compartment model described previously seems adequate to explain the various results obtained on dopaminergic terminals. Moreover, the release experiments have confirmed the view that newly synthesized DA localized in the functional compartment is easily available for release into the synaptic cleft.

ROLE OF NEWLY SYNTHESIZED CA IN FUNCTIONS OF CATECHOLAMINERGIC NEURONS

The role of central catecholaminergic neurons in specific functions of the CNS has often been studied by establishing relationships between modifications of amine metabolism and physiological effects. The specific destruction of CA neurons with intracerebral administration of 6-hydroxy-dopamine represents an interesting model in this regard and has been successfully used to study some of the functions of the nigro-striatal dopaminergic neurons (Ungerstedt and Arbuthnott, 1970; Ungerstedt, 1971a). The inhibition of transmitter synthesis by general or local administration of α-MpT may offer some advantages; amine levels can be restored to their normal steady state levels by peripheral injection of DOPA. On the other hand, amine levels at the receptor sites can be rapidly increased with MAO or reuptake inhibitors. These various procedures and many others have been widely used by various workers to demonstrate the involvement of the tubero infundibular dopaminergic neurons in the control of the ovulation process (Kordon and Glowinski, 1970) and the role of catecholaminergic neurons ascending in the medial forebrain bundle in self-stimulation behavior (Stein, 1962; Poschel and Nintemann, 1966; Wise and Stein, 1969; Stinus, Le Moal, and Cardo, *in preparation*).

We wish to describe two experiments in which the effects of α-MpT on ovulation and self-stimulation have been carefully investigated as a function of time after the drug administration. Particular care was taken to measure the physiological effect of the drug immediately after α-MpT administration. In this situation the synthesis of CA is immediately inhibited, as shown by the marked decrease in the rate of conversion of L-3,5-^{3}H-tyrosine (27 C/mmole) to ^{3}H-DOPA in cortical or striatal slices of α-MpT (200 mg/kg i.p.)-treated animals (Thierry and Blanc, *unpublished observations;* Besson, Cheramy, and Glowinski, 1971). This effect persists for many hours, as shown in *in vivo* studies by measuring the ^{14}C-CA formation from ^{14}C tyrosine (Udenfriend, Zaltzman-Niremberg, Gordon, and Spector, 1966). Furthermore, a marked decline in the amount of transmitter available for release is observed shortly after α-MpT.

Dopamine release from dopaminergic tubero infundibular neurons activates the liberation of luteinizing hormone (LH) from the pituitary. The transmitter may act directly at the level of the median eminence by interfering with the process of LRF secretion and release (Kordon and Glowinski, 1969). This action occurs particularly during the critical period of ovulation control which corresponds to the time interval, in the afternoon of proestrus, during which LH is released. Ovulation can be precisely estimated by counting the number of eggs in the oviducts of 29-day-old rats in which ovulation was induced by treatment with seric gonadotrophin (30 IU s.c. PMS) on day 25 and with chorionic gonadotrophin (5 IU s.c.) at the beginning of the critical period, that is, 25 hr before their sacrifice. As indicated in Fig. 3, the effect of α-MpT (200 mg/kg i.p.) was tested on this preparation by injecting the drug at different times before, during, and after the critical period. The administration of α-MpT during the critical period almost completely blocked the release of the ovulating hormone, probably

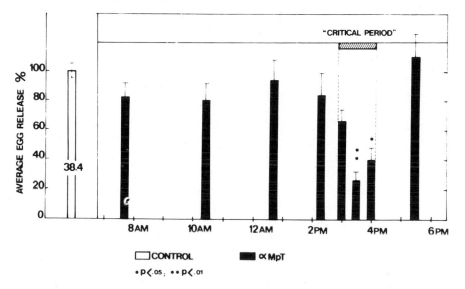

FIG. 3. Effect of αMpT on ovulation process. Groups of 25-day-old rats (6 to 10 animals per group) were injected with gonadotrophin. αMpT was injected intraperitoneally (200 mg/kg) at various time during the proestrus day and the animals were killed 20 to 25 hr after the "critical period." The numbers of ova present in the oviducts were counted; they are represented as vertical bars. The results correspond to the number of ova released per ovulating animal, expressed as percent of the average egg release in the corresponding control (38.4 ± 3.1 ova per animal) (from Kordon and Glowinski, 1969). All data were submitted to variance analysis. The data were analyzed after square root transformation of the variable to approximate a guassian distribution; legitimacy of this operation was confirmed by the low χ^2 values obtained after transformation.

as a result of the immediate diminution of DA release at the synaptic level. Similar and more pronounced effects were seen after the intravenous injection of the drug (50 mg/kg); in this case, the time interval during which α-MpT treatment was effective was limited to 30 min. This suggests, as indicated also by the release experiments, that DA stored in tissues is not available for release shortly after the administration of synthesis inhibitor. However, there seems to be a rapid recovery of LH-release regulation after α-MpT administration, as indicated by the normal or only slightly subnormal ovulatory performances observed when the drug is given one hour or a few hours before the critical period. The recovery of the ovulation process may be attributed to the mobilization of stored DA for release. This implies that DA still present in tissues 30 min or more after α-MpT and mainly localized in the main storage compartment has been transferred to a site from which it can be released and thus be active at the receptor site. From these results it can be assumed that DA in the main storage compartment is available for release 45 to 60 min after the intraperitoneal injection of α-MpT. Such an hypothesis strongly supports the two compartment model proposed for DA storage, but further experiments are needed to investigate the precise latency for the mobilization of the stored DA. Nevertheless, similar interpretations can be made from the results obtained with self-stimulation experiments.

Stinus, LeMoal, and Cardo (1971) have recently studied the effects of various drugs acting on CA metabolism on self-stimulation. In one of their experiments, rats were implanted with bipolar electrodes in the group of DA cell bodies, A 10, which according to Ungerstedt (1971b) mainly innervate the nucleus accumbens and the tuberculum olfactorum. The animals were then trained to press a lever to stimulate their brain electrically during repeated short sessions during a 27-day period (stimulation characteristics: sinusoidal stimulation 100 cps, 200 msec duration and 75 ± 5 μamp intensity). On the day of the experiment, animals were allowed to self-stimulate for 8 hr; self-stimulation sessions of 30 min were regularly alternated, as indicated in Fig. 4, with 30-min rest sessions. The number of self-stimulations made by the animals per 5 min was counted continuously during each 30-min self-stimulation session. Animals were treated with saline or α-MpT (150 mg/kg i.p.) 1 hr after the beginning of the experiment. In the saline-treated animals, the total number of self-stimulations was similar in all self-stimulation sessions; only a very slight decrease in responses was seen as a function of time in each self-stimulation session, probably reflecting slight satiation or fatigue. The record obtained after α-MpT, however, differed markedly, and a few observations can be made. The rate of self-stimulation decreased by almost 50% in the first 30-min session immediately after the intraperitoneal injection of the drug, which again may be attributed to a rapid reduction in the quantities of newly synthesized amines available for release at synapses. The CA, very likely DA, still stored in nerve terminals appeared not to be immediately available for release. As expected, the total number of responses in each self-stimulation session decreased markedly as a function of time during the 6 hr which followed α-MpT injection. Most interestingly, it was found that after each resting session, the number of responses in the initial 5 min was much higher than that estimated at the end of the preceding self-stimulation session. This effect was much more pronounced than in control animals and was a consistent finding. This may be attributed to a partial mobilization during each 30-min resting period of the amine stored in the main storage compartment for subsequent release during self-stimulation. Only small quantities of the transmitter appear to be available for release in this way, as indicated by the

EFFECT OF ∝MpT ON SELF–STIMULATION

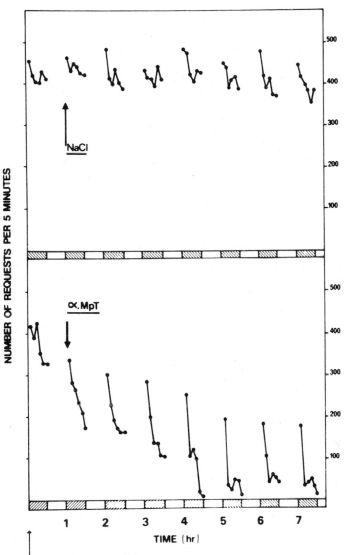

FIG. 4. Effect of αMpT on self-stimulation. Animals were implanted with bipolar electrodes in the group of DA cells A 10 and trained to self-stimulate for 27 days. The figure represents the record obtained after intraperitoneal injection with saline on day 28 and with αMpT (100 mg/kg) on day 29. Animals were allowed to self-stimulate for 30-min periods (hatched horizontal bars) alternating with 30-min rest periods. Each point represents the rate of self-stimulations per 5-min period. Results are the mean of a group of 10 animals (Stinus, Le Moal, and Cardo, 1971).

rapid decrease in the rate of self-stimulation as a function of time in each successive self-stimulation session.

Experiments are in progress to examine more precisely the relationships between the functional and main storage compartment. In any case, these two functional studies clearly show that newly synthesized amines play a major role in events occurring at the receptor level. This is in agreement with earlier speculations of Weissman, Koe, and Tenen (1966) and Rech, Carr, and Moore (1968). The first authors have proposed that the rapid antiamphetamine effect of α-MpT was linked to rapid changes in the levels of CA localized in a functional pool highly susceptible to blockade of synthesis at the tyrosine hydroxylase step. The second group of workers have shown that a small dose of α-MpT markedly impaired avoidance responding, rotarod performance, and motor activity in animals which had been treated 3 days earlier with reserpine to deplete the reserve stores of CA. The authors have suggested that the physiological effects of α-MpT were related to the depletion of newly synthesized amines localized in a functional pool, the only pool detectable in tissues 2 to 3 days after reserpine treatment (Häggendal and Lindqvist, 1963; Glowinski, Iversen, and Axelrod, 1966). It is thus tempting to propose that the functional pool of CA which has been extensively described in this report corresponds to amines associated with newly formed amine storage granules, which are the only ones found in CA terminals 2 to 3 days after reserpine treatment, as suggested by Häggendal and Dahlström (1971).

CONCLUSIONS

Information obtained with a variety of different experimental approaches in physiological or pharmacological situations reveals that newly synthesized CA in the CNS exhibit different properties from older amines stored in the tissue. Briefly, the newly synthesized amines are utilized at a faster rate and are mobilized immediately and preferentially during mild activation of neurons. As shown particularly with dopaminergic neurons, they play a major role in the spontaneous or pharmacological release of the transmitter and seem to contribute predominantly in effects occurring on the receptor cells. There is little doubt that CA are stored heterogenously in central neurons, as previously suggested for peripheral NE (Weiner, 1970). The two-compartment model discussed in this report seems to represent a valid working hypothesis for further studies. It is probably that this simplified representation of the events occurring in nerve terminals will rapidly evolve and change, particularly when new information from morphological or biochemical subcellular studies is obtained. It should also be remembered that another storage compartment, in which the amine has a half-life of about 17 hr, has been described for NE in the CNS (Burack and Draskoćzy, 1964; Glowinski, Kopin, and Axelrod, 1965).

Therefore, in future studies the assumption of a single compartment for the amine storage generally used to calculate the synthesis rate of the amines will have to be revised. Particular attention will have to be given to the role of newly synthesized CA in order to analyze the events occurring at the synaptic level during physiological states or after treatment with small doses of drugs. Moreover, the dynamic metabolic characteristics of the various intraneuronal forms of CA storage will have to be analyzed more extensively. The possible interrelations between these various storage forms raise new and fascinating problems which will also have to be solved in order to finally understand the complex regulatory processes occurring in central CA neurons.

ACKNOWLEDGMENTS

We should like to thank Dr. Cardo and his collaborators from the Laboratoire de Psychophysiologie, Université de Bordeaux, who have kindly allowed some of their recent results to be used for the preparation of this article.

REFERENCES

Besson, M. J., Cheramy, A., Feltz, P., and Glowinski, J. (1969): Release of newly synthesized dopamine from dopamine-containing terminals in the striatum of the rat. *Proceedings of the National Academy of Science*, 62:741–748.

Besson, M. J., Cheramy, A., Feltz, P., and Glowinski, J. (1971): Dopamine: spontaneous and induced release from the caudate nucleus in the cat. *Brain Research*, 32:407–424.

Besson, M. J., Cheramy, A., Gauchy, C., Glowinski, J., and Albe-Fessard, D. Effect of stimulation of substantia nigra and other mesencephalic structures on the release of dopamine from the caudate nucleus of the rat (*in preparation*).

Besson, M. J., Cheramy, A., and Glowinski, J. (1969): Effects of amphetamine and desmethylimipramine on amine synthesis and release in central catecholamine-containing neurons. *European Journal of Pharmacology*, 7:111–114.

Besson, M. J., Cheramy, A., and Glowinski, J. (1971): Effects of some psychotropic drugs on dopamine synthesis in the rat striatum. *Journal of Pharmacology and Experimental Therapeutics*, 177:196–205.

Brodie, B. B., Costa, E., Dlabac, A., Neff, N. H., and Smookler, H. H. (1966): Application of steady state kinetics to the estimation of synthesis rates and turnover time of tissue catecholamines. *Journal of Pharmacology and Experimental Therapeutics*, 154:493–498.

Burack, W. R. and Draskoćzy, P. R. (1964): The turnover of endogenously labelled catecholamine in several regions of the sympathetic nervous system. *Journal of Pharmacology*, 144:66–75.

Cheramy, A., Besson, M. J., and Glowinski, J. (1970): Increased release of dopamine from striatal dopaminergic terminals in the rat after treatment with a neuroleptic: thioproperazine. *European Journal of Pharmacology*, 10:206–214.

Costa, E. and Neff, N. H. (1966): Isotopic and non-isotopic measurements of the rate of catecholamine biosynthesis. In: *Biochemistry and Pharmacology of the Basal Ganglia*, edited by E. Costa, L. J. Côte, and M. D. Yahr. Raven Press, New York, pp. 141–155.

Costa, E. and Neff, N. H. (1970): Estimation of turnover rates to study the metabolic regulation of the steady-state level of neuronal monoamines. In: *Handbook of Neurochemistry*, edited by Lajtha. Plenum Press, New York, Vol IV, pp. 49–90.

Florvall, L. and Corrodi, H. (1970): Dopamine-β-hydroxylase inhibitors. The preparation and the dopamine-β-hydroxylase inhibitory activity of some compounds related to dithiocarbamic and thiuramdisulphide. *Acta Pharmaceutica Suecica*, 7:7–22.

Glowinski, J. and Iversen, L. L. (1966): Regional studies of catecholamines in the rat brain. I. The disposition of ^{3}H-norepinephrine, ^{3}H-dopamine, ^{3}H-DOPA, in various regions of the brain. *Journal of Neurochemistry*, 13:665–669.

Glowinski, J., Iversen, L. L., and Axelrod, J. (1966): Storage and synthesis of norepinephrine in the reserpine-treated rat brain. *Journal of Pharmacology and Experimental Therapeutics*, 151:385–399.

Glowinski, J., Kopin, I. J., and Axelrod, J. (1965): Metabolism of ^{3}H-norepinephrine in the rat brain. *Journal of Neurochemistry*, 12:25–30.

Goldstein, M., Freedman, L. S., and Backstrom, T. (1970): The inhibition of catecholamine biosynthesis by apomorphine. *Journal of Pharmacy and Pharmacology*, 22:715–716.

Goldstein, M., Fuxe, K., Battista, A. F., Backstrom, T., and Nakatani, S. (1970): The effects of antiparkinsonian drugs on striatal dopamine. *Federation Proceedings*, 2445.

Goldstein, M. and Nakajima, K. (1967): The effect of disulfiram on catecholamine levels in the brain. *Journal of Pharmacology and Experimental Therapeutics*, 157:96–102.

Häggendal, J. and Dahlström, A. (1971): The recovery of noradrenaline in adrenergic nerve terminals of the rat after reserpine treatment. *Journal of Pharmacy and Pharmacology*, 23: 81–89.

Häggendal, J. and Lindqvist, M. (1963): Behaviour and monoamine levels during long term administration of reserpine to rabbits. *Acta Physiologica Scandinavica*, 57:431–436.

Iversen, L. L. and Glowinski, J. (1966a): Regional studies of catecholamines in the rat brain. II. Rate of turnover of catecholamines in various brain regions. *Journal of Neurochemistry*, 13:671–682.

Iversen, L. L. and Glowinski, J. (1966b): Regional differences in the rate of turnover of norepinephrine in the rat brain. *Nature*, 210:1006–1008.

Javoy, F. and Glowinski, J. (1971): Dynamic characteristics of the "functional compartment" of dopamine in dopaminergic terminals of the rat striatum. *Journal of Neurochemistry*, 18: 1305–1311.

Kordon, C. and Glowinski, J. (1969): Selective inhibition of superovulation by blockade of dopamine synthesis during the "critical period" in the immature rat. *Endocrinology*, 85: 924–931.

Kordon, C. and Glowinski, J. (1970): Role of brain catecholamines in the control of anterior pituitary functions. In: *Neurochemical Aspects of Hypothalamic Function*, edited by L. Martini and Meites. Academic Press, New York, pp. 85–100.

Persson, T. and Waldeck, B. (1970): Further studies on the possible interaction between dopamine and noradrenaline containing neurons in the brain. *European Journal of Pharmacology*, 11:315–324.

Poschel, B. P. H. and Ninteman, F. W. (1966): Hypothalamic self-stimulation: its suppression by blockade of norepinephrine biosynthesis and reinstatement by metamphetamine. *Life Sciences*, 5:11–16.

Rech, R. H., Carr, L. A., and Moore, K. E. (1968): Behavioral effects of α methyltyrosine after prior depletion of brain catecholamines. *Journal of Pharmacology and Experimental Therapeutics*, 160:326–335.

Sedvall, G. C., Weise, V. K., and Kopin, I. J. (1968): The role of norepinephrine synthesis measured *in vivo* during short intervals: influence of adrenergic nerve impulse activity. *Journal of Pharmacology and Experimental Therapeutics*, 159:274–282.

Spector, S., Sjoerdsma, A., and Udenfriend, S. (1965): Blockade of endogenous norepinephrine synthesis by α-methyl-tyrosine, an inhibitor of tyrosine hydroxylase. *Journal of Pharmacology and Experimental Therapeutics*, 147:86–95.

Stein, L. (1962): Effects and interactions of imipramine, chlorpromazine, reserpine, and amphetamine on self-stimulation: possible neurophysiological basis of depression. *Recent Advances in Biological Psychiatry*, 4:288–308.

Stinus, L., Le Moal, M., and Cardo, B.: Role of newly synthesized CA in self-stimulation. *Physiology and Behaviour* (*in press*).

Svensson, T. H. and Waldeck, B. (1969): On the significance of central noradrenaline for motor activity: experiments with a new dopamine β hydroxylase inhibitor. *European Journal of Pharmacology*, 7.278–282.

Thierry, A. M., Blanc, G., and Glowinski, J. (1971a): Effect of stress on the disposition of catecholamines localized in various intraneuronal storage forms in the brain stem of the rat. *Journal of Neurochemistry*, 18:449–461.

Thierry, A. M., Blanc, G., and Glowinski, J. (1971b): Persistent norepinephrine formation from stored dopamine in central NE terminals of the rat after α-MpT treatment. *Third International Meeting of the International Society for Neurochemistry*.

Thierry, A. M., Blanc, G., and Glowinski, J. (1971c): Dopamine-norepinephrine: another regulatory step of norepinephrine synthesis in central noradrenergic neurons. *European Journal of Pharmacology*, 14:303–307.

Thierry, A. M., Javoy, F., Glowinski, J., and Kety, S. S. (1968): Effects of stress on the metabolism of norepinephrine, dopamine, and serontonin in the central nervous system of the rat. *Journal of Pharmacology and Experimental Therapeutics*, 163:163–171.

Udenfriend, S., Zaltzman-Nirenberg, P., Gordon, R., and Spector, S. (1966): Evolution of the biochemical effects produced *in vivo* by inhibitions of the three enzymes involved in norepinephrine biosynthesis. *Molecular Pharmacology*, 2:95–105.

Ungerstedt, U. (1971a): Adipsia and aphagia after 6-hydroxydopamine induced degeneration of the nigro striatal dopamine system. *Acta Physiologica Scandinavia*, 367 Suppl.: 95–122.

Ungerstedt, U. (1971b): Stereotaxic mapping of the monoamine pathway in the rat brain. *Acta Physiologica Scandinavia*, 367:1–48.

Ungerstedt, U. und Arbuthnott, G. (1970): Quantitative recording of rotational behavior in rats after 6-hydroxy dopamine lesions of the nigro striatal dopamine system. *Brain Research*, 24:485–493.

Weiner, N. (1970): Regulation of NE biosynthesis. *Annual Review of Pharmacology*, 10: 273–290.

Weissman, A., Koe, K. B., and Tenen, S. S. (1966): Antiamphetamine effects following inhibition of tyrosine hydroxylase. *Journal of Pharmacology and Experimental Therapeutics*, 151:339–352.

Wise, C. D. and Stein, L. (1969): Facilitation of brain self-stimulation by control administration of norepinephrine. *Science*, 163:299–301.

Advances in Biochemical Psychopharmacology, Vol. 6
Raven Press, New York © 1972

Isolation of the Cholinergic Receptor Protein of *Torpedo* Electric Tissue

P. B. Molinoff and L. T. Potter

Department of Biophysics, University College of London, London, England

THE CONCEPT OF RECEPTORS AS APPLIED TO NEUROTRANSMITTERS

Nerve cells are highly differentiated cells which have the ability to transmit information over relatively long distances by an all-or-none signal which is electrical in nature (Hodgkin, 1964). When a nerve impulse reaches most synapses in the peripheral and central nervous systems, a chemical mediator is released which interacts with some component of the post-synaptic cell, and thereby initiates the cellular response. The concept that specific "receptive substances" must exist (see Langley, 1907) preceded the first conclusive demonstration of a neurotransmitter (acetylcholine, ACh; Loewi, 1921).

"Receptors" have always been defined operationally in terms of the cellular responses which are initiated when a neurotransmitter interacts with a cell. Once a tissue has been homogenized or otherwise disrupted, its physiological responses are no longer present; thus, the first problem encountered in dealing with the isolation of receptors is to find a suitable and specific *in vitro* assay for them. A complication arises from the fact that receptors are not the only tissue constituents which have affinity for neurotransmitters. In the case of the adrenergic transmitter noradrenaline, there are, in addition to the receptor, two uptake sites, and at least two enzymes which have affinity for the transmitter (*cf.* Molinoff and Axelrod, 1971). In the case of the cholinergic transmitter ACh, the situation is similar. The enzyme acetylcholinesterase is situated at synapses near the receptor, both in muscle (Barrnett, 1962) and in the electric organ of the eel (Massoulie,

111

Reiger, and Tsuji, 1970). Thus, in any attempt to assay for the presence of receptors by interacting them with an agonist or antagonist which seems to have pharmacological specificity, the possibility exists that any one of several proteins will be "seen" by the compound used.

A problem encountered in defining a receptor biochemically is how to decide exactly what should be included in the term. In general, receptor-transmitter interactions lead to a change in the permeability of the post-synaptic membrane to one or several ions. This is the case at vertebrate neuromuscular junctions (Fatt and Katz, 1951) and may also be true for responses mediated through adenyl cyclase (Robison, Butcher, and Sutherland, 1970) which appear to be coupled via an ionophore (Rasmussen, 1970). An adrenergic "receptor" which functions through the activation of adenyl cyclase might be taken to include the specific molecule which interacts with noradrenaline (discriminator), the adenyl cylcase itself (catalytic site), and perhaps one or more molecules involved in translating the activation of the receptor into an increase in cyclase activity (Birnbaumer, Pohl, and Rodbell, 1971). It has been claimed that adenyl cyclase is the adrenergic receptor (see Robison et al., 1970), but it now appears likely that it is separated from the molecule which contains the transmitter recognition site by one or more intermediate molecules. For the purposes of this discussion, the term "receptor" will be used to signify that molecule which itself interacts with the neurotransmitter. The possibility remains, of course, that this molecule may also function as an ion carrier.

RECEPTOR PROPERTIES

Pharmacological Specificity

Receptors are usually classified according to their pharmacological properties. The broad class of cholinergic receptors is subdivided into muscarinic and nicotinic receptors, and for each of these sub-groups a number of specific agonists and antagonists have been described. Curare is a potent blocking agent of nicotinic receptors at neuromuscular junctions, and it also blocks the effect of ACh on *Torpedo* electroplaques (*cf*. Miledi, Molinoff, and Potter, 1971*a*). The fact that many different types of receptor (defined either pharmacologically or in terms of their physiological response) exist for a given transmitter increases the flexibility of chemical neurotransmission, in that a single transmitter can perform different functions (*cf*.

Axelsson, 1971). A good example of this phenomenon comes from work with *Aplysia*, where it has been shown that ACh, released from two branches of the same neuron, is excitatory at one synapse and inhibitory at another (Kandel, Frazier, and Coggeshall, 1967).

The degree of pharmacological specificity possessed by receptors is very great. A given receptor is able to distinguish not only between different excitatory and inhibitory transmitters, but between different isomeric forms of one transmitter. This ability to recognize small molecules with great precision is reminiscent of the behavior of enzymes and has suggested to many workers that receptors might be proteins or proteolipids.

Anatomical Location

It is a reasonable assumption that all neuroreceptors are membrane bound. Most neurotransmitters are ions which would not be expected to diffuse across cell membranes with sufficient speed to account for the physiological effects observed. Muscle cells respond to ACh when it is applied iontophoretically to the outside of the cells, but not if it is applied on the inside of the cell (del Castillo and Katz, 1955). Thus, their receptors appear to be components of the membrane which face the extracellular space. That ACh receptors are membrane bound has been further demonstrated by the observation that the permeability of isolated microsacs to sodium is increased by cholinergic agonists (Kasai and Changeux, 1970). Similarly, the receptors for epinephrine and other hormones are on the membranes of adipose (Birnbaumer and Rodbell, 1970), and liver cells, (Pohl, Birnbaumer, and Rodbell, 1971). The receptor from *Torpedo* electric organ whose partial characterization is described in this chapter is a membrane protein.

In most cases, the location of receptors has been established by the local application of ACh onto specific regions of a sensitive cell. The responsiveness of skeletal muscle, for example, is sharply localized to the region of neuromuscular endplates (Thesleff, 1970), with a smaller amount of sensitivity at the myo-tendon junction (Katz and Miledi, 1964). When skeletal muscles are denervated, the sensitive region spreads (Miledi, 1962) to cover the entire cell. The distribution of receptors, both in normal and denervated muscles, has been confirmed by the use of radioactive ACh antagonists (Lee, Tseng, and Chiu, 1967; Waser, 1970; Miledi and Potter, 1971). A similar focal distribution of sensitivity has been observed at synapses in parasympathetic ganglia (Harris, Kuffler, and Dennis, 1971).

Number of Receptors

The use of radioactively labeled α-bungarotoxin has permitted an estimate of the number of receptors per gram of tissue in *Torpedo* electric tissue (6.6×10^{14}; Miledi et al., 1971a) and per endplate for mouse, rat, and frog muscle (16, 47, and 1,000 million, respectively; Miledi and Potter, 1971). This number is considerably larger than the number of molecules of ACh released by a single nerve impulse (about 3 million in the rat diaphragm; *cf.* Potter, 1970), which is sufficient to depolarize muscle cells. This is consistent with pharmacological evidence that maximal responses of a cell can be produced even when most of its receptors are blocked by an irreversible antagonist (Paton, 1970), and supports the concept that there are many "spare receptors."

The number of receptors is increased up to 20-fold on denervation (Miledi and Potter, 1971), with the increase roughly paralleling the increase in sensitivity to applied ACh (Miledi, 1962). The increase in sensitivity can be prevented by direct electrical stimulation of the muscles (Lømo and Rosenthal, 1972). This suggests that long-term alterations in synaptic efficiency may derive from changes in the number, location, and/or density of receptors. At a higher level of organization, these changes could subserve learning.

Chemical Composition of Receptors

Since the discovery of chemical transmission, it has been apparent that there are molecules with the capacity to recognize and interact with neurotransmitters. The fact that receptors are affected by small molecules suggested that they might, by analogy to enzymes, be proteins (or proteolipids). Support for this hypothesis has come from several sources. (1) Karlin and his collaborators have shown that the ACh receptors of eel electroplaques can be blocked by reagents which reduce S-S bonds to S-H groups and that responsiveness can be restored by the use of oxidizing agents (Karlin, Prives, Deal, and Winnick, 1970). (2) Receptor interactions, measured *in vitro* by equilibrium dialysis, are decreased by proteases (Lee, 1957; Eldefrawi, Eldefrawi, and O'Brien, 1971). (3) A number of different analogs of cholinergic agonists and antagonists have been shown to bind to proteins (Changeux, Kasai, Huchet, and Meunier, 1970; Elde frawi et al., 1971) and to proteolipids (de Robertis, Lunt, and la Torre, 1971). (4) The material whose partial purification is described in this chapter appears to be a lipoprotein or protein.

ISOLATION OF RECEPTOR PROTEINS

The Problem of Specificity

Many attempts have been made to isolate molecules having the receptor site for a neurotransmitter. The major problem has been with regard to the specificity of the agent used to assay the receptor. In several cases there has been far more nonspecific than specific binding [atropine on heart tissue (Clark, 1926), curare on electric tissue (Ehrenpreis, Fleisch, and Mittag, 1969)]. Others have had similar problems using irreversible agents. Takagi and Takahashi (1968) used tritated dibenamine on the isolated muscle strip of the dog small intestine. Even when atropine was used to protect cholinergic receptors during a preliminary treatment with unlabeled dibenamine, the radioactive compound was found to be irreversibly bound to components of all seven protein fractions which were isolated.

Attempts to improve the specificity of labeling reactions have been made in which the alkylating or arylating agent had a high degree of intrinsic affinity for the receptor being studied. For example, p-(trimethylammonium) benzene-diazonium-fluoroborate (Tdf) is a structural analog of phenyltrimethylammonium, which is a potent ACh receptor agonist. Tdf has a reactive diazonum group which forms a covalent bond with the amino acids tyrosine, histidine, and lysine. When an isolated electroplaque was exposed to Tdf, the cell became insensitive to receptor activators (Changeux, Podleski, and Wofsy, 1967). A high concentration of Tdf (10^{-4} M) was required, however, which suggests that much of the agent was bound to nonspecific sites.

Another attempt to label receptors with irreversible affinity labels has been made by Kiefer, Lennox, and Singer (1970), who used photoreactive arylazides (c.f. Singer, 1970). The specificity of these reactions, however, remains to be established. More success with regard to specificity has been achieved by Karlin and his collaborators (Karlin and Bartels, 1966), who have shown that the response of electroplaques to ACh is blocked by the disulfide reducing agent dithiothreitol. This inhibition can be reversed by oxidizing agents or can be made permanent by the use of thiol alkylating agents. Compounds have been synthesized (e.g., 4 maleimidobenzyltrimethylammonium iodide, MBTA) which are affinity labels for reduced receptors (Karlin and Winnik, 1969; Karlin et al., 1970). The binding of MBTA was prevented if the reduced receptors were treated with the affinity oxidizing agent cholinedisulfide, and was considerably decreased when MBTA was added in the presence of hexamethonium. The use of these affinity reagents in sequence, has enabled Karlin et al. (1970) to calculate that there are 26 to 75 $\times$ 10^{-14} moles of receptor per electroplaque cell. This value is similar to the calculated amount of acetylcholinesterase in the cell.

Successful Approaches Using Reversible Agents

It has been suggested that it might be difficult, if not impossible, to isolate receptors without a specific and irreversible receptor label (see discussions in CIBA Symposium, 1970). However, many interesting studies have been carried out with agents which are reversible and which lack the specificity of α-bungarotoxin. For example, Paton and Rang (1965) applied atropine to the abundant muscarinic receptors of gut smooth muscle, and, despite more nonspecific than specific binding, it was possible to correlate the kinetics of binding with receptor blockade. Apparent success has also been achieved with curarine on the cholinergic receptors of the mouse diaphragm (Waser, 1970). The number of curarine molecules bound per endplate was not more than 3 $\times$ 10^6, even at relatively high doses of curarine. This number is somewhat less than the number of α-toxin binding sites (16 million per endplate in the same tissue; Miledi and Potter, 1971).

Comprehensive experiments with membrane fragments and reversible binding agents have been carried out by O'Brien and his co-workers (O'Brien and Gilmour, 1969; Eldefrawi et al., 1971) who have studied the binding of radioactive muscarone, nicotine, decamethonium, dimethyl d-tubocurarine, and atropine to subcellular preparations of Torpedo electroplaques and house-fly brain. Using equilibrium dialysis, it was possible to determine the binding constants for each ligand and the amount bound to each binding site. Binding constants of the order of 1 μM were found. The binding to Torpedo tissue was reduced by trypsin, chymotrypsin, and phospholipase C; binding of the house-fly brain was reduced only by the proteases. This suggests that the former receptor may be a proteolipid, while the latter is a protein. In recent work by Eldefrawi and O'Brien (1971), it was found that binding of ACh itself was autoinhibitory at concentration above 1 μM. The suggestion was made that this result represented the molecular mechanism for desensitization. The amount of muscarone bound to *Torpedo* tissue (10^{-9} moles, or 6×10^{14} molecules per g) (Eldefrawi et al., 1971) is nearly the same as the amount of toxin bound in the same tissue (6.6×10^{14} molecules per g; Miledi et al., 1971*a*).

Evidence that reversible agonists and antagonists are useful for the study of "soluble" neuroreceptors has also been obtained by Changeux and his co-workers (1970). Membrane proteins from the electric tissue of *Electrophorus* were dispersed with the detergent desoxycholate, and receptors were assayed by measuring the binding of labeled decamethonium. The affinity constants for several antagonists were similar to those found with intact electroplaque preparations. Evidence that much of the binding of the decamethonium was to receptors came from the fact that α-bungarotoxin blocked a large fraction of the binding sites. It is interesting that decamethonium binds both to the receptor and to acetylcholinesterase. The binding to the esterase was prevented, however, by flaxedil.

Other experiments using reversible agonists for receptor identification have been carried out by de Robertis and his collaborators, using brain tissue (De Robertis, Fiszer, and Suta, 1967; Fiszer and De Robertis, 1970), and electric tissue from *Torpedo* and *Electrophorus* (la Torre, Lunt, and De Robertis, 1970; De Robertis, 1971). In many of their experiments, proteolipids were isolated which had a high affinity for one or another transmitter (or transmitter analog). These experiments were carried out in relatively nonionic media or in nonpolar solvents, and, under these conditions, compounds such as ACh, methylhexamethonium, and dimethyltubocurarine, as well as adrenergic blocking agents and serotonin, were bound irreversibly. Since these compounds normally act reversibly, it has not been possible to determine affinity constants. Extensive efforts have been made, without success, to return material extracted into chloroform-methanol to an aqueous medium. If this could be done, it might be possible to determine by conventional means if the extracts actually contained receptors.

Successful Approaches Using Irreversible Agents

The compound benzilylcholine mustard (BCM) was found to be a long-lasting inhibitor of muscarinic receptors, which suggested that it would be a useful label for these receptors (Gill and Rang, 1966; Rang, 1967). The compound has a high affinity for these receptors, forming a complex which is initially reversible. Alkylation occurs rapidly, however, and the receptors are thus labeled covalently. When strips of guinea pig ileum were exposed to ^{3}H-BCM (2×10^{-9} M), there was about a 95% receptor blockage. More than two-thirds of the binding was blocked in the presence of 30 nM atropine. After solubilization of muscle proteins with 1% sodium dodecyl sulfate, polyacrylamide gel electrophoresis revealed peaks of labeled protein with apparent molecular weights of 23 and 50 thousand, plus a variable amount of material which was too large to enter the gel (Fewtrell and Rang, *in press*). It is probable that the membrane protein which binds BCM is largely muscarinic receptors.

The α-toxins of *Bungarus multicinctus* (Chang and Lee, 1963) and *Naja nigricollis* (Boquet, Izard, Jounnet and Meaume, 1966) are irreversible inhibitors of cholinergic receptors which have recently come into extensive use. These toxins have been used to study the cholinergic receptors of *Torpedo* (Miledi et al., 1971*a*; Potter and Molinoff, *in press*) and *Electrophorus* electric tissue (Changeux, Kasai, and Lee, 1970; Meunier, Olsen, Menex, Morgat, Fromageot, Ronseray, Boquet, and Changeux, 1971), and of skeletal muscle (Miledi and Potter, 1971; Berg, Kelly, Sargent, Williamson, and Hall, 1972). The results of experiments in which α-bungarotoxin was used to purify the cholinergic receptor protein from *Torpedo* electric tissue are reported below. In general, it can be said that this toxin binds specifically and irreversibly to those nicotinic receptors which are blocked by curarine. Binding to *Torpedo* and *Electrophorus* membranes is antagonized by cholinergic agonists and antagonists, and preliminary purification of the receptor from both sources has been carried out. The behavior of the toxin-labeled receptor(s) on molecular sieves, in the centrifuge, and, in the case of the *Torpedo* receptor, on ion-exchange resins has been studied.

STUDIES OF THE CHOLINERGIC RECEPTOR OF *TORPEDO* ELECTRIC TISSUE

Torpedo Marmorata

The electric organs of these bottom-feeding elasmobranchs (skates) are embryologically similar to skeletal muscle. The organs are relatively large, making up about 25% of the body weight of the fish, which vary from about 5 cm across to more than a meter in diameter. The fish are readily caught in nets in shallow coastal bays, in the Mediterranean basin and on both sides of the Atlantic. Their electric output (only 20 to 60 V, but up to 50 amp in a large fish) is probably used to stun shrimp and other food. The small fish used in these experiments, less than 30 cm in diameter, are relatively easy to handle and are not capable of producing dangerous shocks. Their ready availability and ability to survive in cold sea water without feeding for many weeks makes them a convenient starting material from which to purify nicotinic receptors.

Each electric organ consists of about 500 stacks or columns of cells which run from dorsal to ventral skin. Through the ventral skin, the hexagonal borders of the individual stacks can be seen. Each column consists of hundreds to thousands of thin flat cells (5 to 10 μm in thickness and 1 to 10 mm in diameter). Each cell is innervated over most of its ventral surface (Sheridan, 1965; Nickel and Potter, 1970) by cholinergic nerve terminals (Feldberg and Fessard, 1942; Israel, 1970). The ventral membrane is only excitable chemically (Bennett, 1961) in contrast to the less densely innervated membrane of *Electrophorus*, which is excitable both chemically and electrically. The dorsal non-innervated membrane of *Torpedo* is morphologically distinguishable from the innervated membrane by the presence of large numbers of tubular infoldings.

Alpha-Bungarotoxin

The venom of the Formosan krait (*Bungarus multicinctus*) has components which are active both pre- and postsynaptically. The curare-like action of this venom was first analyzed in detail by Chang (1960). The crude venom was then separated into four fractions by starch block electrophoresis (Chang and Lee, 1963, 1966). One, called α-bungarotoxin, made up 61% of the total protein. Its curare-like effects on neuromuscular transmission were similar to those of cobra α-neurotoxin and included depression of endplate potentials, without any effect on resting potentials, muscle action potentials, or terminal nerve spikes. The effect of α-toxin, which was prevented by *d*-tubocurarine, was irreversible. Using toxin labeled with ^{131}I, Lee et al. (1967) showed by radioautography that neurotoxin accumulates on the motor endplate of the mouse diaphragm. After cutting the phrenic nerve, the radioactivity was observed over most of the denervated muscle.

To obtain the pure α-toxin used in these experiments, several grams of dried venom was subjected to chromatography on Sephadex G-50 fine, and then Sephadex CM-25 at pH 7.5 (Miledi and Potter, *unpublished*). Twelve pure proteins were obtained, including four which blocked the action of ACh at neuromuscular junctions in the frog sartorius, and six which blocked release of ACh from the motor nerves. One of the two remaining proteins was acetylcholinesterase and one was physiologically inactive at these junctions. Although the major component which was active postsynaptically made up only 20 to 25% of the protein in the venom, it had the properties described for α-bungarotoxin (Chang and Lee, 1963), and was so designated. It gives a single band by polyacrylamide gel electrophoresis, with or without pretreatment with 1% sodium dodecyl sulfate and 1% β-merceptoethanol. Its molecular weight, as estimated by molecular sieving, and by gel electrophoresis is 8,000. The amino acid sequence of pure α-toxin has recently been determined (Mebs, Karita, Iwanaga, Samejuma, and Lee, 1971). It has 74 amino acid residues, including 10 half-cystines. Approximately 50% of the residues are homologous to those of the α-neurotoxin of *Naja nivea*.

Alpha-bungarotoxin has been labeled with carrier-free ^{131}I of the highest available specific activity, using nitrite as an oxidizing agent (Pressman and Eisen, 1950). The labeled protein, after separation from unreacted iodine on a column of Sephadex G-25, has an initial specific activity of about 23 C per mmole. Even maximal iodination has no effect on the potency of the toxin.

Binding of α-Toxin to Membranes

When homogenates of fresh or frozen electric tissue are made in isotonic or hypotonic media, some of the membrane fragments produced are capable of binding ^{131}I-α-toxin. Over 90% of the toxin-labeled membranes and of the cholinesterase can be sedimented in 10 min at 20,000 × g. With subsaturating amounts of toxin, at least 80% of the toxin added will become bound to large molecular weight proteins (Miledi et al., 1971a; Potter and Molinoff, *in press*). The binding of toxin to these membrane fragments is a time-dependent process, which is inhibited by curare and carbachol. The degree of inhibition of binding by these agents is similar with a crude membrane fraction and with detergent-dispersed membrane proteins. The membranes from 1 g of electric tissue can bind, at saturation, 7.43 μg of toxin. We have calculated that a gram of tissue has 6.6×10^{14} binding sites, and that, taking into account the molecular weight of acetylcholinesterase, the number of active sites per molecule and its turnover number, there are 6.3×10^{14} active sites per gram of tissue (Miledi et al., 1971a).

Isolation of Receptor-Rich Membrane Fragments

The isolation procedure is summarized in Table 1. ^{131}I-α-toxin is added to an initial homogenate of electric tissue in 0.4 M NaCl. After the receptor is labeled, the membranes are sedimented by centrifugation. Soluble proteins are discarded, and the membrane pellet is sonicated in dilute buffer.

TABLE 1. *Purification schema used for the preparation of dispersed membrane proteins from Torpedo electric tissue*

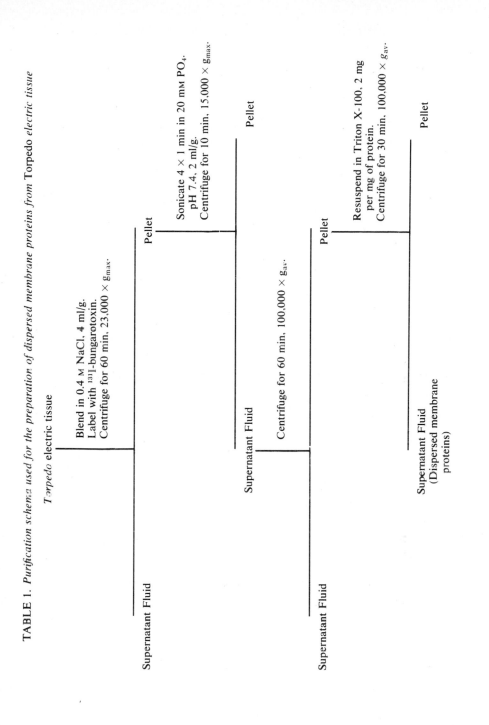

Torpedo electric tissue

Blend in 0.4 M NaCl, 4 ml/g.
Label with ^{131}I-bungarotoxin.
Centrifuge for 60 min. 23,000 × g_{max}.

Supernatant Fluid

Pellet

Sonicate 4 × 1 min in 20 mM PO$_4$.
pH 7.4, 2 ml/g.
Centrifuge for 10 min, 15,000 × g_{max}.

Supernatant Fluid

Pellet

Centrifuge for 60 min, 100,000 × g_{av}.

Supernatant Fluid

Pellet

Resuspend in Triton X-100, 2 mg
per mg of protein.
Centrifuge for 30 min, 100,000 × g_{av}.

Supernatant Fluid
(Dispersed membrane
proteins)

Pellet

The rationale for this procedure is to prepare the initial homogenate in salt to try to solubilize as much protein as possible, while sonication is done in hypotonic media to disrupt maximally membrane structures. In several experiments, the sonicated material has been fractionated on linear sucrose density gradients (10 to 50%, w/w; Potter and Molinoff, 1972). Most of the radioactivity is associated with a band of particles isodense with 37% sucrose; electron microscopy of this fraction shows small vesicles and membrane fragments. A small percentage of the radioactivity is seen along with about 75% of the protein in a band at 42% sucrose; this fraction contains recognizable pieces of dorsal cell membrane. There is usually no radioactivity associated with an intermediate band of mitochondria, or with less dense bands of myelin and microsomes. Since the percentage of radioactivity found in the fastest moving peak decreases with the duration of sonication, we believe that the radioactivity of this fraction is trapped with pieces of dorsal, and perhaps other, membrane particles. This experiment is important in that it shows that there are at least five subcellular fractions which do not bind significant amounts of toxin.

A surprising result in these experiments was the localization of acetylcholinesterase. We expected to find this enzyme associated with the same membrane fraction as the radioactive toxin. Eighty percent of the enzyme was found, however, with the bulk of the membrane proteins at 42% sucrose despite several attempts to minimize redistribution of either the enzyme or the receptor. Although redistribution of the receptor or the esterase cannot be excluded, we are coming to the conclusion that the receptor is on a different piece of membrane than is acetylcholinesterase, in the *Torpedo*. In the electric eel, the esterase and toxin-binding material are on the same surface of the electroplaque cell (Bourgeois, Tsuji, Boquet, Pillot, Ryter, and Changeux, 1971). Further, when a homogenate of electric organ from the eel is spun into a density gradient, esterase-containing membranes are well separated from ATPase-containing membranes (Bauman, Changeux, and Benda, 1970), and it is the esterase-rich membrane fraction which contains the receptors (Changeux, Kasai, Huchet, and Meunier, 1970).

After sonication of the membrane suspension, microsomes are collected by differential centrifugation. When these microsomes were subjected to density-gradient centrifugation, the large peak toward the bottom of the gradient was absent, while the particle peak associated with the labeled toxin was unchanged. It thus appears that sonication of *Torpedo* membranes generates microsomes which are smaller or less dense than fragments produced from other membranes of the tissue. Isolation of these artifactual microsomes, produced by sonication, results in a major purification of the receptor.

Solubilization of Toxin-Labeled Protein

Several different means of dissolving toxin-tagged receptors from the partially purified membranes were investigated (Potter and Molinoff, 1972). Sonication in dilute buffer did not remove any of the radioactive label. Treatment of the material with 2 M NaCl removed a small (1 to 2%) amount of the toxin, whereas treatment with high concentrations of NaBr, NaI, urea, or sodium dodecyl sulfate (SDS) partially or fully disassociated the toxin from its binding sites. Treatment with NaI, urea, or SDS prevented subsequent binding of toxin to the receptor, even after the agent in question was removed by dialysis or passage through a Sephadex G-25 column. Of the procedures we tried, the most success has been achieved with Triton X-100. The sedimented microsomes are resuspended by brief sonication, and then 2 mg of Triton is added per mg of protein. After 30 min at 4°C, this suspension is ultracentrifuged, and the pellet, which contains about one-third of the protein but only 10% of the radioactivity, is discarded.

Attempts to Solubilize with Chloroform-Methanol

After mechanical blending of labeled membranes with chloroform-methanol (two phase suspension), most of the protein and ^{131}I were found at the interface, and none was in the organic phase. Several experiments were carried out with freeze-dried membranes, using methods described by la Torre et al. (1970). In the first of these experiments, toxin-labeled membranes were lyophilized and then blended with chloroform-methanol (2:1). After low-speed centrifugation (500 × g for 5 min), less than 10% of the radioactivity was in the supernatant fluid. In another experiment, toxin-labeled membranes were lyophilized to dryness and then blended in chloroform-methanol. The total contents of the tube were dried under reduced pressure and then the residue was taken up in Triton X-100 (1.5% in buffer). Most (79%) of the radioactivity was sedimented by low-speed centrifugation, although nearly all of the toxin-receptor was solubilized by this procedure in the absence of pretreatment with chloroform-methanol. An aliquot of the supernatant fluid which contained 21% of the original radioactivity was run through a small column of Sephadex G-50 to see whether the radioactive toxin was associated with protein or was free in solution. All of the toxin in the supernatant fluid was retarded on the column, as is free toxin.

It was concluded that treatment of labeled membranes with chloroform-methanol denatures the toxin-binding material and results in the liberation of some (10 to 20%) of the toxin. It is possible, however, that the binding of toxin to the receptor alters its properties such that it cannot be extracted into chloroform-methanol. To investigate this possibility, 5 g of frozen tissue was homogenized in 50 ml of water in a blender for three 1-min periods. The homogenate was then frozen and lyophilized to dryness overnight. The powder obtained from 1 g of tissue was blended with 15 ml of chloroform-methanol (2:1, v/v), following the procedure of de Robertis et al. (1971). The total contents of the tube, which must have included the receptor, was then dried under vacuum. After dissolving the residue in Triton, ^{131}I-α-toxin was added. An aliquot was chromatographed on a column of Sephadex-G-50. All of the radioactivity was retarded on the column, as was free α-toxin run in control experiments. When tissue was carried through the procedure described above, except for exposure to chloroform-methanol, all of the radioactivity was associated with a large molecular weight substance, so that it came out in the void volume (determined in each run with Dextran Blue–2000). These experiments suggest that, at least as far as toxin binding is concerned, the receptor is denatured by treatment with chloroform-methanol. It is still possible, as claimed by De Robertis, that the receptor is able to bind ACh, after being exposed to chloroform-methanol.

Molecular Sieving of the Toxin-Binding Material

When Triton-dispersed membrane proteins, labeled with radioactive toxin, were subjected to molecular sieving on Sepharose 6B, about half of the radioactivity was found in the void volume, while the rest was retarded by the column and eluted in a broad peak. The radioactivity was thus associated with material which varied in apparent molecular weight from over a million down to the approximate size (assuming a globular shape) of acetylcholinesterase (260,000; Millar and Grafius, 1970). This indicates that treatment with Triton does not produce monodisperse receptor-toxin complex. The facts that the esterase ran on Separose as a single narrow peak and that this peak was in the expected position for a globular protein of molecular weight 260,000 indicated that cholinesterase was soluble and monodisperse under these conditions.

The elution profiles in Triton show that the receptor and the enzyme acetylcholinesterase are entirely separate molecules (Miledi et al., 1971a; Meunier et al., 1971). This is consistent with the fact that they were found on different membrane fragments as discussed above, and with the fact that the two proteins can be separated by ultracentrifugation. A second conclusion which was drawn from these studies was that the protein to which the α-toxin is bound is larger than many of the other proteins in the preparation. This conclusion was supported by experiments in which samples of Triton-dispersed protein were subjected to prolonged centrifugation in 20 mM phosphate buffer. After 10 hr of centrifugation, 91% of the receptor, but only 48% of the protein, had sedimented. These results indicate that the complex is larger and/or more dense than much of the membrane protein.

In an attempt to disrupt salt linkages, and hopefully to obtain a homogeneous preparation of toxin-receptor complex, increasing amounts of NaCl were added to the Triton-solubilized protein, and the material was chromatographed on a column of Sepharose 6B. As the salt concentration was increased, the peak of protein and labeled receptor in the void volume disappeared, and both were eluted in a peak almost coincident with that of acetylcholinesterase (mol. wt. 260,000; Fig. 1A). It can be seen that in the presence of a high concentration of salt the peak of protein and of radioactivity were nearly superimposed on that of the esterase, although the slightly increased width of the radioactive peak still suggested some heterogeneity.

No significant purification of the receptor was obtained on Sepharose either before treatment with or in the presence of salt. However, when Triton-dispersed proteins were exposed to a high concentration of salt and then the salt was removed (Fig. 1B), a two- to threefold purification resulted from molecular sieving on Sepharose 6B. Under these conditions, both protein and radioactivity were eluted from Sepharose in a pattern which was distinctly different from that seen before salt treatment, or in the presence of salt (Fig. 1A). Approximately 40% of the protein was in the void volume while another 20 to 25% ran as if it were smaller than the receptor. Standardization of the Sepharose column with Dextran Blue 2000, β-galactosidase, catalase, and free ^{131}I-α-toxin indicated that the receptor-toxin complex in the post-salt state behaved as would a globular protein with a molecular weight about 400,000.

It is likely that the toxin-receptor complex is composed of sub-units. The results of preliminary experiments with polyacrylamide gel electrophoresis (Meunier et al., 1971) suggest that a labeled sub-unit exists of molecular weight about 50,000 Daltons. These experiments, however, included treatment with SDS, which removes most of the toxin from the receptor protein. We originally reported that, after addition of cold 0.5% SDS to Triton-dispersed material, a small amount of radioactivity was eluted from Sephadex G-200 in a position that would correspond to that of a globular protein of molecular weight 88,000, and we suggested that this smaller peak might represent a subcomponent of the receptor polymer (Miledi et al.,

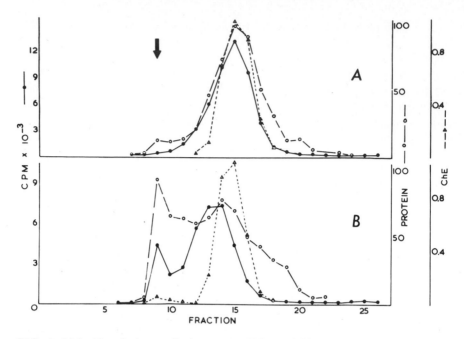

FIG. 1. Molecular sieving on Sepharose 6B. Triton-solubilized labeled membrane proteins were exposed to 2.0 M NaCl for 12 hr. Part of this material (1 ml corresponding to about 5 g of original tissue) was layered onto a 1 × 50 cm column of Sepharose 6B (1-ml fractions were collected). The column was equilibrated with buffer containing 1.5% Triton with (*A*) and without (*B*) 1.0 M NaCl. The void volume (arrow) was determined with Dextran Blue 2000 included in each sample. Radioactivity is in cpm/50 μl, protein in μg per 400 μl, cholinesterase (ChE) as the change in OD$_{412}$ per min when a 20 μl sample was incubated with 2.5 ml of 1 mM acetylthiocholine iodide, 1 mM dithionitrobenzoate in 100 mM phosphate buffer.

1971*a*). Further experiments showed that α-toxin behaves anomalously on Sephadex in the presence of SDS, and it is probable that this small peak represented α-toxin which had been dissociated from the receptor by SDS. After treatment of toxin-labeled membranes with 1% SDS at 37°C for 15 min or longer, with or without Triton and β-mercaptoethanol, most of the radioactivity was eluted from Sephadex G-200 in this anomalous position for α-toxin.

Ultracentrifugation of the Toxin-Receptor Complex

Molecular sieving on Sepharose separates molecules on the basis of their diffusion into the gel beads, i.e., on the apparent Stokes radii of the protein molecules. Ultracentrifugation affords further information about the size (as well as the shape and density) of protein molecules, but, because the molecules tumble during centrifugation, their rate of movement is inversely proportional to their maximum rather than minimum diameter. When a sample of Triton-dispersed material was subjected to centrifugation, the labeled protein(s) had a higher sedimentation rate than did most of the remaining proteins.

The sedimentation properties of the labeled receptor were compared before treatment of the material with NaCl (Fig. 2A), in the presence of salt (Fig. 2C), and after the salt had been removed by dialysis (Fig. 2B). The gradients used were designed to cover the same range of densities, and, as expected, acetylcholinesterase was found in approximately the same position after centrifugation in all three gradients. In contrast to the results on Sepharose, the behavior of the radioactively labeled material was the same after being exposed to salt (Fig. 2B) as it was before such exposure (Fig. 2A). However, the sedimentation rate of the toxin-receptor complex was greater in the presence of salt than either before or after salt treatment. The increase in the sedimentation velocity of the toxin receptor complex in the presence of NaCl (compare Fig. 2B and C) indicates that the complex has aggregated with other protein, has become more dense, or has a smaller overall diameter, than material which has not been exposed to salt or which has been pretreated with salt and then dialyzed free of salt.

In the three gradients depicted in Fig. 2, the labeled protein moved in two major peaks. In other experiments, we have observed only a single major peak (*cf.* Miledi et al., 1971*a*) or a central peak with shoulders on one or on both sides. These multiple peaks demonstrate heterogeneity in the size and/or density of toxin-receptor complexes. In all cases where the centrifugation has been carried out in media of low ionic strength (Fig. 2A and C), the labeled protein peaks have appeared between those of acetylcholinesterase (mol. wt. 260,000) and of β-galactosidase (mol. wt. 540,000), and the central or major peak has moved as would a globular protein having a molecular weight of approximately 400,000 (Sw, 20° of the major peak in Fig. 2B is 13.8).

Ion-Exchange Chromatography

In 20 mM sodium phosphate buffer containing 1.5% Triton X-100, most of the soluble protein and all of the labeled protein was adsorbed to DEAE-Sephadex by anion exchange at and above pH 6.4, and to CM-Sephadex by cation exchange below pH 5. The toxin-receptor complex,

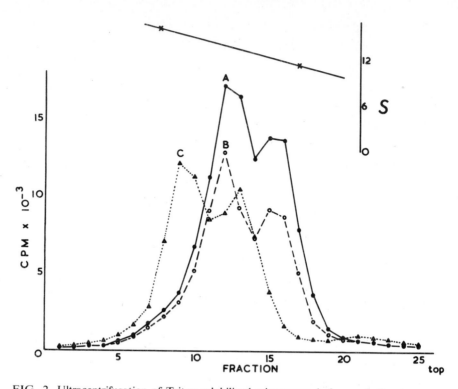

FIG. 2. Ultracentrifugation of Triton-solubilized microsomes before and after treatment with salt, and in the presence of salt. Linear gradients were prepared that covered the same range of densities (15 to 24% sucrose, w/w for *A* and *B* and 5 to 14% sucrose plus 1 M NaCl for *C*). A sample of 0.4 ml of Triton-solubilized membrane proteins was layered onto each gradient. Those for *A* had undergone no prior treatment, while those in *B* and *C* had been exposed to 2.0 M salt prior to centrifugation. The sample in *B* was dialyzed free of salt before being applied to the gradient. All samples were diluted 1:1 with 20 mM phosphate buffer, containing 1.0% Triton before being layered on the gradients. The sucrose solutions contained 1.0% Triton and 20 mM buffer. Radioactivity is in cpm per 50 μl. The Sw, 20° for β-galactosidase activity (determined by measuring the change in absorbance at 420 nm/min when 50 μl of the gradient was added to 2.5 ml o-nitrophenyl-β-D-galacto-pyranoside in 100 mM sodium phosphate buffer, pH 7.5) and cholinesterase (as in Fig. 1) are taken as 16.0 and 11.3, respectively. The peak of cholinesterase activity was in tube 17 in all gradients. β-galactosidase activity was maximal in tube 8 in the absence of salt (*A* and *B*) and in tube 2 in the presence of salt (*C*).

after treatment with 2 M salt, and passage over a Sepharose 6B column in the absence of salt, was tightly bound to a column of DEAE-Sephadex at pH 6.6. When gradient elution was performed with an increasing concentration of NaCl, the labeled material was eluted as a single peak between 0.2 and 0.4 M salt. This procedure yielded a further twofold purification.

Similar results were also obtained with material that had not been exposed to salt or passed over a column of Sepharose (Potter and Molinoff, 1971).

CONCLUSIONS

The α-toxin prepared from the venom of *Bungarus multicinctus* appears to bind specifically and (for practical purposes) irreversibly to cholinergic receptors of skeletal muscles and electric organs. The binding of α-bungarotoxin occurs at the endplates of skeletal muscles (Lee et al., 1967; Miledi and Potter, 1971; Barnard, Wieckowski, and Chiu, 1972), and the binding of the α-toxin of *Naja* occurs at the innervated surface of *Electrophorus* (Bourgeois et al., 1971). Further evidence of the specificity of the interaction comes from the finding that neither release of endogenous ACh, nor the electrical properties of the postsynaptic cell are affected by the presence of toxin. In addition to this physiological and anatomical specificity, we have shown that the binding of toxin to both membrane fragments and to detergent-dispersed material can be inhibited by the cholinergic ligands curare and carbachol.

The above considerations show that nicotinic receptors are labeled by the toxin. The question remains, however, whether the toxin labels other proteins as well. There is evidence from work with muscles (Miledi and Potter, 1971; Berg, Kelly, Sargent, Williamson, and Hall, 1972) that about 15% of the toxin is bound nonspecifically. We have not been able to determine conclusively the biochemical specificity of the toxin-receptor complex of *Torpedo*. Most of the techniques which have been used, including ultracentrifugation and chromatography on Sepharose 6B, both before and after treatment of the proteins with salt, routinely yield more than one peak of radioactivity. On the other hand, only a single ionic species is seen on DEAE-Sephadex chromatography. It is necessary to determine whether the several peaks in the ultracentrifuge and on Sepharose represent aggregates of similar or different subcomponents, or of pieces of incompletely dispersed membrane material. It is known that a particulate preparation from *Torpedo* electroplaque binds ACh reversibly and with high affinity at two sites (Eldefrawi and O'Brien, 1971). Moreover, only half of the toxin-binding sites in frog muscle appear to be protected by curare (Miledi and Potter, 1971). It is possible that there are two or more kinds of sites which can bind α-toxin, and that we are seeing a partial separation of these sites.

It is difficult to know how to relate the properties of the partially purified receptor to those of the receptor *in vivo*. This is a problem with most membrane proteins, but it is a particularly difficult question in this case, since some of the procedures used, including in particular treatment with salt, cause irreversible changes in some of the properties of the receptor-toxin complex. It appears likely that the receptor is assuming a rod-like configuration after exposure to Triton, but we cannot be certain of its native size, shape, or state of aggregation.

Before treatment of the material with salt, most of the toxin-binding material behaved on Sepharose as would globular proteins of molecular weight ranging from about 500 thousand to 2 million. In the ultracentrifuge, on the other hand, the Triton-solubilized material had a sedimentation rate between those of acetylcholinesterase and β-galactosidase. The two most likely explanations for this difference are that the toxin-binding material has a large lipid content (which would decrease its density), or a high axial ratio (which would increase its Stokes radius). In the presence of salt, the sedimentation rate increases while the Stokes radius decreases. After the salt has been removed, the sedimentation coefficient is the same as it was before salt treatment. This suggests that exposure to salt has not resulted in an irreversible alteration in the primary structure of the toxin-binding material. Sedimentation coefficients are, however, relatively insensitive to changes in shape. The results obtained with Sepharose demonstrate that the Stokes radius of the toxin-binding material is decreased by exposure to a high concentration of salt, and that this decrease is only partially reversible. The simplest interpretation of these results is that the toxin-binding material has a high axial ratio, and that this ratio is decreased by exposure to salt.

An unexplained finding concerns the behavior of the membrane proteins in the presence of salt. In the ultracentrifuge, the toxin-labeled material had a higher sedimentation coefficient than did most other proteins, even if the centrifugation was carried out in the presence of 1 M salt. Thus, the sedimentation coefficients of the proteins solubilized from the postsynaptic membranes of *Torpedo* cover a wide range from about 15S down to about 6S. On the other hand, all of these proteins, including the toxin-labeled material, have, in the presence of a high concentration of salt, approximately the same Stokes radius. One possible explanation for the difference in the results obtained in the ultracentrifuge from those obtained on Sepharose is that the proteins are of similar size and shape but differ in their content of lipid (density). Alternative explanations based on the shape of the protein molecules are also possible, however.

From the number of binding sites for the toxin (6.6×10^{17} per kg of electric tissue) and our estimate of the area of postsynaptic membrane (70 m²/kg), it is possible to estimate roughly the number of receptors in the membrane as $10,000/\mu^2$ (Miledi et al., 1971a). This suggests that a significant fraction of the area of postsynaptic membranes is taken up by receptors, and perhaps by other large molecules which may be required to subserve the conductance mechanisms of synaptic potentials. It appears likely that the postsynaptic membrane is actually crowded with the protein molecules which subserve neurotransmission.

The striking similarity in the number of active sites of esterase with the number of toxin-binding sites requires explanation (Miledi et al., 1971a; Barnard et al., 1971). One possibility is that the receptor and the esterase are linked, perhaps as part of a polymer in the membrane and/or basement membrane. Alternatively, the synthesis of receptor molecules may be linked with that of esterase molecules. Our observation that the esterase and the receptor appear to be associated with different membrane fragments makes an explanation of the quantitative relationship even more difficult.

ACKNOWLEDGMENTS

Support for this research was generously provided by the British Medical Research Council. During these studies, P.B.M. was a Fellow of the John Simon Guggenheim Memorial Foundation, and then of the National Institute of Neurologic Disease and Stroke (1 F 10 NS 2282–01 NSRB).

REFERENCES

Axelson, J., (1971): Catecholamine functions. *Annual Review of Physiology,* 33:1–30.

Barnard, E. A., Wieckowski, J., and Chiu, T. H. (1971): Cholinergic receptor molecules and cholinesterase molecules at mouse skeletal muscle junctions. *Nature,* 234:207–209.

Barrnett, R. J., (1962): The fine structural localization of acetylcholinesterase at the myoneural junction. *Journal of Cell Biology,* 12:247–262.

Bauman, A., Changeux, J.-P., and Benda, P. (1970): Purification of membrane fragments derived from the non-excitable surface of the eel electroplax. *FEBS Letters,* 8:145–148.

Bennett, M. V. L. (1961): Modes of operation of electric organs. *Annals of the New York Academy of Science,* 94:458–509.

Berg, D. K., Kelly, R. B., Sargent, P. B., Williamson, P., and Hall, Z. W. (1972): Binding of α-bungarotoxin to acetylcholine receptors in mammalian muscle. *Proceedings of the National Academy of Sciences,* 69:147–152.

Birnbaumer, L., and Rodbell, M. (1970): Adenyl cyclase in fat cells. *Journal of Biological Chemistry,* 244,3477–3482.

Birnbaumer, L., Pohl, S. L., and Rodbell, M. (1971): The glucagen-sensitive adenyl cyclase system in plasma membranes of rat liver. II. Comparison between glucagen and fluoride-stimulated activities. *Journal of Biological Chemistry,* 246:1857–1860.

Boquet, P., Izard, Y., Jouannet, M., and Meaume, J. (1966): Etude de deux antigenes toxiques du venom de *Naja nigricolis. Comptes Rendus de l'Academie des Sciences,* 262, Serie D: 1134–1137.

Bourgeois, J. P., Tsuji, S., Boquet, P., Pillot, J., Ryter, A., and Changeux, J.-P. (1971): Localization of the cholinergic receptor protein by immunofluorescence in eel electroplax. *FEBS Letters*, 16:92–94.

del Castillo, S., and Katz, B. (1955): On the localization of acetylcholine receptors. *Journal of Physiology*, 128:157–181.

Chang, C. C. (1960): Studies on the mechanism of curare-like action of *Bungarus multicinctus* venom. I. Effect on the phrenic nerve-diaphragm preparation of the rat. *Journal of Formosan Medical Association*, 59:315–322.

Chang, C. C., and Lee, C. Y. (1963): Isolation of neurotoxins from the venom of *Bungarus multicinctus* and their modes of neuromuscular blocking action. *Archives Internationales de Pharmacodynamie et de Therapie*, 144:241–257.

Changeux, J.-P., Kasai, M., Huchet, M., and Meunier, J.-C. (1970): *In vitro* studies with the cholinergic receptor of the eel electroplax. *Perspectives in Virology*, 7:33–47.

Changeux, J.-P., Kasai, M., and Lee, C.-Y. (1970): Use of a snake venom toxin to characterize the cholinergic receptor protein. *Proceedings of the National Academy of Sciences*, 67:1241–1247.

Changeux, J.-P., Meunier, J. C., and Huchet, M. (1971): Studies on the cholinergic receptor protein of *Electrophorus electricus*. 1. An essay *in vitro* for the cholinergic receptor site and solubilization of the receptor protein from electric tissue. *Molecular Pharmacology*, 7:538–553.

Changeux, J.-P., Podleski, T. R., and Wofsy, J. (1967): Affinity labelling of the acetylcholine-receptor. *Proceedings of the National Academy of Sciences*, 58:2067.

CIBA Symposium: (1970): Molecular Properties of Drug Receptors, edited by A. Porter and M. O'Connor, J & A. Churchill, London.

Clark, A. J. (1926): The antagonism of ACh by Atropine. *Journal of Physiology*, 61:547.

Ehrenpreis, S., Fleisch, J. H., and Mittag, T. W. (1969): Approaches to the molecular nature of pharmacological receptors. *Pharmacological Review*, 21:131–181.

Eldefrawi, M. E., Eldefrawi, A. T., and O'Brien, R. D. (1971): Binding of five cholinergic ligands to house-fly brain and *Torpedo* electroplax. *Molecular Pharmacology*, 7:104–110.

Eldefrawi, M. E., and O'Brien, R. D. (1971): Autoinhibition of acetylcholine binding to *Torpedo* electroplax; a possible molecular mechanism for desensitization. *Proceedings of the National Academy of Sciences*, 68:2006–2007.

Fatt, P., and Katz, B. (1951): An analysis of the end-plate potential recorded with an intracellular electrode. *Journal of Physiology*, 115:320–370.

Feldberg, W., and Fessard, A. (1942): The cholinergic nature of the nerves to the electric organ of the *Torpedo*. *Journal of Physiology*, 101:200–215.

Fewtell, C., and Rang, H. P. (1971): Distribution of bound ^{3}H-benzilylcholine mustard in subcellular fractions of smooth muscle from guinea-pig ileum. *British Journal of Pharmacology*, 43:417–418 p.

Fiszer, S., and De Robertis, E. (1969): Subcellular distribution and chemical nature of the receptor for 5-hydroxytryptamine in the central nervous system. *Journal of Neurochemisty*, 16:1201.

Gill, E. W., and Rang, H. P. (1966): An alkylating derivitive of benzilylcholine with specific long-lasting parasympatholytic activity. *Molecular Pharmacology*, 2:284–287.

Harris, A. J., Kuffler, S. W., and Dennis, M. S. (1971): Differential chemosensitivity of synaptic and extrasynaptic areas on the neural surface in parasympathetic neurons of the frog, tested by microapplication of acetylcholine. *Proceedings of the Royal Society of London, B*, 177:541–553.

Hodgkin, A. L. (1964): The conduction of the nerve impulse. *The Sherrington Lectures*, VII, Liverpool University Press.

Israel, M. (1970): Localisation d'acetylcholine des synapses myoneurales et nerf-electro-plaques. *Archives d'Anatomie Microscopique et de Morphologie Expérimentale*, 59:67–98.

Kandel, E. R., Frazier, W. T., and Coggeshall, R. (1967): Opposite synaptic actions by different branches of identifiable interneuron in Aplysia. *Science*, 155:364–379.

Karlin, A. (1969): Chemical modification of the active site of the acetylcholine receptor. *Journal of General Physiology*, 54:245–264.

Karlin, A., and Bartels, E. (1966): Effects of sulphydryl groups and of reducing disulfide bonds on the acetylcholine-activated permeability system of the electroplax. *Biochemica et Biophysica Acta*, 126:525–535.

Karlin, A., Prives, J., Deal, W., and Winnik, M. (1970): Counting acetylcholine receptors in the electroplax. In: CIBA Symposium *Molecular Properties of Drug Receptors*, edited by A. Porter and M. O'Connor; J. & A. Churchill, London, pp. 247–261.

Karlin, A., and Winnik, M. (1968): Reduction and specific alkylation of the receptor for acetylcholine. *Proceedings of the National Academy of Sciences*, 60:668–674.

Katz, B., and Miledi, R. (1964): Further observations on the distribution of acetylcholine-reactive sites in skeletal muscle. *Journal of Physiology*, 170:379.

Kiefer, H., Lindstrom, J., Lennox, E. S., and Singer, S. J. (1970): Photo-affinity labelling of specific acetylcholine binding sites on membranes. *Proceedings of the National Academy of Sciences*, 67:1688–1694.

Langley, J. N. (1906): On the contraction of muscle, chiefly in relation to the presence of "receptive" substances. Part I. *Journal of Physiology*, 36:347–384.

Lee, C. Y., and Chang, C. C. (1966): Modes of actions of purified toxins from Elapid venoms on neuromuscular transmission. *Mems. Institute Butantan*, 33:555–572.

Lee, C. Y., Tseng, L. F., and Chiu, T. H. (1967): Influences on denervation on localization of neurotoxins from Elapid venoms in rat diaphragm. *Nature*, 215:1177–1178.

Loewi, O. (1921): Über humorale Veberagbarkeit der Herzennervenwirkung. *Pflügers Archives der gesamte Physiologie*, 189:239–242.

Lømo, T., and Rosenthal (1972): Control of acetycholine sensitivity by muscle activity in the rat. *Journal of Physiology*, 221:493–513.

Massoulie, J., Rieger, J., and Tsuji, S. (1970): Solubilisation de l'acetylcholinesterase des organes electriques de gymnote action de la trypsine. *European Journal of Biochemistry*, 14:430–439.

Mebs, D., Karita, K., Iwanaga, S., Samejuma, Y., and Lee, C. Y. (1971): Amino acid sequence of α-Bungarotoxin from the venom of *Bungarus multicinctus*. *Biochemical and Biophysical Research Communications*, 44:711.

Meunier, J.-C., Olsen, R., Menez, A., Morgat, J.-L., Fromageot, P., Ronseray, A.-M., Boquet, P., and Changeux, J.-P. (1971): Quelques propriétés physiques de la protéine réceptrice de l'acétylcholine étudiées a l' aide d' une neurotoxine radioactive. *Comptes Rendus De L' Academie des Sciences*, Serie D, 595–598.

Meunier, J.-C., Huchet, M., Boquet, P., and Changeux, J.-P. (1971): Separation de la protéine receptrice de l'acetylcholine et de l' acetylcholinesterase. *Comptes Rendus De L' Academie des Sciences*, 272, Serie D: 117–120.

Miledi, R. (1962): Induction of receptors. In: CIBA Symposium, *Enzymes and Drug Action*, edited by J. L. Morgan and Aus de Rueck. Little, Brown & Co, Boston, pp. 220–235.

Miledi, R., Molinoff, P., and Potter, L. T. (1971a): Isolation of the cholinergic receptor protein of *Torpedo* electric tissue. *Nature*, 229:554–557.

Miledi, R., and Potter, L. T. (1971): Acetylcholine receptors in muscle fibers. *Nature*, 233:599–603.

Miller, D. B., and Grafius, M. A. (1970): The subunit molecular weight of acetylcholinesterase. *FEBS Letters*, 12:61–64.

Molinoff, P. B., and Axelrod, J. (1971): Biochemistry of catecholamines. *Annual Review of Biochemistry*, 40:465–500.

Nickel, E., and Potter, L. T. (1970): Synaptic vesicles in freeze-etched electric tissue of *Torpedo*. *Brain Research*, 23:95–100.

O'Brien, R. D., and Gilmour, L. P. (1969): A muscarone-binding material in electroplax and its relation to the acetylcholine receptor. A centrifugal assay. *Proceedings of the National Academy of Sciences*, 63:496–503.

Paton, W. D. M. (1970): Receptors as defined by their pharmacological properties. In: CIBA

Symposium on *Molecular Properties of Drug Receptors*, edited by R. Porter and M. O'Connor: J. & A. Churchill, London, pp. 3–30.

Paton, W. D. M., and Rang, H. P. (1965): The uptake of atropine and related drugs by intestinal smooth muscle of the guinea pig in relation to acetylcholine receptors. *Proceedings of the Royal Society B*, 163:1–44.

Pohl, S. L., Birnbaumer, L., and Rodbell, M. (1971): The glucagon-sensitive adenyl-cyclase system in plasma membranes of rat liver. *Journal of Biological Chemistry*, 276:1849–1856.

Potter, L. T., and Molinoff, P. B. (1972): Isolation of cholinergic receptor proteins in *Recent Advances in Neuropharmacology: A tribute to Julius Axelrod*, edited by S. Snyder, Oxford University Press, Oxford.

Pressman, D., Eisen, H. N. (1950): Zone of localization of antibodies, Part V. An attempt to saturate antibody binding sites in mouse kidney. *Journal of Immunology*, 64:273–279.

Rang, H. P. (1967): The uptake of atropine and related compounds by smooth muscle. *Annals of the New York Academy of Science*, 144:756–767.

Rasmussen, H. (1970): Cell communication, calcium ion and cyclic adenosine monophosphate. *Science*, 170:404–412.

De Robertis, E. (1971): Molecular biology of synaptic receptors. *Science*, 171:963–971.

De Robertis, E., Fiszer, S., and Soto, E. F. (1967): Cholinergic binding capacity of proteolipids from isolated nerve-ending membranes. *Nature*, 158:928–9.

De Robertis, E., Lunt, G. S., and la Torre, J. L. (1971): Multiple binding sites for acetylcholine in a proteolipid from electric tissue. *Molecular Pharmacology*, 7:97–103.

Robison, G. A., Butcher, R. W., and Sutherland, E. W. (1970): On the relation of hormone receptors to adenyl cyclase. In: *Fundamental Concepts in Drug Receptor Interactions*, edited by J. P. Danielli, D. J. Triggle, and J. F. Moran. Academic Press, New York.

Sheridan, M. N. (1965): The fine structure of the electric organ of the *Torpedo marmarata*. *Journal of Cell Biology*, 24:129–141.

Singer, S. J. (1970): Affinity labeling of protein active sites. In: CIBA Symposium, *Molecular Properties of Drug Receptors*, edited by R. Porter and M. O'Connor. J. & A. Churchill, London, p. 229.

Takagi, K., and Takahashi, A. (1969): Studies of separation and characterization of acetylcholine receptor labeled with tritiated dibenamine. *Biochemical Pharmacology*, 17:1609–1618.

la Torre, L. J., Lunt, G. S., and de Robertis, E. (1970): Isolation of a cholinergic proteolipid receptor from electric tissue. *Proceedings of the National Academy of Sciences*, 65:716–720.

Thesleff, S. (1970): The cholinergic receptor in skeletal muscle. In: CIBA Symposium, *Molecular Properties of Drug Receptors*, edited by R. Porter and M. O'Connor. J. & A. Churchill, London, pp. 33–39.

Waser, P. G. (1970): On receptors in the postsynaptic membrane of the motor endplate. In: CIBA Symposium, *Molecular Properties of Drug Receptors*, edited by R. Porter and M. O'Connor. J. & A. Churchill, London, pp. 59–69.

Advances in Biochemical Psychopharmacology, Vol. 6
Raven Press, New York © 1972

Drugs Affecting Monoamines in the Basal Ganglia

G. Bartholini and A. Pletscher

*Research Department, F. Hoffmann-La Roche & Co. Ltd.,
Basle, Switzerland*

The present review deals with -3,4-dihydroxyphenylalanine (L-DOPA) as well as with neuroleptics of the chlorpromazine and haloperidol type. These drugs have been chosen because today they are in the center of clinical interest, as they exert pronounced effects on the basal ganglia, although not exclusively.

L-DOPA

General Metabolism

In animal and man, this amino acid represents the immediate precursor of dopamine (DA), which is formed through the action of the decarboxylase of L-aromatic amino acids. Further metabolic transformations of DA lead to accumulation in several tissues of phenolcarboxylic acids (PCA), i.e., homovanillic acid (HVA) and dihydroxyphenylacetic acid (DPAA) and of some norepinephrine (NE) (Fig. 1).

Administered L-DOPA is rapidly metabolized mainly in the extra-cerebral organs, i.e., liver, kidney, heart (Bartholini and Pletscher, 1968). The biological half-life of DOPA is about 30 and 45 min in rat and man, respectively (Bartholini, Pletscher, and Kuruma, 1970c) (Fig. 2). On oral administration, a large part of L-DOPA is decarboxylated already in the gastrointestinal tract (Bartholini and Pletscher, 1968). As a consequence, only a limited amount of the unaltered amino acid penetrates into the brain, where it leads to a small formation of catecholamines (Bartholini and

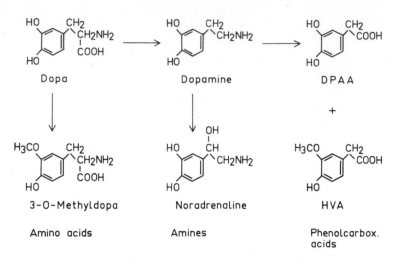

FIG. 1. Major metabolic pathways of L-DOPA.

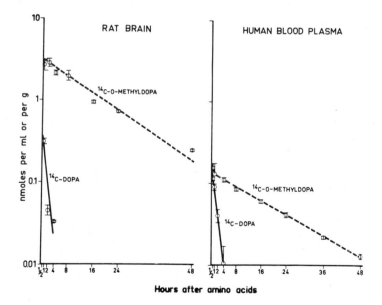

FIG. 2. Half-life of ¹⁴C-DOPA and ¹⁴C-OM-DOPA in brain of rat and in the blood plasma of man. Rats were injected i.p. with either 5 mg/kg L-¹⁴C-DOPA or 1 mg/kg L-¹⁴C-OM-DOPA. Averages with SE of three or four experiments. Humans received 100 μg/kg L-¹⁴C-DOPA (2 individuals) or 26 μg/kg L-¹⁴C-OM-DOPA (4 individuals) i.v. Averages with SE. *Ordinate:* concentration of ¹⁴C-DOPA or ¹⁴C-OM-DOPA in nmoles per g brain or per ml blood plasma (Bartholini et al., 1970c).

Pletscher, 1968; Pletscher, Bartholini, Gey, and Jenni, 1970; Wurtmann, Rose, Matthysse, Stephenson, and Baldessarini, 1970) (Fig. 3).

Cerebral Metabolism

The catecholamines formed in the brain from L-DOPA consist mainly of DA and partially of NE; their relative amounts depend on the dose of L-DOPA administered. With low doses of the amino acid mainly NE is formed. Higher amounts of L-DOPA increase the cerebral content of DA more markedly than that of NE (Bartholini and Pletscher, 1968) possibly due to a saturation of the enzyme DA-β-hydroxylase, which seems to be the rate-limiting step in the synthesis of NE.

After relatively large amounts of L-DOPA, the catecholamines (mainly

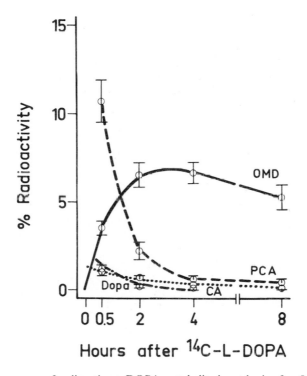

FIG. 3. Time curves of radioactive L-DOPA metabolite in rat brain after 5 mg/kg L-^{14}C-DOPA i.p. *Ordinate:* Radioactivity of the various metabolites per g brain in percent of the radioactivity administered per g body weight. Averages with SE of three or four experiments. CA = catecholamines; PCA = phenolcarboxylic acids; OMD = O-methyl-DOPA (Pletscher et al., 1970).

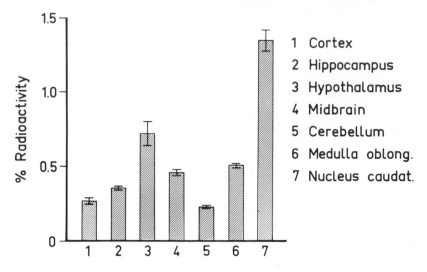

FIG. 4. Distribution of labeled catecholamines in various regions of the rat brain. L-^{14}C-DOPA (5 mg/kg) was administered i.p. 2 hr before sacrifice. Average with SE of two experiments each performed with a pool of three to six brain regions. *Ordinate:* Radioactivity per g brain in percent of the radioactivity administered per g body weight (Pletscher et al., 1970).

DA) accumulate preferentially in the basal ganglia (e.g., caudate nucleus). Other brain areas—e.g., cortex, cerebellum, medulla oblongata—however, show only a small increase in the amines (Fig. 4) (Pletscher et al., 1970; Kuruma, Bartholini, Tissot, and Pletscher, 1972). The preferential accumulation of DA in the striatum is probably due to the fact that in this structure the blood-brain barrier for DOPA (i.e., the DOPA-decarboxylase of the endothelial cells of the brain capillaries) (Bertler, Falck, Owman, and Rosengrenn, 1966) is less active than in other regions of the brain, leading to an enhanced penetration of the amino acid. In fact, it has been demonstrated with the histofluorimetric method of Falck, Hillarp, Thieme, and Thorp (1962) that Ro 4–4602[1] (see below), a selective inhibitor of the decarboxylase in the extracerebral organs (including that of the brain capillaries), inhibits this enzyme more markedly in the capillaries of the striatum than in those of other brain areas like the cortex (Constantinidis, Bartholini, Geissbühler, and Tissot, 1970). In addition, the preferential accumulation of DA in the striatum might be due to a relatively high activity of decarboxylase in this structure (Bogdanski, Weissbach, and Udenfriend, 1957).

---

[1] (N-(DL-seryl)-N′-(2,3,4-trihydroxybenzyl) hydrazine) • HCl; synthetized by Dr. B. Hegedüs, Dept. of Chemistry, F. Hoffmann-La Roche & Co. Ltd., Basle.

In addition to DA, relatively high levels of PCA (mainly HVA) and small amounts of DOPA are found in the brain after L-DOPA administration (Bartholini and Pletscher, 1968; Pletscher et al., 1970). The rise of the level of PCA, similarly to that of DOPA, is rapid and of rather short duration, but the concentrations of the acidic metabolites attain maximal values about three to four times higher than those of DOPA (Fig. 3). The relatively marked rise of PCA in the brain suggests that greater amounts of DA than those actually found have been formed intermediately in this organ. In fact, the main precursor of cerebral HVA and DPAA is probably DA, since transamination of DOPA seems to be a minor metabolic pathway. In addition, the cerebral PCA cannot have their main origin in the blood because these compounds have been shown not to penetrate in relevant amounts into the brain (Bartholini, Pletscher, and Tissot, 1966). It remains, however, to be elucidated how much of the cerebral DA and PCA accumulating after L-DOPA administration is localized within the capillary walls of the brain. The latter have been demonstrated to accumulate and metabolize DOPA and DA (Bertler et al., 1966).

Cerebrospinal Fluid (CSF)

In man and animals, L-DOPA administration leads to a rise of HVA in the CSF (Bartholini et al., 1966; Pletscher, Bartholini, and Tissot, 1967a). As previously demonstrated, this increase cannot be due to a direct penetration of HVA from the blood into the CSF but must have its origin in structures in the central nervous system (Bartholini et al., 1966; Pletscher et al., 1967a). Experiments with Ro 4–4602 (see above) in combination with L-DOPA indicate, however, that the increased HVA in the CSF probably derives not only from the parenchyma but also from the capillaries of the brain. Ro 4–4602 inhibits the decarboxylase in the extracerebral organs (including that in the brain capillaries). As a consequence, this inhibitor enhances the L-DOPA-induced increase of DOPA in the blood and thus the supply of L-DOPA to the brain. In this organ, DOPA is decarboxylated to DA, since the cerebral enzyme is not affected by Ro 4–4602. In fact, Ro 4–4602 enhances the L-DOPA-induced increase of DA and its main metabolite HVA in the brain (Bartholini, Bates, Burkard, and Pletscher, 1967; Bartholini and Pletscher, 1968; Constantinidis, Bartholini, Tissot, and Pletscher, 1968; Bartholini, Tissot, and Pletscher, 1969; Tissot, Bartholini, and Pletscher, 1969; Bartholini et al., 1970c). However, the HVA of CSF does not show a concomitant rise in animals and in man. This missing increase is probably due to inhibition by Ro 4–4602 of the formation of

TABLE 1. *Effect of ³H-L-DOPA alone and in combination with Ro 4–4602 on various metabolite fractions in the striatum and CSF of rabbits*

Fraction	L-DOPA	Ro 4–4602 + L-DOPA
	Striatum	
Phenolcarboxylic acids	15.16 ± 1.91	21.66 ± 1.84[a]
Amino acids	13.76 ± 3.18	73.35 ± 6.34[a]
Catecholamines	9.30 ± 1.75	26.93 ± 1.21[a]
	Cerebrospinal fluid	
Phenolcarboxylic acids	2.27 ± 0.33	2.22 ± 0.24[b]
Amino acids	2.09 ± 0.30	10.72 ± 1.17[a]

L-³H-DOPA (5 μg/kg) was administered i.v. 2 hr before sacrifice. Ro 4–4602 (100 mg/kg) was injected i.p. 15 min prior to and 1 hr after L-³H-DOPA. The values indicate the radio-activity per g tissue or per ml cerebrospinal fluid in percent of the radioactivity injected per g body weight. Averages with SE of 3–4 experiments: (a) $p < 0.01$. (b) $p > 0.05$ (Bartholini et al., 1971).

HVA in the brain capillaries (Bartholini, Tissot, and Pletscher, 1971) (Table 1). These results therefore confirm that part of the HVA appearing after L-DOPA administration in the CSF originates in the capillaries of the brain.

3-O-Methyl-DOPA (OM-DOPA)

A further important metabolite of DOPA in animals and man is 3-O-methyl-DOPA (OM-DOPA) formed through the action of the catechol-O-methyl-transferase, mainly in the liver but probably also in several other organs including the brain (Pletscher et al., 1967a; Bartholini and Pletscher, 1968; Kuruma, Bartholini, and Pletscher, 1970). OM-DOPA accumulates to a large extent in many tissues (Bartholini, Kuruma, and Pletscher, 1970b). The labeled O-methylated amino acid has a relatively long biological half-life (12 and 15 hr in rat and man, respectively) (Fig. 2) which might be due to the fact that it is slowly metabolized and poorly excreted. Thus, in rats about 10 percent of the administered radioactivity is eliminated in the feces mainly as metabolic end products, and 46 percent is excreted in the urine within 24 hr (Bartholini et al., 1970b). The urinary radioactivity is composed of about 10% of unchanged OM-DOPA, 0.70% of catecholamines, and 85% of acidic metabolites (Bartholini et al., 1970c; Bartholini, Kuruma, and Pletscher, *in preparation*). The main metabolites of L-OM-DOPA found in the urine as well as in the various organs and the blood are HVA and 3-methoxy-4-hydroxyphenyllactic acid (Bartholini et al., 1970b). The latter is probably formed by transamination of OM-DOPA via 3-methoxy-4-hydroxyphenylpyruvic acid. Part of HVA seems to derive from direct decarboxylation of OM-DOPA (which is, however, a poor substrate for the decarboxylase compared to DOPA) (Ferrini and Glässer, 1964). Another part of HVA probably derives from DOPA which has been formed by demethylation of OM-DOPA. Thus, minor amounts of labeled dihydroxylated metabolites—i.e., DOPA, DA, DPAA—have been found in the urine, as well as DA in the brain of rats after administration of L-^{14}C-OM-DOPA, indicating that this amino acid is partly converted into DOPA (Bartholini et al., 1970c; Kuruma, Bartholini, Tissot, and Pletscher, 1971).

Accumulation in the tissues of OM-DOPA formed from DOPA and slow demethylation of the O-methylated intermediate may explain the sustained (days to weeks) effect of L-DOPA after its discontinuation in parkinsonian patients (Rao, 1970). This persistence of the therapeutic action is probably not due to the presence of DOPA in the brain, since this amino acid has been shown to have a very short biological half-life.

For various reasons discussed elsewhere (Hornykiewicz, 1968; Pletscher et al., 1970), it can be assumed that the therapeutic action of L-DOPA in parkinsonian patients is due to the DA newly formed in the basal ganglia. Other possibilities must, however, be considered. For instance, L-DOPA has been shown to decrease the content of endogenous 5-hydroxytryptamine (Bartholini, Da Prada, and Pletscher, 1968; Everett and Borcherdiry, 1970) and S-adenosylmethionine in the brain (Wurtmann et al., 1970) as well as to activate the transamination of tyrosine *in vivo* (Bartholini, Gey, and Pletscher, 1970). In addition, the possible consequence of the cerebral accumulation of OM-DOPA and the formation of NE needs further investigation.

NEUROLEPTICS

In animals, chlorpromazine (CPZ) is known to increase markedly the level of endogenous methylated catecholamines as well as of HVA in the brain without affecting the concentration of DA (Carlsson and Lindqvist, 1963; Andén, Roos, and Werdinius, 1964; Laverty and Sharman, 1965; Roos, 1965; Da Prada and Pletscher, 1966; Pletscher, Gey, and Burkard, 1967b). Among the psychotropic drugs, this effect seems to be specific for the neuroleptics. In fact, chlorprothixene and haloperidol, like CPZ, markedly increase HVA, whereas thymoleptics such as imipramine and amitriptyline, tranquilizers such as meprobamate, chlordiazepoxide, and diazepam, and hypnotics such as phenobarbital, have no significant effect

TABLE 2. *Effects of various psychotropic drugs on the level of*
endogenous HVA and 5HIAA in the brain stem of rats

Drug	Dose (mg/kg)	HVA	Dose (mg/kg)	5HIAA
Chlorpromazine	10	314 ± 21	20	119 ± 3
Chlorprothixene	10	300 ± 17	20	125 ± 4
Haloperidol	5	340 ± 8	10	122 ± 5
Imipramine	10	91 ± 9	20	72 ± 3
Amitriptyline	10	125 ± 17	20	82 ± 5
Meprobamate	50	115 ± 8	50	130 ± 6
Chlordiazepoxide	50	83 ± 5	50	132 ± 7
Diazepam	10	83 ± 8	10	124 ± 5
Phenobarbital	50	100 ± 17	50	111 ± 5
Hexobarbital	50	100 ± 17	50	120 ± 14

The drugs were injected i.p. 2 to 3 hr before sacrifice. The values are expressed in percent of controls (= 100%) and represent averages with SE of four to ten experiments (Da Prada and Pletscher, 1966).

(Laverty and Sharman, 1965; Roos, 1965; Pletscher et al., 1967b) (Table 2).

The neuroleptic-induced rise of HVA in the basal ganglia is not due to liberation and subsequent metabolism of DA, since these drugs do not markedly influence the DA content of the striatum of some species, e.g., the rat. Neither is hypothermia involved, since CPZ also elevates HVA if the animals are kept normothermic (Pletscher et al., 1967b). Finally, a delayed disappearance of HVA from the brain is unlikely, since CPZ neither influences the clearance of HVA, increased by previous administration of monoamine releasers, nor affects the cerebral content of another phenolcarboxylic acid, i.e., 5-hydroxyindolacetic acid (5HIAA) (Pletscher et al., 1967b) (Table 2). However, good evidence exists that neuroleptics enhance the turnover of striatal DA. Thus, CPZ accelerates the α-methyl-*p*-tyrosine-induced decrease of endogenous DA (Neff and Costa, 1966) as well as the disappearance of labeled DA which has accumulated in the brain after previous administration of L-^{14}C-DOPA (Pletscher et al., 1967b). Furthermore, CPZ increases in the basal ganglia the synthesis of labeled catecholamines from L-^{14}C-tyrosine administered intravenously (Burkard, Gey, and Pletscher, 1966, 1967; Nybäck and Sedvall, 1968; Pletscher et al., 1967b) or into the cerebral ventricles (Bartholini and Pletscher, 1969). The latter experiment excludes a peripheral effect such as an enhanced penetration of tyrosine or of DOPA into the brain, due to neuroleptics.

Neuroleptics do not seem to activate directly the hydroxylation of tyrosine as indicated by *in vitro* experiments (Pletscher et al., 1967b). Therefore, the increased turnover of DA may be due to a positive feedback mechanism which, however, has not yet been elucidated. There are two main hypotheses concerning its nature. First, it is possible that the activation of tyrosine-hydroxylase is connected with a decrease of the concentration of cytoplasmatic DA. Thus, evidence exists that CPZ inhibits the uptake of biogenic amines at the level of cytoplasmatic membranes (Gey and Pletscher, 1964; Thoenen, Hürlimann, and Haefely, 1965; Pletscher et al., 1967b).

Assuming that inhibition of DA reuptake by neuroleptics occurs at the level of the dopaminergic synapses in the basal ganglia, the concentration of free DA within the neurons might be decreased, leading to a reduction of the end product inhibition on tyrosine-hydroxylase. This mechanism has been claimed to be involved in the rapid regulation of CA syntheses (Costa and Neff, 1966; Alousi and Weiner, 1966).

The second hypothesis claims that a primary blockade of the dopaminergic receptors in the striatum by the neuroleptics might cause an activation of a neuronal pathway leading to an increased activity of the nigrostriatal neurons and, therefore, to an enhanced DA turnover (Carlsson and Lindqvist, 1963; Andén et al., 1964). However, the localization of this neuronal pathway is unknown. A striato-nigral system has been described in monkeys (Poirier, Bouvier, Bédard, Boucher, La Rochelle, Olivier, and Singh, 1969), but its role in the control of DA turnover remains to be investigated.

There is some evidence that the pathway through which the positive feedback operates might be cholinergic. Thus, intraperitoneal administration of anticholinergic drugs such as atropine, scopolamine, and Ditran® markedly counteracts the rise of HVA in the striatum induced by neuroleptics (O'Keefe, Sharman, and Vogt, 1970; Andén and Bédard, 1971). In addition, atropine alone also reduces the level of HVA in the brain without affecting the DA concentration (Fig. 5) (Andén and Bédard, 1971; Bartholini and Pletscher, 1971). This probably indicates a reduction of the turnover of the amine, although a shift in its metabolism cannot be excluded. These findings, therefore, support the hypothesis that a cholinergic input might stimulate the activity of the nigro-striatal neurons.

On the other hand, administration of atropine into the lateral ventricles of the rat brain (Fig. 6) leads to a marked increase of endogenous HVA in the striatum without changing the DA concentration. This finding remains to be further investigated. The effect of intraventricularly administered atropine is probably not due to a blockade of DA reuptake into the striatal synapses, since injection of atropine into the striatum does not affect the levels of either cerebral DA or HVA. Neither does atropine inhibit the transport of HVA from the brain, as shown by experiments with the benzoquinolizine deriva-

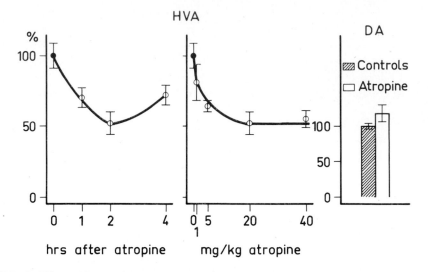

FIG. 5. Effect of intraperitoneal administration of atropine on the content of endogenous HVA and DA of the rat brain. HVA was measured at various time intervals after administration of 20 mg/kg atropine (*left*) or 2 hr after various doses of the drug (*middle*). DA was determined 2 hr after 40 mg/kg atropine (right). The values are expressed in percent of controls (= 100%; point O on the abscissa). Average with SE of two to five experiments (Bartholini and Pletscher, 1971).

tive Ro 4–1284.[2] This drug, due to a rapid liberation of endogenous DA in the brain, causes a marked rise of cerebral HVA. This increase is further enhanced by probenecid, a known inhibitor of the transport of the PCA, but not by atropine (Bartholini and Pletscher, 1971). As a tentative hypothesis, it may be assumed that a second inhibitory cholinergic system modulates the activity of the nigro-striatal neurons. Blockade of this system by atropine would lead to an enhanced turnover of DA.

In conclusion, two cholinergic systems, one inhibitory, the other excitatory, seem to be involved in the regulation of DA turnover in the nigro-striatal neurons. The inhibitory cholinergic input, on the one hand, might act at the level of the dopaminergic cell bodies in the substantia nigra. Thus, in preliminary experiments supranigral injection of atropine causes an increase of HVA without changing the DA concentration in the striatum (Bartholini, Pieri, and Pletscher, *in preparation*). On the other hand, the excitatory cholinergic system, which is inhibited by systemic administration of anticholinergic drugs, might be connected with other brain regions, for instance,

---

[2]2-hydroxy-2-ethyl-3-isobutyl-9,10-dimethoxy-1,2,3,4,6,7-hexahydro-11bH-benzo(a)quinolizine.

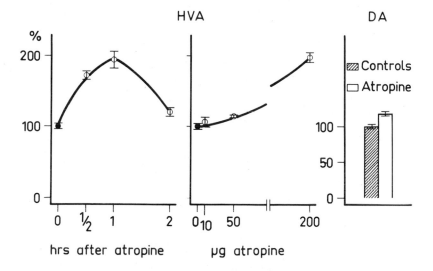

FIG. 6. Effect of intraventricular administration of atropine on the levels of endogenous HVA and DA in the rat brain. Atropine was injected into the right lateral ventricle of the brain. The animals were sacrificed at various time intervals after 200 μg (*left*) or at 1 hr after various doses of the drug (*middle*). DA was measured 1 hr after 200 μg atropine (*right*). The values are expressed in percent of controls (= 100%; point O on the abscissa) and represent averages with SE of two to five experiments. All the values of HVA are significantly different from controls ($p < 0.01$) with the exception of that obtained after 10 μg atropine ($p > 0.05$) (Bartholini and Pletscher, 1971).

the nucleus centromedianus of the thalamus, which has been demonstrated by McLennan (1964) to liberate DA in the striatum during electrical stimulation. It remains to be elucidated, however, why intraperitoneal injection of atropine seems to diminish, whereas intraventricular administration of the drug probably enhances the turnover of brain DA. The bivalent action of atropine may be explained by differences in the distribution of the drug in the brain. After intraperitoneal injection, the distribution of atropine might be such that the stimulatory system is preferentially inhibited, whereas on intraventricular administration the drug interferes mainly with the inhibitory projection.

SUMMARY

Two types of drugs known to interfere with the function of the basal ganglia are discussed.

(1) L-DOPA, due to a rapid extracerebral metabolism, penetrates only

in small amounts into the brain, where it is decarboxylated into dopamine (DA). This amine preferentially accumulates in the striatum. The major metabolite of DA is homovanillic acid, which also appears in the cerebrospinal fluid and which seems to be partly formed in the wall of the brain capillaries. Part of the L-DOPA is also transformed into 3-O-methyl-DOPA. This metabolite, because of its long biological half-life, accumulates in the tissues and undergoes slow, partial 3-O-demethylation.

(2) Neuroleptics of the chlorpromazine and haloperidol type enhance the turnover of DA in the basal ganglia. This seems to be due to a positive feedback mechanism as a possible consequence of blockade of dopaminergic receptors and of an inhibition of DA reuptake. Atropine intraperitoneally counteracts the increase of the cerebral DA turnover caused by neuroleptics. The anticholinergic drug alone decreases the cerebral DA turnover if administered intraperitoneally, but increases this turnover if injected into the cerebral ventricles. This opposite action of atropine may be due to the existence of two cholinergic systems, one excitatory and one inhibitory, regulating the activity of the nigro-striatal dopaminergic neurons.

REFERENCES

Alousi, A. and Weiner, N. (1966): The regulation of norepinephrine synthesis in sympathetic nerves: effect of nerve stimulation, cocaine and catecholamine-releasing agents. *Proceedings of the National Academy of Sciences,* 56:1491–1496.

Andén, N. E., Roos, B. E., and Werdinius, B. (1964): Effect of chlorpromazine, haloperidol, and reserpine on the levels of phenolic acids in rabbit corpus striatum. *Life Sciences,* 3: 149–158.

Andén, N. E. and Bédard, P. (1971): Influences of cholinergic mechanisms on the function and turnover of brain dopamine. *Journal of Pharmacy and Pharmacology,* 23:460–462.

Bartholini, G., Pletscher, A., and Tissot, R. (1966): On the origin of homovanillic acid in the cerebrospinal fluid. *Experientia,* 22:609–610.

Bartholini, G., Bates, H. M., Burkard, W. P., and Pletscher, A. (1967): Increase of cerebral catecholamines caused by 3,4-dihydroxyphenylalanine after inhibition of peripheral decarboxylase. *Nature,* 215:852–853.

Bartholini, G., Da Prada, M., and Pletscher, A. (1968): Decrease of cerebral 5-hydroxytryptamine by 3,4-dihydroxyphenylalanine after inhibition of extracerebral decarboxylase. *Journal of Pharmacy and Pharmacology,* 20:228–229.

Bartholini, G. and Pletscher, A. (1968): Cerebral accumulation and metabolism of ^{14}C-DOPA after selective inhibition of peripheral decarboxylase. *Journal of Pharmacology and Experimental Therapeutics,* 161:14–20.

Bartholini, G. and Pletscher, A. (1969): Enhancement of tyrosine hydroxylation within the brain by chlorpromazine. *Experientia,* 25:919–920.

Bartholini, G., Tissot, R., and Pletscher, A. (1969): Selective increase of cerebral dopamine: a therapeutic possibility in parkinsonism. In: *Third Symposium on Parkinson's Disease, Edinburgh, May 1968,* edited by F. J. Gillingham and I. M. L. Donaldson. E. & S. Livingstone Ltd., Edinburgh.

Bartholini, G., Gey, K. F., and Pletscher, A. (1970a): Enhancement of tyrosine transamination *in vivo* by catecholamines. *Experientia,* 26:980–981.

Bartholini, G., Kuruma, I., and Pletscher, A. (1970b): Distribution and metabolism of L-3-O-methyldopa in rats. *British Journal of Pharmacology*, 40:461–467.
Bartholini, G., Pletscher, A., and Kuruma I. (1970c): Metabolism of L-DOPA after inhibition of extracerebral decarboxylase and metabolic fate of L-3-O-methyldopa. In: *Proceedings of IV Bel Air Symposium Monoamines et noyaux gris centraux, Geneva, September 1970*, edited by J. de Ajuriaguerra. George et Masson, Geneva.
Bartholini, G., Tissot, R., and Pletscher, A. (1971): Brain capillaries as a source of homovanillic acid in cerebrospinal fluid. *Brain Research*, 27:163–168.
Bartholini, G., and Pletscher, A. (1971): Atropine-induced changes of cerebral dopamine turnover. *Experientia* 27:1302–1303.
Bertler, A., Falck, B., Owman, C. H., and Rosengrenn, E. (1966): The localization of monoaminergic blood-brain barrier mechanism. *Pharmacological Reviews*, 18:369–385.
Bogdanski, D. F., Weissbach, H., and Udenfriend, S. (1957): The distribution of serotonin, 5-hydroxytryptophan decarboxylase, and monoamine oxidase in brain. *Journal of Neurochemistry*, 1:272–278.
Burkard, W. P., Gey, K. F., and Pletscher, A. (1966): Neuroleptika als Aktivatoren der Tyrosinhydroxylierung *in vivo*. *Helvetica Physiologica Pharmalogica Acta*, 24:c78–80.
Burkard, W. P., Gey, K. F., and Pletscher, A. (1967): Activation of tyrosine hydroxylation in rat brain *in vivo* by chlorpromazine. *Nature*, 213:732–733.
Carlsson, A., and Lindqvist, M. (1963): Effect of chlorpromazine or haloperidol on formation of 3-methoxytyramine and normetanephrine in mouse brain. *Acta Pharmacologia Toxicologica (Copenhagen)*, 20:140–144.
Constantinidis, J., Bartholini, G., Tissot, R., and Pletscher, A. (1968): Accumulation of dopamine in the parenchyma after decarboxylase inhibition in the capillaries of brain. *Experientia*, 24:130–131.
Constantinidis, J., Bartholini, G., Geissbühler, F., and Tissot, R. (1970): La barrière capillaire enzymatique pour la DOPA au niveau de quelques noyaux du tronc cérébral du rat. *Experientia*, 26:381–383.
Costa, E., and Neff, N. H. (1966): Isotopic and non-isotopic measurements of the rate of catecholamine biosynthesis. In: *Biochemistry and Pharmacology of the Basal Ganglia*, edited by E. Costa, L. J. Côté, and M. D. Yahr. Raven Press, New York.
Da Prada, M. and Pletscher, A. (1966): On the mechanism of chlorpromazine-induced changes of cerebral homovanillic acid levels. *Journal of Pharmacy and Pharmacology*, 18:628–630.
Everett, G. M. and Borcherdiry, J. W. (1970): L-DOPA: Effect on concentration of dopamine, norepinephrine, and serotonin in brains of mice. *Science*, 168:849–850.
Falck, N., Hillarp, A., Thieme, G., and Thorp, A. (1962): Fluorescence of catecholamines and related compounds condensed with formaldehyde. *Journal of Histochemistry and Cytochemistry*, 10:348–354.
Ferrini, R., and Glässer, A. (1964): *In vitro* decarboxylation of new phenylalanine derivatives. *Biochemical Pharmacology*, 13:798–800.
Gey, K. F., and Pletscher, A. (1964): Effects of chlorpromazine on the metabolism of dl-2-^{14}C-DOPA in the rat. *Journal of Pharmacology and Experimental Therapeutics*, 145:337–343.
Hornykiewicz, O. (1968): Gegenwärtiger Stand der biochemisch-pharmakologischen Erforschung des extrapyramidal-motorischen Systems. *Pharmakopsychiatrie, Neuro-Psychopharmakologie*, 1:6–17.
Kuruma, I., Bartholini, G., and Pletscher, A. (1970): L-DOPA-induced accumulation of 3-O-methyl-DOPA in brain and heart. *European Journal of Pharmacology*, 10:189–192.
Kuruma, I., Bartholini, G., Tissot, R., and Pletscher, A. (1971): The metabolism of L-3-O-methyl-DOPA, a precursor of DOPA in man. *Clinical Pharmacology and Therapeutics*. 12:678–682.
Kuruma, I., Bartholini, G., Tissot, R., and Pletscher, A. (1972): Comparative investigation of inhibitors of extracerebral DOPA-decarboxylase in man and rat. *Journal of Pharmacy and Pharmacology*, 24:289–296.

Laverty, R., and Sharman, D. F. (1965): Modification of drugs of the metabolism of 3,4-di-hydroxyphenylethylamine, noradrenaline and 5-hydroxytryptamine in the brain. *British Journal of Pharmacology and Chemotherapy*, 24:759–772.

McLennan, H. (1964): The release of acetylcholine and of 3-hydroxytyramine from the caudate nucleus. *Journal of Physiology*, 174:152–161.

Neff, N. H. and Costa, E. (1966): Effect of tricyclic antidepressants and chlorpromazine on brain catecholamine synthesis. *Proceedings of the First International Symposium on Anti-depressant Drugs*. Excerpta Medica International Congress, Series No. 122.

Nybäck, H. and Sedvall, G. (1968): Effect of chlorpromazine on accumulation and disappearance of catecholamines formed from tyrosine-^{14}C in brain. *Journal of Pharmacology and Experimental Therapeutics*, 162:294–301.

O'Keefe, R., Sharman, D. F., and Vogt, M. (1970): Effect of drugs used in psychoses on cerebral dopamine metabolism. *British Journal of Pharmacology*, 38:287–304.

Pletscher, A., Bartholini, G., and Tissot, R. (1967a): Metabolic fate of L-^{14}C-DOPA in cerebrospinal fluid and blood plasma of humans. *Brain Research*, 4:106–109.

Pletscher, A., Gey, K. F., and Burkard, W. P. (1967b): Effect of neuroleptics on the cerebral metabolism of catecholamines. In: *Proceedings of the European Society for the Study of Drug Toxicity, Vol. 9. Toxicity and Side Effects of Psychotropic Drugs*. Paris, February 1967, pp. 98–106. Excerpta Medica International Congress, Series 145.

Pletscher, A., Bartholini, G., Gey, K. F., and Jenni, A. (1970): Die biochemischen Grundlagen für die Behandlung des Parkinson-Syndroms mit L-DOPA. *Schweizerische Medizinische Wochenschrift*, 19:797–804.

Poirier, L. J., Bouvier, G., Bédard, P., Boucher, R., La Rochelle, L., Olivier, A., and Singh, P. (1969): Essai sur les circuits neuronaux impliqués dans le tremblement postural et l'hypokinésie. *Revue Neurologique*, 120:15–40.

Rao, N. S. (1970): Effect of withdrawing DOPA in Parkinson's disease. *Lancet*, 2:470–471.

Roos, B. E. (1965): Effect of certain tranquillizers on the level of homovanillic acid in the corpus striatum. *Journal of Pharmacy and Pharmacology*, 17:820–821.

Thoenen, H., Hürlimann, A., and Haefely, W. (1965): On the mode of action of chlorpromazine on peripheral adrenergic mechanisms. *International Journal of Neuropharmacology*, 4:79–89.

Tissot, R., Bartholini, G., and Pletscher, A. (1969): Drug-induced changes of extracerebral DOPA metabolism in man. *Archives of Neurology*, 20:187–190.

Wurtmann, R. J., Rose, C. M., Matthysse, S., Stephenson, J., and Baldessarini, R. (1970): L-dihydroxyphenylalanine: Effect on S-adenosylmethionine in brain. *Science*, 169:395–397.

Advances in Biochemical Psychopharmacology, Vol. 6
Raven Press, New York © 1972

Molecular Basis of Inhibition of Monooxygenases by p-Halophenylalanines

E. M. Gál

Division of Neurobiochemistry, Department of Psychiatry, University of Iowa College of Medicine, Iowa City, Iowa

The use of halo-amino acid analogs as metabolic antagonists as well as their ability to incorporate into microbial protein are well established (Shive and Skinner, 1963). Following the observation of a selective reduction of cerebral serotonin (5-HT) by chloroamphetamine derivatives (Pletscher, Burkard, Bruderer, and Gey, 1963; Fuller, Hines, and Mills, 1965), Koe and Weissman (1966) described specific depletion of brain 5-HT by p-chlorophenylalanine (PCP) and by p-chlorophenylpyruvic acid (PCPPA). Subsequently, Jequier, Lovenberg, and Sjoerdsma (1967) demonstrated that the selective depletion of 5-HT was due to irreversible inactivation of cerebral tryptophan-5-hydroxylase by PCP. The inactivation of this enzyme by PCPPA *in vivo* was shown to be the result of very active transamination of PCPPA to PCP (Gál, Roggeveen, and Millard, 1970). A statistically significant decrease in the transport of both tryptophan and 5-hydroxytryptophan into brain was also noted as a consequence of PCP administration.

Further studies in our laboratory with intraperitoneally administered radioactive PCP established the incorporation of this amino acid analog into cerebral tryptophan-5-hydroxylase and hepatic phenylalanine-4-hydroxylase (Gál et al., 1970). These two monooxygenases were irreversibly inactivated. It was found that the reappearance of enzymic activity was functional to the disappearance of radioactivity in the enzyme protein.

However, a mechanistically similar enzyme, cerebral tyrosine hydroxylase, in spite of the demonstration of incorporation of (^{14}C)p-halophenylalanines, was not inactivated. This led us to postulate that the irreversible inactivation *in vivo* of the two monooxygenases by the p-halophenylalanines

149

was primarily due to their incorporation into the enzyme protein near or at the active site (Gál and Millard 1971).

During this work, we isolated enzymatically and electrophoretically pure samples of phenylalanine-4-hydroxylase in quantities sufficient to study the nature of PCP-produced inactivation at the molecular level (Gál and Millard, *submitted for publication*). This chapter discusses, therefore, some of the changes in the nature of the enzyme thus inactivated.

INCORPORATION OF HALO-SUBSTITUTED AMINO ACIDS INTO PROTEIN

The evidence for the incorporation of halo-substituted amino acids is well established, particularly with respect to the protein of bacterial origin. Even though similar studies with proteins of mammalian sources are considerably less extensive, the few examples given in Table 1 are sufficiently corroborative to establish the presence of a mechanism enabling incorporation of these analogs via the existing pathways of protein synthesis. To this date, only two examples exist where incorporation of a halo-amino acid will lead to functional impairment of an enzyme from mammalian tissues (see Table 1.).

The irreversible inactivation of these monooxygenases as a result of *p*-halophenylalanine administration is of about 1-week's duration as measured for cerebral tryptophan-5-hydroxylase in the $30,000 \times g$ super-

TABLE 1. *Some studies of incorporation of halo-substituted amino acids into protein*

Compound	System	Effect	Reference
Fluorotryptophans	*E. coli* — wild	Inhibits growth	Browne, Kenyon, and
	E. coli — mutant	Stimulates growth and incorporates	Hegeman (1970)
p-Fluorophenylalanine	Rabbit muscle aldolase	No enzyme inhibition with incorporation	Westhead and Boyer (1961)
p-Fluorophenylalanine	Plasma and pancreas protein	Incorporation	Dolan and Godin (1966)
p-Chlorophenylalanine	Lipoyl dehydrogenase	No effect	Millard, Kubose, and
	Transhydrogenase	No effect	Gál (1969)
	Succinic dehydrogenase		
	Tyrosine 3-hydroxylase	No effect	Gál and Millard (1971)
	Tryptophan 5-Hydroxylase	Inactivation	
	Phenylalanine 4-Hydroxylase	Inactivation	

natant (Jequier et al., 1967) and in the purified enzyme (Gál and Roggeveen, *submitted for publication*). A similar pattern is obvious from the time-course experiments with purified labeled phenylalanine-4-hydroxylase (AlC$_\gamma$ stage) (Fig. 1). It is apparent from these time-course studies that the maximum incorporation of ^{14}C-PCP coincides with maximal inactivation of the enzyme and that 6 days later, when the enzymic activity is approaching the original level, the radioactive values indicate an 80% drop compared to the maximal incorporation. In agreement with Guroff (1969), the half-life of phenylalanine-4-hydroxylase in the rat is 48 hr.

To assess the actual irreversible nature of the inactivation as distinguished from competitive or noncompetitive inhibition, it is critical to probe the activity with the purified enzyme rather than with the tissue supernatants. During the first 48 hr, the free drug may still be present at an inhibitory concentration. For instance, following intraperitoneal administration of PCP (300 mg/kg) to rats, the $100,000 \times g$ supernatant of liver and

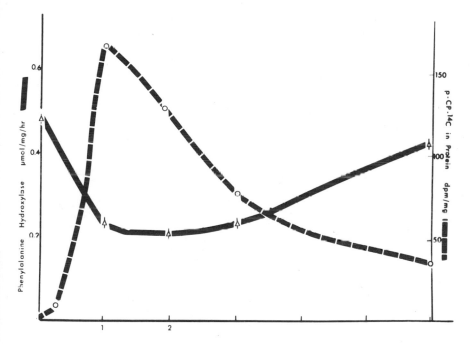

FIG. 1. Phenylalanine hydroxylase activity and *p*-chloro-(^{14}C)phenylalanine (^{14}C)*p*-CP in phenylalanine hydroxylase purified to the AlC$_\gamma$ stage. *p*-chloro-(^{14}C)phenylalanine (300 mg/kg, 90 μC/kg) was administered intraperitoneally at day 0. Enzyme was purified from the combined livers of three rats and assays were run in duplicate. From Gál and Millard (1971), reproduced by permission of *Biochimica et Biophysica Acta*.

TABLE 2. *Effect of cycloheximide on the incorporation of (2-¹⁴C) p-CP and (¹⁴C) tyrosine into rat liver and brain protein*

Compounds injected[a]	Radioactivity recovered							
	Liver				Brain			
	AA[b] (dpm/mg)	RNA-AA[c] (dpm/mg RNA)	S-RNA-AA[d] (dpm/mg RNA)	Protein (dpm/mg)	AA[b] (dpm/mg)	RNA-AA[c] (dpm/mg RNA)	S-RNA-AA[d] (dpm/mg RNA)	Protein (dpm/mg)
Tyrosine (1)	6,940	619	–	209	4,284	913	–	98
Tyrosine + cyclo-heximide (1)	29,100	230	–	17	11,700	284	–	7
p-CP (2)	42,000	230	14	23	26,250	302	21	16
p-CP + cyclohexi-mide (2)	43,000	93	< 1	< 1	20,000	104	< 1	< 1

[a] Cycloheximide (2.0 mg), 2 μC ¹⁴C-tyrosine, and 1.8 μC ¹⁴C-p-CP were injected intraperitoneally at 0, 1, 2, and 3 hr; cycloheximide (400 μg) was also injected into each cortical hemisphere at 0 hr. Animals were sacrificed at 4 hr. Number of animals in parentheses.
[b] Free amino acid (cold HClO₄ extract).
[c] Amino acid esterified to total RNA (hot HClO₄ extract).
[d] Amino acid esterified to soluble RNA (hot HClO₄ extract).
From Gal and Millard (1971), reproduced by permission of *Biochimica et Biophysica Acta*.

TABLE 3. *Effect of cycloheximide on inhibition of hepatic phenylalanine-4-hydroxylase by p-CP*

Exp. no.	Cycloheximide (mg/kg)	Time (hr)	Step of enzyme purification	Control	Cycloheximide	p-CP	p-CP[a] + cycloheximide
					(μmole tyrosine mg/hr ± S.E.)		
1	4	24	(NH$_4$)$_2$SO$_4$	0.16 ± 0.01	0.16 ± 0.01	0.08 ± 0.01	0.12[b]
2	3	24	(NH$_4$)$_2$SO$_4$	0.17 ± 0.01	—	0.06 ± 0.01	0.13 ± 0.01
			AlC$_\gamma$	0.34 ± 0.02		0.05 ± 0.01	0.22 ± 0.02
4	3	48	(NH$_4$)$_2$SO$_4$	0.18 ± 0.01	0.16 ± 0.01	0.09 ± 0.01	0.15 ± 0.01
			AlC$_\gamma$	0.50 ± 0.01	0.48 ± 0.02	0.20 ± 0.02	0.40 ± 0.01

Enzyme purified from combined livers of three animals; duplicate enzyme assays.
[a] p-CP (300 mg/kg) administered i.p. 2 hr after cycloheximide.
[b] Liver from single animal due to high mortality at 4 mg/kg cycloheximide.
From Gál and Millard (1971), reproduced by permission of Biochimica et Biophysica Acta.

brain contained about 1 to 5×10^{-4} M PCP ($K_i = 3 \times 10^{-4}$ M) over a 48-hr period.

Further evidence was obtained for the active incorporation of p-halophenylalanines by demonstrating that pretreatment of the animals with puromycin aminonucleoside or with cycloheximide prior to injection of the inhibitor substantially reduced incorporation (Table 2). Following inhibition of incorporation of PCP, substantial reduction in the inactivation of the enzyme took place (Table 3).

We have also measured ^{14}C-phenylalanine esterified to total RNA and these studies *in vivo* also indicate that phenylalanine-t-RNA formation has outstripped p-chlorophenylalanyl-t-RNA by about a three-to-one ratio. This difference might be interpreted in terms of the results obtained by Dunn and Leach (1967) with p-fluorophenylalanine in a cell-free *Escherichia coli* system. According to these authors, the accessibility of the two codons for the natural amino acid is limited to one codon for the p-halophenylalanines. Experimental evidence was offered to show that a decrease in incorporation of p-fluorophenylalanine into protein was functionally related to the increased UC copolymers in the incubation system. The cross-reactivity of AAA and GAA anticodons of phenylalanine is, therefore, not available to p-halophenylalanines since the GAA-t-RNA was not charged by p-fluorophenylalanine on the enzyme. This is consistent with the hypothesis that for p-halophenylalanines AAA-t-RNA is the only anticodon reacting with UUU codon.

PREPARATIVE AND ANALYTICAL DISC GEL
ELECTROPHORESIS OF PHENYLALANINE-4-
HYDROXYLASE

Pure phenylalanine-4-hydroxylase was isolated by preparative gel electrophoresis of the enzyme protein which was carried through the calcium phosphate gel stage of purification (Kaufman and Fisher, 1970). The protein was run at 4°C with 2.5% Tris–2.9% glycine buffer, pH 8.5, in the electrophoresis unit and 0.02 M Tris acetate buffer, pH 7.3, in the elution chamber according to the method described by Gál and Millard (*submitted for publication*). The design of the preparative gel electrophoresis unit was that of Orr, Blakley, and Panagou (1972). There was no significant difference between the elution volumes for the enzymes from control and PCP-treated rats. The purity of the enzyme protein obtained from the livers of control and PCP-treated rats was assessed by measuring its specific enzymic activity and by analytical gel electrophoresis. Figure 2 shows that

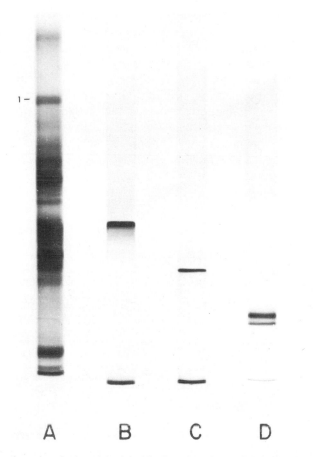

FIG. 2. Electrophoresis of phenylalanine-4-hydroxylase on polyacrylamide gel (13%). Electrophoresis was carried out at 6°C at 5 mamp/tube. Gel length was 18 cm. After the gels were fixed in 20% trichloroacetic acid for 1 hr, the protein bands were localized by staining the gels with 0.1% amido black. Gels—*A:* Enzyme (0.4 mg) (CaPO$_4$-gel step) run 22 hr. Electrolyte was 0.02 M Tris-glycine buffer, pH 8.75. Band 1 has the enzyme activity. *B:* Pure enzyme (0.1 mg) after 16 hr. *C:* Pure enzyme (0.05 mg) (from liver of PCP-treated rats) run 20 hr. *D:* Enzyme (0.05 mg) run 10 hr. Samples *B, C,* and *D* were run in 0.05 M phosphate buffer, pH 7.0.

even on overloading the gel with 100 μg of enzyme protein (control), a single band was obtained corresponding to the enzyme activity. The extent of purification is especially striking when one compares it to the electrophoretic pattern of the protein at the calcium phosphate gel stage.

Chromatographic analysis of hydrolysates of purified ^{14}C-PCP-labeled phenylalanine-4-hydroxylase established the presence of radioactivity as

[14]C-PCP in the enzyme protein (Gál et al., 1970). Subsequent analysis of the pure protein indicates that in the event of complete inactivation, one residue of PCP per molecule of enzyme is incorporated (Table 4). The amount of label that can be recovered in a molecule of the pure enzyme protein is almost functional to the degree of the inhibition measurable at the first step of purification [ethanol or $(NH_4)_2SO_4$ fractionation]. The specific radioactivity of the enzyme protein remains fairly constant from the calcium phosphate gel stage through either AlC_γ or preparative gel purification. [14]C-*p*-Fluorophenylalanine is not suitable for quantitative studies of incorporation since almost 50% will be converted into tyrosine *in vivo* (Dolan and Godin, 1966; Gál et al., 1970).

TABLE 4. *Recovery of Radioactive PCP in pure phenylalanine-4-hydroxylase*

Step of enzyme purification	Time of sacrifice (hr)	Specific activity		Inhibition (%)	^{14}C-PCP (dpm/mg)	Mole PCP per mole enzyme
		Control (mmole/mg/min)	PCP			
$(NH_4)_2SO_4$	24[a]	0.012	0.006	50	170	
Prep. gel		0.44	0.018	96	314	0.48
$(NH_4)_2SO_4$	48[b]	0.015	0.005	70	250	
Prep. gel		0.48	0.024	95	400	0.77

Injected intraperitoneally [a]1.75×10^8 and [b]1.4×10^8 dpm of ^{14}C-DL-PCP, respectively.

Proteins can be separated by analytical gel electrophoresis in the presence of an anionic detergent such as sodium dodecyl sulfate (SDS). The separation is an expression of the molecular weights of the polypeptide chains (Shapiro, Viñuela, and Maizel, 1967). Pure phenylalanine hydroxylase from livers of control and PCP-injected animals (as shown in Fig. 2) after incubation for 4 hr in 0.1 M phosphate containing 1% mercaptoethanol and 1% SDS at 37°C, and following dialysis for 15 hr, invariably yielded four major bands for the control on SDS-polyacrylamide gels and three bands for the PCP-enzyme protein. The disappearance of band 5 (Fig. 3) from the PCP enzyme is striking. At present, no explanation of this can be offered without knowing the nature of this peptide from the control sample. Additionally, the gels C and D which depict the pattern of difference between the control and PCP enzymes after 2 weeks of storage seem to reveal possible differences in the lability of the enzyme subunits.

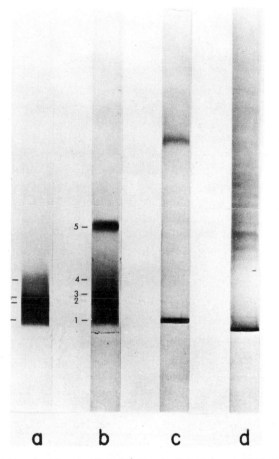

FIG. 3. Electrophoresis of pure phenylalanine hydroxylase on SDS (0.1%)-containing polyacrylamide gels. The enzyme proteins were prepared by incubation of the native enzymes in phosphate buffer containing 1% mercaptoethanol and 1% SDS for 3 hr at 37°C. Samples were dialyzed overnight. Gels—*a:* PCP enzyme (120 μg). *b:* Control enzyme (120 μg). Electrolyte was 0.05 M phosphate buffer at pH 7.0. Samples were run 8 hr at 25°C at 8 mamp/tube. After being fixed in 20% TCA, the gels were stained with 0.05% Coomassie blue for 3 hr and destained with 20% acetic acid. *c, d:* 100-μg samples of control and PCP enzyme, respectively, after 3 weeks of storage at −24°C. Samples were run in 0.02 M Tris-glycine, pH 8.75, for 23 hr at 6°C. After fixing, the gels were stained with 0.1% amido black and destained electrolytically.

AMINO ACID ANALYSES AND MEASUREMENT
OF CONFORMATIONAL CHANGES

Samples (5 mg) of pure enzyme protein from control and PCP-treated rats were hydrolyzed with 6 N HCl for 24 hr at 110°C and submitted to amino acid analyses (Gál and Millard, *submitted for publication*) (Table 5). The results of molecular weight determinations indicate that the enzyme may be a monomer, dimer, or tetramer (Kaufman and Fisher, 1970). Our preliminary measurements of the molecular weight of this enzyme suggest that the dimer is about 134,000 as compared to 110,000 as determined by Kaufman and Fisher (1970), and this value was used in calculating some of the physicochemical parameters of the enzyme protein.

We suspected that the differences obtained by SDS electrophoresis and after storage were the consequences not only of changes in the primary structure of the enzyme but also of those of higher order due to the incorporation of PCP *in vivo*. Accordingly we have undertaken to investi-

TABLE 5. *Amino acid composition of phenylalanine-4-hydroxylase*

Amino acid	mmole/100 g protein	
	Control	PCP
Lysine	9.8	11.1
Histidine	3.7	4.1
Arginine	8.1	8.1
Aspartic acid	15.9	18.1
Threonine	8.7	10.1
Serine	10.5	11.2
Glutamic acid	19.0	20.0
Proline	8.7	9.8
Glycine	11.7	14.4
Alanine	12.4	13.7
Half-cystine	1.5	1.5
Valine	10.9	12.7
Methionine	3.4	4.4
Isoleucine	8.4	8.9
Leucine	15.7	15.0
Tyrosine	5.5	5.3
Phenylalanine	7.3	7.0
Tryptophan[a]	2.2	2.9

[a] Measured by the method of Edelhoch (1967).

gate some of the differences due to possible changes in conformation that may have occurred as a consequence of PCP incorporation. Measurement of the excitation and emission spectra as well as changes in the intensity of fluorescence at various wavelengths revealed no difference between the PCP-labeled enzyme protein and that of the control; i.e., at 273 nm excitation, the emission maximum was at 325 nm. In order to separate the possible tyrosine and tryptophan components, we have investigated the relative fluorescence intensities at 275, 285, and 295 nm excitation with emission monochromators set at 308, 325, and 350 nm as suggested by Weber (1961). There is apparently no detectable contribution from tyrosine in either sample of enzyme protein.

Next we examined the possible conformational changes with optical rotatory dispersion (ORD) and CD with a Cary Model 60, along with the ultraviolet spectrum. First we looked at the CD of L-phenylalanine and L-PCP. At equimolar concentration, there is not only an increase of intensity of L-PCP but also a change in both position and number of the bands, although in both instances the bands remain positive (Fig. 4). The appearance of a new band owing to the 4-chloro-substitution with a maximum at 273.5 nm is particularly marked. In view of the differences in the CD spectrum between L-phenylalanine and L-p-chlorophenylalanine (Fig. 4), it was possible that incorporation of this analog into the protein might affect the optical properties of the enzyme. The circular dichroism of the two species of the enzyme protein measured at pH 7.4 with 0.025 M Tris acetate buffer (Fig. 5) revealed only minor differences, the significance of which is under further investigation.

The ORD expressed as the mean residual specific rotation $[m']_{230}^{22°}$ was $-4,208$ for control and $-3,538$ for the PCP-incorporated enzyme.

MODE OF ACTION OF PCP AND PCA

Recently it was shown that some of the p-chloro-substituted amines affect the activity of tryptophan hydroxylase from rat brain stem during the first 24 hr after their administration without affecting the enzyme activity in assays *in vitro* (Sanders-Bush and Bushing, 1971). We have confirmed this but find that the mode of action is quite different from that of the p-halophenylalanines. For instance, there is no inhibition of hepatic phenylalanine-4-hydroxylase, nor is the time course of the inhibition of the cerebral tryptophan hydroxylase comparable to that caused by PCP (Fig. 6). Sanders-Bush and Bushing (1971) could not reverse the inhibition by

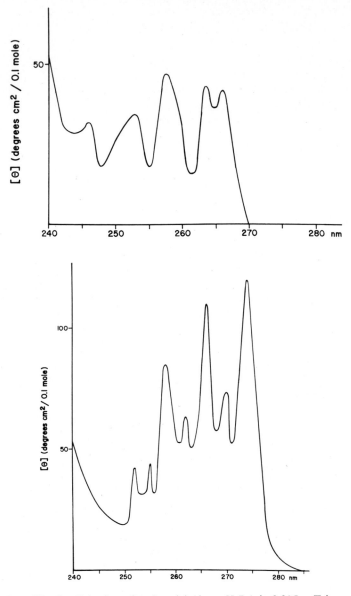

FIG. 4. *Top:* Circular dichroism of ʟ-phenylalanine, pH 7.4, in 0.025 ᴍ Tris-acetate buffer. Spectra were obtained on solutions containing 3.1 mg/ml in a 1.0 cm cell. Measurement at 23°C.

Bottom: Circular dichroism of ʟ-*p*-chlorophenylalanine at pH 7.4. Conditions as above.

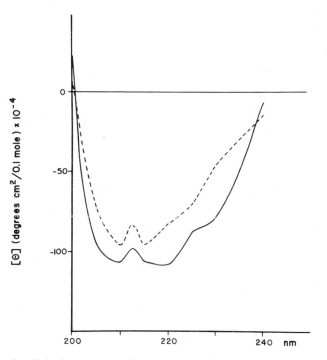

FIG. 5. Circular dichroism spectra of pure phenylalanine-4-hydroxylase at pH 7.4 in 0.05 M Tris-acetate buffer. Enzyme protein was 0.06% from control (–●–●–) and 0.18% from PCP-treated animals (–○–○–) in a 0.5-cm cell at 23°C.

dialysis, and they postulate the formation of an "active metabolite" of *p*-chloroamphetamine (PCA). This is unlikely. We have demonstrated that the effect of dialysis is difficult to interpret because of the sensitivity of cerebral tryptophan-5-hydroxylase to dialysis *per se* (Gál et al., 1970). Furthermore, the dialyzed tryptophan-5-hydroxylase requires the addition of an endogenous factor (Gál, 1971) as well as one of the known pteridine cofactors for activity.

The data reviewed in this chapter lend further support to the concept that the *p*-halophenylalanines cause irreversible inactivation of some of the monooxygenases by changes in the primary structure of the enzyme protein near or at the active site.

Now that we can prepare pure phenylalanine-4-hydroxylase in amounts necessary for peptide sequencing, the testing of the above hypothesis has become feasible.

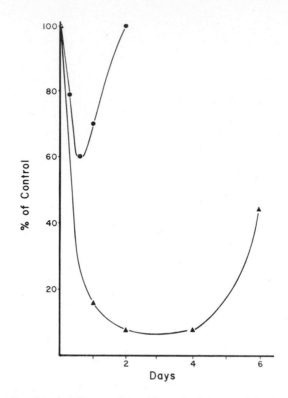

FIG. 6. Tryptophan-5-hydroxylase activity of rat brain stems following intraperitoneal administration of *p*-chloroamphetamine (10 mg/kg) (–●–●–) or *p*-chlorophenylalanine (300 mg/kg) (–▲–▲–).

REFERENCES

Browne, D. T., Kenyon, G. L., and Hegeman, G. D. (1970): Incorporation of monofluoro-tryptophans into protein during the growth of *Escherichia coli*. *Biochemical and Biophysical Research Communications*, 39:13–19.

Dolan, G., and Godin, C. (1966): *In vivo* formation of tyrosine from *p*-fluorophenylalanine. *Biochemistry*, 5:922–925.

Dunn, T. F., and Leach, F. R. (1967): Incorporation of *p*-fluorophenylalanine into protein by a cell-free system. *Journal of Biological Chemistry*, 242:2693–2699.

Edelhoch, H. (1967): Spectroscopic determination of tryptophan and tyrosine in proteins. *Biochemistry*, 6:1948–1954.

Fuller, R. W., Hines, C. W., and Mills, J. (1965): Lowering of brain serotonin levels by chlor-amphetamines. *Biochemical Pharmacology*, 14:483–488.

Gál, E. M. (1971): Stimulation of cerebral hydroxylases by a new factor. *Federation Proceedings*, 30:1085 Abs.

Gál, E. M. and Millard, S. A. (1971): The mechanism of inhibition of hydroxylases *in vivo* by p-cholorophenylalanine: The effect of cycloheximide. *Biochimica et Biophysica Acta,* 227: 32–41.

Gál, E. M., and Millard, S. A.: Inactivation of hepatic phenylalanine 4-hydroxylase by *p*-chlorophenylalanine: Molecular aspects *(submitted for publication).*

Gál, E. M., and Roggeveen, A. E. (1972): Purification and properties of cerebral tryptophan-5-hydroxylase *(submitted for publication).*

Gál, E. M., Roggeveen, A. E., and Millard, S. A. (1970): DL-[2-¹⁴C] *p*-Chlorophenylalanine as an inhibitor of tryptophan 5-hydroxylase. *Journal of Neurochemistry,* 17:1221–1235.

Guroff, G. (1969): Irreversible in vivo inhibition of rat liver phenylalanine hydroxylase by *p*-chlorophenylalanine. *Archives of Biochemistry and Biophysics,* 134:610–611.

Hedrick, J. L., and Smith, A. J. (1968): Size and charge isomer separation and estimation of molecular weights of proteins by disc gel electrophoresis. *Archives of Biochemistry and Biophysics,* 126:155–164.

Jequier, E., Lovenberg, W., and Sjoerdsma, A. (1967): Tryptophan hydroxylase inhibition: The mechanism by which *p*-chlorophenylalanine depletes rat brain serotonin. *Molecular Pharmacology,* 3:274–278.

Kaufman, S., and Fisher, D. B. (1970): Purification and some physical properties of phenylalanine hydroxylase from rat liver. *Journal of Biological Chemistry,* 245:4745–4750.

Koe, B. K., and Weissman, A. (1966): *p*-Chlorophenylalanine: Specific depletor of brain serotonin. *Journal of Pharmacology and Experimental Therapeutics,* 154:499–516.

Millard, S. A., Kubose, A. and Gál, E. M. (1969): Brain lipoyl dehydrogenase: Purification, properties and inhibitors. *Journal of Biological Chemistry,* 244:2511–2515.

Orr, M. D., Blakley, R. L., and Panagou, D. (1972): Discontinuous buffer systems for analytical and preparative electrophoresis of enzymes on polyacrylamide gels. *Analytical Biochemistry* 45.68–85.

Pletscher, A., Burkard, W. P., Bruderer, H., and Gey, K. F. (1963): Decrease of cerebral 5-hydroxytryptamine and 5-hydroxyindoleacetic acid by an arylalkylamine. *Life Sciences,* 2:828–833.

Sanders-Bush, E., and Bushing, J. A. (1971): Inhibition of cerebral tryptophan hydroxylase by *p*-chloroamphetamine (PCA). *Federation Proceedings,* 30:381.

Shapiro, A. L., Vinuela, E., and Maizel, J. V. (1967): Molecular weight estimation of polypeptide chains by electrophoresis in SDS-polyacrylamide gels. *Biochemical and Biophysical Research Communications,* 28:815–820.

Shive, W., and Skinner, C. G. (1963): Amino acid analogs. In: *Metabolic Inhibitors* Vol. I, pp. 1–73, edited by R. M. Hochster and J. H. Quastel. Academic Press, New York.

Weber, G. (1961): Enumeration of components in complex systems by fluorescence spectrophotometry. *Nature,* 190:27–29.

Westhead, E. W. and Boyer, P. D. (1961): The incorporation of p-fluorophenylalanine into some rabbit enzymes and other proteins. *Biochimica et Biophysica Acta,* 54:145–156.

Advances in Biochemical Psychopharmacology, Vol. 6
Raven Press, New York © 1972

Glutamic Acid and Primary Afferent Transmission

Richard Hammerschlag and Daniel Weinreich

*Division of Neurosciences, City of Hope National Medical Center,
Duarte, California 91010*

Glutamic acid is the leading candidate for a role as an excitatory transmitter at two synapses widely differing in both phylogenetic localization and neural function: the primary afferent synapse of vertebrates and the neuromuscular junction of arthropods. This situation points up the neurochemical curiosity that while vertebrate motoneurons are cholinergic and sensory neurons are not, the reverse pattern of transmitter coding exists in crustacea and insects where sensory neurons appear to traffic in acetylcholine (ACh) (Florey, 1967).

The present review will focus on the vertebrate primary afferent synapse in the spinal cord. A pharmacology of this synapse, which may begin to approach the array of therapeutic agents developed for modifying the cholinergic neuromuscular synapse, depends largely on establishing the identity of the "sensory" transmitter. At the same time, a comparison of the chemical and physiological mechanisms underlying these two types of excitatory synapses will help to define the unique properties of primary afferent transmission which may be pharmacologically modified. Brief descriptions of the anatomy and pharmacology of the primary afferent system will set the stage for a comparison of glutamate receptors in the spinal cord subserving excitation and uptake and for an assessment of the evidence for glutamate as the primary afferent transmitter.

ANATOMY

Primary afferent neurons serve to convey information from various types of somatic and visceral sensory transducers directly into the CNS for synaptic relay. Study of the cell bodies of these neurons is facilitated by their anatomical packaging into discrete ganglia lying just outside the spinal cord. Apparently no integration of afferent signals occurs at these soma since there is neither morphological nor physiological evidence of any synaptic contacts within the ganglia. The cell bodies, moreover, are not located in the usual place between dendrites and axon. Rather, primary afferent neurons are classified as unipolar since the axon bifurcates shortly after leaving the soma (Ha, 1970). The central branch enters the cord via the dorsal root, while the peripheral branch travels in the spinal nerve until it ramifies near its peripheral receptor sites. Both branches are considered to be axons, and both are frequently myelinated. The peripheral and central ramifications (dendrites and nerve endings, respectively), however, are always unmyelinated. Degeneration studies have shown that such central endings exhibit the clusters of vesicles and synaptic cleft typically associated with a chemical synapse (Ralston, 1968). The vesicle hypothesis may apply to the primary afferent synapse, since monosynaptic transmission of dorsal root impulses to spinal motoneurons occurs in quantal steps (Kuno, 1964).

Each dorsal root fiber, once in the cord, divides into ascending and descending branches which course in the dorsal funiculus; the ascending branch can travel without interruption as far as the medulla oblongata. Both branches send off numerous collaterals which synapse with spinal neurons to initiate intra- and intersegmental reflexes. Primary afferent fibers synapse with three types of neurons: motoneurons (cells whose axons can be traced out the ventral root), interneurons (cells which function in polysynaptic pathways between sensory and motoneurons), and sensory relay neurons (e.g., cells of Clarke's column nuclei, or the medullary cuneate and gracilis nuclei which relay afferent information to higher regions of the brain). Such primary afferent synapses are diverse in terms of their localization on the postsynaptic neuron (Rall, Burke, Smith, Nelson, and Frank, 1967), and in terms of their bouton size: axodendritic primary afferent endings on Clarke's column neurons, which form the largest synapses in the cord (Szentágothai and Albert, 1955), are about 10 times greater in diameter than primary afferent boutons on motoneurons (Haggar and Barr, 1950). Another type of synapse that may be relevant to primary afferent function is the axoaxonal synapse which appears to terminate on the afferent ending (Gray, 1962; Conradi, 1969). The possible significance of this finding as a basis for presynaptic inhibition will be discussed later.

The dorsal roots of the cat have been estimated to contain some one million fibers (Duncan and Keyser, 1938). These fibers vary in terms of sensory modality, diameter, degree of myelination, and synaptic localization and terminal size. In spite of this heterogeneous morphology, the current neurochemical assumption is that there is only one primary afferent excitatory transmitter substance. Perhaps, until proven wrong, we may consider this assumption as a "primary collateral" of Dale's law.

NEUROPHARMACOLOGY

No pharmacological agent has yet been shown to have its locus of action uniquely on one of the processes underlying primary afferent transmission. Drug studies, therefore, have been of little value in the identification of the substance(s) released from these terminals. This lack of specific antagonists does not imply that this particular synapse is resistant to pharmacological manipulation: short-acting depressants, such as thiopental, can reduce the amount of transmitter released by each afferent volley (Weakley, 1969); conversely, convulsant phenolic substances exert strong facilitory effects at the primary afferent synapse, presumably by increasing the amount of excitatory transmitter released by impulses in the primary afferent nerve (Banna and Jabbur, 1970).

It may also be possible to manipulate transmitter release by drugs acting at sites remote from those involved in quantal release. Eccles (1964) has proposed that the quantity of excitatory transmitter released from primary afferent terminals can be diminished via inhibitory axoaxonal synapses localized on primary afferent terminals. In his postulated mechanism of presynaptic inhibition, the inhibitory transmitter is released onto the primary afferent terminal membrane, initiating a depolarization. This action results in a diminution of the afferent nerve action potential and thereby reduces the quantity of excitatory transmitter released. Although there is considerable evidence for the existence of primary afferent depolarization (PAD), there remains some doubt concerning the origin of this phenomenon (Wall, 1964).

Since there appears to be a causal relationship between depolarization of the presynaptic fiber and inhibition of primary afferent transmission, several pharmacological investigations have dealt with the actions of drugs on these two processes (Eccles, 1964). The convulsant drug picrotoxin can simultaneously depress PAD and presynaptic inhibition, whereas strychnine, metrazol, and other convulsants lack direct effects (Eccles, Schmidt, and Willis, 1963). It can also be shown that certain anesthetics intensify both presynaptic inhibition and PAD. More thorough pharmacological investigations, however, have revealed that depolarization of afferent terminals and presynaptic inhibition can be dissociated (Miyahara, 1966a,b).

Both ethanol and procaine produced an increase in inhibition associated not with an increase in depolarization, but with a diminution in PAD. A similar dissociation of the two phenomena was noted after the administration of nonanesthetic agents such as diphenylhydantoin, tetrodotoxin, and guanidine. These findings led Miyahara to conclude that depolarization of primary afferent terminals is not the principal mediator of presynaptic inhibition. Whatever the mechanism(s) of presynaptic inhibition (Curtis and Felix, 1971), these results clearly demonstrate that synaptically mediated alterations of primary afferent terminal excitability can be modified by drugs.[1]

MOLECULAR PHARMACOLOGY

To map out a working model of a glutaminergic primary afferent synapse, we need to view two types of terrain. The first comprises two functionally distinct receptor sites for glutamate: a postsynaptic site which triggers a specific conductance change, and a site which may be pre- or postsynaptic or glial, which transports the amino acid out of the synaptic cleft. The second type of terrain is even less clearly marked and consists of sites through which transmitter-receptor interactions may be modified indirectly.

Comparison of Excitation and Uptake Sites

When glutamate is presumably released into the synaptic cleft, a portion of the transmitter reversibly combines with the postsynaptic receptors associated with ionic conductances before it too diffuses from the cleft or is actively transported into cells. It is of interest in terms of developing potential pharmacological antagonists to determine whether the receptors that subserve excitation are structurally different from those for uptake.

Considerable information about a glutamate excitatory receptor has been obtained by studying the effects of a series of acidic amino acid analogs on spinal neurons of the cat (Curtis and Watkins, 1960, 1963) and toad (Curtis, Phillis, and Watkins, 1961). By extensively modifying chain length and charged groups and by making the reasonable assumptions that the

---

[1] Recent studies in cat (Curtis, Duggan, Felix, and Johnston, 1971) and in frog (Davidoff, 1972) have demonstrated a specific blocking action of bicuculline on presynaptic inhibition. Use of this alkaloid may be to advantage in attempts to identify the primary afferent transmitter released by nerve stimulation.

compounds (unmetabolized) are all acting at a common membrane site, a three-point receptor was postulated as the best fit for the data. Since the acidic amino acid analogs were ranked in order of their efficacy of excitation, we could then test many of the same compounds for their ability to inhibit the uptake of glutamate into spinal cord slices (Hammerschlag, Potter, and Vinci, 1971). Because no evidence was found in cord for more than one glutamate uptake mechanism, we considered that the general property shared by all neural tissue to transport glutamate might also be utilized at the primary afferent synapse to terminate transmitter action. Again, on the supposition that those acidic amino acids which are actively taken up into cells are transported at a common site (Blasberg and Lajtha, 1965), it appeared that a three-point receptor model also fit the uptake site. Glutamate derivatives in which the polarity of any of the three charged moieties was modified were without effect on glutamate uptake when tested at a 40:1 molar ratio of analog:glutamate. A precise steric requirement is also indicated because α-Me-L-glutamate, α-NH$_2$-L-adipate, and DL-homocysteate, compounds with unsubstituted polar groups but possessing an additional carbon, were also without effect on glutamate uptake. L-Aspartate and L-cysteate, compounds which are similar in excitatory potency to L-glutamate, were the most effective competitive inhibitors tested of glutamate uptake, both having K_i values similar to the K_m for glutamate (Table 1). However, a 40-fold molar excess of N-Me-DL-aspartate or DL-homocysteate, compounds that are considerably more potent excitatory agents than glutamate, had a negligible effect on glutamate uptake. Since structurally

TABLE 1. *Comparison of excitatory potency of amino acids with their ability to competitively inhibit glutamate uptake*

Amino acid	Relative excitatory potency[a]	K_i (mM) for inhibition of L-glutamate uptake[b]
N-Me-D-Aspartate	100	[c]
N-Me-DL-Aspartate	45–65	[d]
DL-Homocysteate	30–55	[d]
L-Glutamate		0.020 (K_m)
L-Cysteate	8–20	0.010
L-Aspartate		0.009
D-Aspartate	4–10	0.012
D-Glutamate		1.20
γ-Methylene-L-glutamate	[c]	0.13

[a] Cat spinal neurons (Curtis and Watkins, 1963).
[b] Slices of rat spinal cord (Hammerschlag, Potter, and Vinci, 1971).
[c] Not tested.
[d] No significant inhibition at 40:1 molar ratio of test agent:L-glutamate.

similar amino acids are transported by a common carrier mechanism, the lack of inhibition by these analogs suggests that they are taken up into cord tissue to a very slight extent. A longer extracellular half-life for N-Me-DL-aspartate and DL-homocysteate would help to explain the pharmacological observation (Curtis and Watkins, 1960, 1963) that these compounds have a longer duration of action as well as a more potent excitatory effect on spinal neurons than do the parent L-amino acids, aspartate, cysteate, and glutamate. The observation that *p*-chloromercuriphenylsulfonate enhances L-glutamate- and L-aspartate-induced spinal excitation to a much greater extent than N-Me-DL-aspartate- or DL-homocysteate-induced excitation suggests that the effects of the mercurial may be on the uptake receptor rather than on the excitatory receptor (Curtis, Duggan, and Johnston, 1970). The neurotoxin β-N-oxalyl-L-α,β-diamino-propionate, the most potent L-amino acid excitant of spinal neurons (Watkins, Curtis, and Biscoe, 1966), was also without effect on glutamate uptake (Haskell and Hammerschlag, *unpublished observations*).

D-glutamate has a lower affinity for the uptake receptor than does either L-glutamate or both isomers of aspartate, as indicated by the relative K_i values (Table 1). This ranking is somewhat different than that found for the relative excitatory potency of these compounds on spinal neurons, where D-asparate and D-glutamate are each slightly less potent than their respective L-isomers (Curtis and Watkins, 1963), but is the same ranking as was found for excitation of cortical cells (Krnjević, 1970*b*).

Thus the two functionally distinct membrane sites for glutamate appear to contain different structural and sterochemical features. While several compounds (e.g., DL-homocysteate) interact with the excitatory receptor without significantly affecting uptake, an agent has yet to be found which will inhibit glutamate uptake and which itself does not produce excitation. The various intensities of excitation produced following the administration of acidic amino acids may reflect, in part, differential affinities for the membrane sites. It would thus be of considerable interest to compare the relative excitatory or competitive inhibitory potencies of these compounds under conditions where one site or the other has been inactivated. One might predict, for example, a shift in rank-order of excitatory potency when the amino acids are tested in tissue slices where the uptake mechanism has been inactivated by lowering the temperature. Of the few compounds that inhibit uptake, but have yet to be tested on excitable tissues, the most interesting is the antibiotic, avenaciolide, which was recently brought to our attention by Dr. Graham Johnston. This drug, although nonpolar, is isosteric with glutamate (McGiven and Chappell, 1970) and has been shown to inhibit uptake into both brain and spinal cord slices. Since the antibiotic is only effective if the tissue is pretreated, a "K_i" for comparison with aspartate inhibition cannot be determined. Gamma-methylene-L-glutamate, an ionic analog of avenaciolide, also inhibits glutamate uptake (Table 1).

Secondary Sites

In addition to developing drugs which may selectively alter the affinity of glutamate for excitatory or uptake receptor sites, future research will very likely describe the existence of additional pre- and postsynaptic sites through which primary afferent transmission may be pharmacologically modified. This second class of sites would be analogous to the regulatory sites of enzymes, through which additional substrate molecules, reaction products, metabolites, cofactors or hormones indirectly affect the enzymatic "active" or catalytic site.

Evidence for regulatory sites at vertebrate synapses is sparse (Florey, 1967); however, several studies suggesting such sites at the presumptive glutaminergic neuromuscular junction of arthropods offer experimental leads for further mapping of the vertebrate primary afferent synapse. Both neuron- and glutamate-induced excitatory postsynaptic potentials (EPSPs) recorded from the crayfish walking-leg muscle are potentiated by the addition of 5'-AMP or 5'-GMP (Ozeki and Sato, 1970). It was suggested that these agents selectively facilitated the interaction between glutamate and the postsynaptic receptors. An example of presynaptic regulation might be an apparent amplifier action of glutamate in increasing the frequency of miniature end-plate potentials at several arthropod nerve-muscle preparations (Usherwood and Machili, 1966; Kerkut and Walker, 1967; Florey and Woodcock, 1968). These observations imply that glutamate was enhancing the release of transmitter quanta. This amplification effect of glutamate may have a parallel in the vertebrate CNS during the initiation of spreading depression (van Harreveld and Fifková, 1970). The physiological significance of this phenomenon, however, is still controversial because no evidence has yet been obtained for a presynaptic effect of glutamate at a specific CNS synapse (Curtis, 1965).

EVIDENCE FOR GLUTAMIC ACID AS THE PRIMARY AFFERENT TRANSMITTER

In the course of formulating his now famous "law," Dale (1935) suggested that the substance inducing peripheral vasodilation following stimulation of sensory nerves might be the same substance released by these nerves in the CNS. On this basis ATP, histamine, and substance P, each of which is vasodilatory and is present in sensory nerve bundles, have been studied as CNS transmitter candidates (Crossland, 1962). Evidence that the primary afferent transmitter is not ACh was provided by the lack of effect of ACh or prostigmine on synaptic potentials set up by dorsal root volleys (Eccles, 1947). More recently, glutamic acid has been proposed as the transmitter of these cells (Graham, Shank, Werman, and Aprison, 1967) because of its excitatory action on spinal neurons and because of its distribution pattern in the cord. Since glutamate, unlike ACh, also functions as a key intermediate metabolite, studies of a putative glutaminergic synapse will necessitate reevaluating several of the criteria for transmitter identification that have been formulated largely from studies at peripheral cholinergic junctions. In terms of a functional sequence, these criteria involve presynaptic synthesis, storage, and release of transmitter, and a specific interaction with the postsynaptic membrane that is both rapid and reversible.

Synthesis and Storage

The occurrence of ACh in the nervous system appears to be restricted to those fiber tracts where it has a synaptic function. The identification of cholinergic fibers is also facilitated by the presence of the unique synthetic enzyme choline acetyltransferase (ChA) which has a distribution paralleling that of its transmitter product. By contrast, glutamic acid, together with at least three enzymes capable of its synthesis—glutamic dehydrogenase, aspartate aminotransferase, and glutaminase—is present in high concentration in all neural tissue (van den Berg, 1970).

With respect to the primary afferent system, the activities of these three glutamate enzymes in dorsal roots of cat are comparable to the levels in ventral roots (Graham and Aprison, 1969), whereas ChA activity as well as ACh levels are negligible in dorsal roots[2] and highly concentrated in ventral roots (MacIntosh, 1941; Wolfgram, 1954; Hebb and Silver, 1956). The distribution of glutamate, although ubiquitous, is not uniform; it is unique among the free amino acids in that its concentration is 50 to 200% higher in dorsal roots than in peripheral sensory nerve (Duggan and Johnston, 1970; Johnson and Aprison, 1970), suggesting a specific transport mechanism for glutamate from the unipolar cell body to the central nerve ending. The levels of glutamate in ventral roots are comparable to those in peripheral nerves, while within the spinal cord glutamate maintains a distribution con-

---

[2] See recent findings of Welsch, Schmidt, and Dettbarn (1972).

sistent with a sensory transmitter, higher in dorsal gray than in ventral gray, and high in the gracilis, cuneate, and trigeminal nuclei, sites rich in primary afferent endings (Graham et al., 1967; Johnson and Aprison, 1970).

A parallel situation concerning relative concentrations of transmitter candidates exists at the crustacean neuromuscular junction. Gamma-amino-butyric acid (GABA), the probable inhibitory transmitter, is present at two orders of magnitude greater concentration in inhibitory than in excitatory axons, while glutamate, the leading excitatory transmitter candidate, is found in excitatory axons at only a 30% molar excess over the levels in inhibitory axons (Kravitz, Molinoff, and Hall, 1965). It will be of interest to determine if the excess glutamate in vertebrate dorsal roots and in crustacean excitatory nerves may represent a separate metabolic pool of glutamate not present in other neural tissue.

Although glutamate is not restricted to specific fibers, the cholinergic model would at least have the amino acid compartmentalized in a manner that allows release of the transmitter to occur in quantal steps. While no studies have been reported to date on primary afferent synaptosomes, glutamate does not appear to be significantly concentrated in synaptosomal or synaptic vesicle fractions of brain relative to cytoplasmic markers (Ryall, 1964; Mangan and Whittaker, 1966; Kuriyama, Roberts, and Kakefuda, 1968). However, when ^{3}H-glutamate was taken up into brain slices, it was found to be associated predominantly with the same subcellular fraction as ^{3}H-norepinephrine, a synaptosomal marker (Kuhar and Snyder, 1970). In terms of the concentration of glutamate required for postsynaptic excitation, it can be argued that vesicles need not concentrate, but only package, the transmitter. Glutamate is present in primary afferent regions at a level of 4 to 6 mM, and since it appears more concentrated in neurons than glia (Tower, 1960; Rose, 1968; Mokrasch, 1971), this can be considered a conservative estimate of its concentration in nerve endings. Since the threshold concentration of iontophoretically applied glutamate (which is most likely to be higher than the concentration of glutamate released at a synapse) is 0.1 to 1.0 mM for depolarization of spinal neurons (Curtis and Watkins, 1965), the presynaptic glutamate concentration is above this level, even allowing for the possibility that as little as 10% of the total glutamate may contribute to the transmitter pool.

The fact remains that extensive neurochemical studies have found no substances other than glutamate and aspartate which are neuroexcitatory and present in neural tissue in sufficient quantities to be considered as excitatory transmitter candidates. Excitatory actions of ATP (Holton, 1959) may now be explained by the general property of such substances to chelate calcium (Galindo, Krnjević, and Schwartz, 1967).

Release

The demonstrated release of ACh from the vertebrate neuromuscular junction following nerve stimulation was the major piece of evidence in establishing its transmitter role. Two difficulties have prevented a similar approach for glutamate as well as for other CNS transmitter candidates. First, the central localization of primary afferent synapses makes it difficult not only to collect substances released by nerve stimulation but also to precisely determine the site of release of any substance that might be collected. Second, pharmacology has yet to isolate from the bark of a tree or from the skin of a toad, or yet to synthesize, an "eserine" for the putative glutamate synapse—that is, a drug which will specifically block the mechanism(s) inactivating synaptically released glutamate and thereby facilitate attempts to identify this compound as a central transmitter. To date, stimulus-induced release of glutamate has been demonstrated from peripheral nerve (Wheeler, Boyarsky, and Brooks, 1966; DeFeudis, 1969), from cerebral cortex (Jasper, Khan, and Elliott, 1965; Jasper and Koyama, 1969), from brain slices (Katz, Chase, and Kopin, 1969), and from isolated brain synaptosomes (Bradford, 1970). These experiments suggest that a release of glutamate can occur during nerve activity, but whether these observations are related to a transmitter function for glutamate remains unknown. Future attempts at demonstrating a stimulus-induced release of glutamate from primary afferent nerve endings may thus be hampered by a high background efflux of this amino acid from conducting axons as well as from depolarized dendrites or soma.

Postsynaptic Action

Although glutamate does excite such primary afferent target sites as spinal interneurons, motoneurons (Curtis, Phillis, and Watkins, 1960), and secondary sensory neurons in the cuneate and gracilis nuclei (Galindo et al., 1967), it has, with few exceptions, a similar excitatory action on all central neurons (Curtis and Watkins, 1965; Krnjević, 1965; Phillis, 1970). This excitatory effect is seemingly nonspecific to the degree that such a receptor site triggering depolarization may be a functional part of all neuronal membranes. Although this nonspecificity has been cited as evidence against a specific transmitter role for glutamate, the same argument is not heard in the case of GABA, which shows a similar degree of nonspecificity in its inhibitory effect on central neurons (Curtis and Watkins, 1965), yet is well on its way to being accepted as an inhibitory transmitter at a number of specific CNS sites (Krnjević, 1970*a*).

Once a transmitter candidate is shown to mimic qualitatively the substance released by nerve action potentials, several more vigorous tests of identity of action should be applied, involving comparisons of both the potential and conductance changes exerted on the postsynaptic membrane. To this end, the equilibrium potential for glutamate depolarization of spinal motoneurons was found to occur at a more polarized level than that of the EPSP (Curtis, 1965), a fact which was at first entered on the debit side of the glutamate transmitter ledger. But these findings are what would be predicted if glutamate is released near the recording electrode in the soma, while a large proportion of the primary afferent synapses have a remote dendritic localization (Jack, Miller, Porter, and Redman, 1970).

A stronger case for the involvement of glutamate in primary afferent transmission would be made if it were shown that similar changes in neuronal membrane resistance resulted during synaptic activation and during iontophoretic application of glutamate as the ionic environment of the neuron was altered (Werman, 1966).

Inactivation

Although the time course of decay of the primary afferent EPSP is similar to that for the cholinergic endplate potential, there is no evidence for an enzymatic inactivation mechanism for transmitter glutamate. Pretreatment with inhibitors of enzymes which metabolize glutamate — e.g., aminooxyacetic acid to block glutamic decarboxylase, methionine sulfoximine to block glutamine synthetase, or isoniazid to block aspartate amino transferase — had no effect on the decay-time of glutamate-induced excitation of spinal neurons (Curtis, Phillis, and Watkins, 1960). The similarity of the time course of the excitatory action of the L- and D-isomers of glutamate is also cited as evidence against an enzymatic mechanism for terminating the synaptic action of glutamate.

An alternative route for removing transmitter molecules from the synaptic cleft is via active uptake into pre- or postsynaptic regions or into perisynaptic glial elements.[3] Such a mechanism has been proposed for the inac-

---

[3] For discussion of glial uptake see Henn and Hamberger (1971).

tivation of several transmitter substances (Iversen, 1970), including glutamate at the arthropod neuromuscular junction (Faeder and Salpeter, 1970).
Spinal cord shares with other neural tissue the capacity for active transport
of glutamate (Quastel, 1970). Using slices of rat spinal cord, we have
shown this uptake mechanism to have a saturable component that is dependent on temperature, cell metabolism, and external sodium ions. The
positive correlation observed in various brain regions between the rate of
glutamate uptake and its tissue concentration (Kandera, Levi, and Lajtha,
1968) can be extended to spinal cord since both parameters are lower in
cord than in any brain region (Levi and Lajtha, 1965). We have also found
this correlation to hold when these two measurements were carried out on
slices prepared from dorsal and ventral regions of rat spinal cord (Hammerschlag, 1971). The rate of uptake of glutamate was found to be 2–3 times
greater in dorsal than in ventral cord; K_m values were similar in both
regions, but the difference was reflected in the relative V_{max} values. Thus
there may be no difference in the nature of the glutamate uptake sites in
these two regions, but the dorsal cord may contain more sites. At the cockroach neuromuscular junction, the technique of electron microscope autoradiography has been utilized to demonstrate an uptake of glutamate that
was approximately doubled by nerve stimulation (Faeder and Salpeter,
1970). As yet, similar correlations have not been attempted between the intensity of primary afferent synaptic activity and glutamate uptake.

CONCLUSIONS

Glutamate, then, has not yet been established as the excitatory transmitter released from primary afferent endings, although it remains the only
real candidate for the role. We can also conclude that several of the criteria
for transmitter identification cannot be strictly applied in the case of glutamate.

Since the terms cholinergic and adrenergic imply a localization of synthesis and storage of transmitter to specific fibers, we need to redefine a
biochemical criterion relevant to the glutaminergic fiber. This criterion
would be the demonstration of a mechanism in primary afferent fibers for
"mobilizing" a portion of the cellular glutamate for use as a transmitter.
Such a mechanism, e.g., a metabolic or structural compartment, and the
membrane or macromolecular specificity required to achieve it, would *not*
be present in other neurons which use glutamate only as an intermediate
metabolite.

ACKNOWLEDGMENTS

This review was written during the tenure of NIH grant NS09885–01 (R.H.) and NSF postdoctoral fellowship 41059 (D.W.).

REFERENCES

Banna, N. R., and Jabbur, S. J. (1970): Increased transmitter release induced by convulsant phenols. *Brain Research*, 20:471–473.

Blasberg, R., and Lajtha, A. (1965): Substrate specificity of steady-state amino acid transport in mouse brain slices. *Archives of Biochemistry and Biophysics*, 112:361–377.

Bradford, H. F. (1970): Metabolic response of synaptosomes to electrical stimulation: release of amino acids. *Brain Research*, 19:239–247.

Conradi, S. (1969): Ultrastructure of dorsal root boutons on lumbosacral motoneurons of the adult cat, as revealed by dorsal root section. *Acta Physiologica Scandinavica*, Supplement 332:85–115.

Crossland, J. (1962): Some possible mediators of non-cholinergic central transmission. In: *Neurochemistry*, edited by K. A. C. Elliott, I. H. Page, and J. H. Quastel. Charles C Thomas, Springfield.

Curtis, D. R. (1965): The actions of amino acids upon mammalian neurones. In: *Studies in Physiology*, edited by D. R. Curtis and A. K. McIntyre. Springer-Verlag, Heidelberg.

Curtis, D. R., Duggan, A. W., and Johnston, G. A. R. (1970): The inactivation of extracellulary administered amino acids in the feline spinal cord. *Experimental Brain Research*, 10:447–462.

Curtis, D. R., and Felix, D. (1971): GABA and prolonged spinal inhibition. *Nature* New Biology 231:187–188.

Curtis, D. R., Phillis, J. W., and Watkins, J. C. (1960): The chemical excitation of spinal neurones by certain acidic amino acids. *Journal of Physiology*, 150:656–682.

Curtis, D. R., Phillis, J. W., and Watkins, J. C. (1961): Actions of amino-acids on the isolated hemisected spinal cord of the toad. *British Journal of Pharmacology*, 16:262–283.

Curtis, D. R., and Watkins, J. C. (1960): The excitation and depression of spinal neurones by structurally related amino acids. *Journal of Neurochemistry*, 6:117–141.

Curtis, D. R., and Watkins, J. C. (1963): Acidic amino acids with strong excitatory actions on mammalian neurones. *Journal of Physiology*, 166:1–14.

Curtis, D. R., and Watkins, J. C. (1965): Pharmacology of amino acids related to aminobutyric acid (GABA). *Pharmacological Reviews*, 17:347–391.

Curtis, D. R., Duggan, A. W., Felix, D., and Johnston, G. A. R. (1971): Bicucullin, an antagonist of GABA and synaptic inhibition in the spinal cord of the cat. *Brain Research*, 32:69–96.

Dale, H. H. (1935): Pharmacology and nerve endings. *Proceedings of the Royal Society of Medicine*, 28:319–332.

Davidoff, R. A. (1972): Gamma-aminobutyric acid antagonism and presynaptic inhibition in the frog spinal cord. *Science*, 175:331–332.

DeFeudis, F. V. (1969): Glutamate fluxes in peripheral nerve. *Abstracts of Second Meeting, International Society for Neurochemistry*, Milan.

Duggan, A. W., and Johnston, G. A. R. (1970): Glutamate and related amino acids in cat spinal roots, dorsal root ganglia, and peripheral nerves. *Journal of Neurochemistry*, 17:1205–1208.

Duncan, D., and Keyser, L. L. (1938): Further determinations of the numbers of fibers and cells in the dorsal roots and ganglia of the cat. *Journal of Comparative Neurology*, 68:479–490.

Eccles, J. C. (1947): Acetylcholine and synaptic transmission in the spinal cord. *Journal of Neurophysiology*, 10:197–204.

Eccles, J. C. (1964): *The Physiology of Synapses*. Springer-Verlag, Berlin.

Eccles, J. C., Schmidt, R., and Willis, W. D. (1963): Pharmacological studies on presynaptic inhibition. *Journal of Physiology*, 168:500–530.

Faeder, I. R., and Salpeter, M. M. (1970): Glutamate uptake by a stimulated insect nerve muscle preparation. *Journal of Cell Biology*, 46:300–307.

Florey, E. (1967): Neurotransmitters and modulators in the animal kingdom. *Federation Proceedings*, 26:1164–1178.

Florey, E., and Woodcock, B. (1968): Presynaptic excitatory action of glutamate applied to crab nerve-muscle preparations. *Comparative Biochemistry and Physiology*, 26:651–661.

Galindo, A., Krnjević, K., and Schwartz, S. (1967): Micro-iontophoretic studies on neurones in the cuneate nucleus. *Journal of Physiology*, 192:359–377.

Graham, L. T., Jr., and Aprison, M. H. (1969): Distribution of some enzymes associated with the metabolism of glutamate, aspartate, γ-aminobutyrate, and glutamine in cat spinal cord. *Journal of Neurochemistry*, 16:559–566.

Graham, L. T., Jr., Shank, R. P., Werman, R., and Aprison, M. H. (1967): Distribution of some synaptic transmitter suspects in cat spinal cord. *Journal of Neurochemistry*, 14:465–472.

Gray, E. G. (1962): A morphological basis for pre-synaptic inhibition? *Nature*, 193:82–83.

Ha, H. (1970): Axonal bifurcation in the dorsal root ganglion of the cat: a light and electron microscopic study. *Journal of Comparative Neurology*, 140:227–240.

Haggar, R. A., and Barr, M. L. (1950): Quantitative data on the size of synaptic end-bulbs in the cat's spinal cord. *Journal of Comparative Neurology*, 93:17–35.

Hammerschlag, R. (1971): *In vitro* uptake of ^{14}C-glutamate into dorsal and ventral spinal cord of rat. *Abstracts of the Third International Meeting, International Society for Neurochemistry, Budapest.*

Hammerschlag, R., Potter, L. T., and Vinci, J. M. (1971): *In vitro* uptake of ^{14}C-glutamate by rat spinal cord. *Transactions of the American Society for Neurochemistry*, 2:78.

Hebb, C. O., and Silver, A. (1956): Choline acetylase in the central nervous system of man and some other mammals. *Journal of Physiology*, 134:718–728.

Henn, F. A., and Hamberger, A. (1971): Glial cell function: uptake of transmitter substances. *Proceedings of the National Academy of Sciences*, 68:2686–2690.

Holton, P. (1959): The liberation of adenosine triphosphate on antidromic stimulation of sensory nerves. *Journal of Physiology*, 145:494–504.

Iversen, L. L. (1970): Neuronal uptake processes for amines and amino acids. In: *Advances in Biochemical Psychopharmacology*, edited by E. Costa and E. Giacobini, Raven Press, New York, 2:109–132.

Jack, J. J. B., Miller, S., Porter, R., and Redman, S. J. (1970): The distribution of group Ia synapses on lumbosacral spinal motoneurons in the cat. In: *Excitatory Synaptic Mechanisms*, edited by P. Andersen and J. K. S. Jansen. Universitetsforlaget, Oslo.

Jasper, H. H., Khan, R. T., and Elliott, K. A. C. (1965): Amino acids released from the cerebral cortex in relation to its state of activation. *Science*, 147:1448–1449.

Jasper, H. H., and Koyama, I. (1969): Rate of release of amino acids from the cerebral cortex in the cat as affected by brainstem and thalamic stimulation. *Canadian Journal of Physiology and Pharmacology*, 47:889–905.

Johnson, J. L., and Aprison, M. H. (1970): The distribution of glutamic acid, a transmitter candidate, and other amino acids in the dorsal sensory neuron of the cat. *Brain Research*, 24:285–292.

Kandera, J., Levi, G., and Lajtha, A. (1968): Control of cerebral metabolite levels: II. Amino acid uptake and levels in various areas of rat brain. *Archives of Biochemistry and Biophysics*, 126:249–260.

Katz, R. I., Chase, T. N., and Kopin, I. J. (1969): Effect of ions on stimulus-induced release of amino acids from mammalian brain slices. *Journal of Neurochemistry*, 16:961–967.

Kerkut, G. A., and Walker, R. J. (1967): The effect of iontophoretic injection of L-glutamic acid and γ-amino-N-butyric acid on the miniature end-plate potentials and contractures of the coxal muscles of the cockroach *Periplaneta americana L. Comparative Biochemistry and Physiology,* 20:999–1003.

Kravitz, E. A., Molinoff, P. B., and Hall, Z. W. (1965): A comparison of the enzymes and substrates of gamma-aminobutyric acid metabolism in lobster excitatory and inhibitory axons. *Proceedings of the National Academy of Sciences,* 54:778–782.

Krnjević, K. (1965): Actions of drugs on single neurones in the cerebral cortex. *British Medical Bulletin,* 21:10–14.

Krnjević, K. (1970a): Glutamate and γ-aminobutyric acid in brain. *Nature,* 228:119–124.

Krnjević, K. (1970b): Central excitatory transmitters in vertebrates. In: *Excitatory Synaptic Mechanisms,* edited by P. Andersen and J. K. S. Jansen. Universitetsforlaget, Oslo.

Kuhar, M. J. and Snyder, S. H. (1970): The subcellular distribution of free ^{3}H-glutamic acid in rat cerebral cortical slices. *Journal of Pharmacology and Experimental Therapeutics,* 171:141–152.

Kuno, M. (1964): Quantal components of excitatory synaptic potentials in spinal motoneurones. *Journal of Physiology,* 175:81–99.

Kuriyama, K., Roberts, E., and Kakefuda, T. (1968): Association of the γ-aminobutyric acid system with a synaptic fraction from mouse brain. *Brain Research,* 8:132–152.

Levi, G., and Lajtha, A. (1965): Cerebral amino acid transport *in vitro.* II. Regional differences in amino acid uptake by slices from central nervous system of the rat. *Journal of Neurochemistry,* 12:639–648.

MacIntosh, F. C. (1941): The distribution of acetylcholine in the peripheral and the central nervous system. *Journal of Physiology,* 99:436–442.

Mangan, J. L., and Whittaker, V. P. (1966): The distribution of free amino acids in subcellular fractions of guinea-pig brain. *Biochemical Journal,* 98:128–137.

McGiven, J. D., and Chappell, J. B. (1970): Avenaciolide: a specific inhibitor of glutamate transport in rat liver mitochondria. *Biochemical Journal,* 116:37P–38P.

Miyahara, J. T., Esplin, D. W., and Zablocka, B. (1966a): Differential effects of depressant drugs on presynaptic inhibition. *Journal of Pharmacology and Experimental Therapeutics,* 154:119–127.

Miyahara, J. T. (1966b): A physiological and pharmacological analysis of the mechanism of presynaptic inhibition. Ph.D. Thesis, Department of Pharmacology, The University of Utah, Salt Lake City.

Mokrasch, L. C. (1971): Free amino acid content of normal and neoplastic rodent astroglia. *Brain Research,* 25:672–676.

Ozeki, M., and Sato, M. (1970): Potentiation of excitatory junctional potentials and glutamate-induced responses in crayfish muscle by 5′-ribonucleotides. *Comparative Biochemistry and Physiology,* 32:203–218.

Phillis, J. W. (1970): *The Pharmacology of Synapses.* Pergamon Press, Oxford.

Quastel, J. H. (1970): Transport processes at the brain cell membrane. In: *Neurosciences Research,* edited by S. Ehrenpreis and O. C. Solnitzsky, 3:1–41. Academic Press, New York

Rall, W., Burke, R. E., Smith, T. G., Nelson, P. G., and Frank, K. (1967): Dendritic location of synapses and possible mechanisms for the monosynaptic EPSP in motoneurons. *Journal of Neurophysiology,* 30:1169–1193.

Ralston, H. J. (1968): Dorsal root projections to dorsal horn neurons in the cat spinal cord. *Journal of Comparative Neurology,* 132:303–329.

Rose, S. P. R. (1968): The biochemistry of neurones and glia. In: *Applied Neurochemistry,* edited by A. N. Davison and J. Dobbing. Blackwell, Oxford.

Ryall, R. W. (1964): The subcellular distribution of acetylcholine, substance P, 5-hydroxytryptamine, γ-aminobutyric acid, and glutamic acid in brain homogenates. *Journal of Neurochemistry,* 11:131–145.

Szentágothai, J., and Albert, A. (1955): The synaptology of Clarke's column. *Acta Morphologica Hungaricae,* 5:43–51.

Tower, D. B. (1960): The neurochemistry of asparagine and glutamine. In: *The Neurochemis-*

try of Nucleotides and Amino Acids, edited by R. O. Brady and D. B. Tower. John Wiley, New York.

Usherwood, P. N. R., and Machili, P. (1966): Chemical transmission at the insect excitatory neuromuscular synapse. *Nature,* 210:634–636.

van den Berg, C. J. (1970): Glutamate and glutamine. In: *Handbook of Neurochemistry,* Vol. III, edited by A. Lajtha. Plenum Press, New York.

van Harreveld, A., and Fifková, E. (1970): Glutamate release from the retina during spreading depression. *Journal of Neurobiology,* 2:13–29.

Wall, P. D. (1964): Presynaptic control of impulses at the first central synapse in the cutaneous pathway. In: *Progress in Brain Research,* Vol. 12, edited by J. C. Eccles and J. P. Schade. Elsevier, Amsterdam.

Watkins, J. C., Curtis, D. R., and Biscoe, T. J. (1966): Central effects of β-N-oxalyl-α, β-diaminopropionic acid and other *Lathyrus* factors. *Nature,* 211:637.

Weakly, J. N. (1969): Effect of barbiturates on "quantal" synaptic transmission in spinal motoneurons. *Journal of Physiology,* 204:63–77.

Welsch, F., Schmidt, D. E., and Dettbarn, W.-D. (1972): Acetylcholine, choline acetyltransferase and cholinesterases in motor and sensory nerves of the bull frog. *Biochemical Pharmacology,* 21:847–856.

Werman, R. (1966): A review: criteria for identification of a central nervous system transmitter. *Comparative Biochemistry and Physiology,* 18:745–766.

Wheeler, D. D., Boyarsky, L. L., and Brooks, W. H. (1966): The release of amino acids from nerve during stimulation. *Journal of Cellular Physiology,* 67:141–148.

Wolfgram, F. J. (1954): Relative amounts of choline acetylase and cholinesterases in dorsal and ventral roots of cattle. *American Journal of Physiology,* 176:505–507.

Advances in Biochemical Psychopharmacology, Vol. 6
Raven Press, New York © 1972

An Approach to the Study of the Biochemical Pharmacology of Cholinergic Function

I. Hanin, R. Massarelli, and E. Costa

Laboratory of Preclinical Pharmacology, National Institute of Mental Health, Saint Elizabeths Hospital, Washington, D.C. 20032

The turnover rate of a neurotransmitter is defined, according to the general concepts proposed by Zilversmit (1960), as the amount of transmitter stored in neurons which is being renewed per unit of time.

Turnover rates of brain acetylcholine have not been measured using the principles of steady-state kinetics, mainly because an efficient labeling of choline and acetate pools functioning in this tissue as precursors of acetylcholine has not been readily obtainable. Two further complications are encountered in such studies. (1) Cholinergic neurons in brain are distributed in a ubiquitous manner with little or no polarization in any particular brain structure (e.g., MacIntosh, 1941; Crossland and Merrick, 1954; Takahashi and Aprison, 1964; Giarman and Pepeu, 1964; Campbell and Jenden, 1970). This obviously creates problems in interpreting turnover rate measurements of brain acetylcholine in functional terms. (2) Until recently, adequate chemical techniques for the simultaneous assay of acetylcholine and choline specific activity had not been developed.

The goal of this chapter is to discuss possible approaches to the study of acetylcholine turnover *in vivo* and to present the rat salivary glands as a simple biochemical model for initiating a kinetic study to provide valid estimates of the turnover rates of acetylcholine in neurons. We have also attempted to use this model to evaluate the effect of various pharmacological agents acting on cholinergic mechanisms, and have applied physiological perturbations to this biological model in order to gain some understanding of the various processes involved in the regulation of cholinergic mechanisms. Our interest in these studies stems from the necessity to establish if changes of turnover rates measured *in vivo* can be used to study how nerve function regulates the availability of the transmitter, and how drugs affect cholinergic function by mechanisms other than change of steady-state levels of acetylcholine.

To define our attempts more clearly, it may be in order to give some relevant background and to describe how the study of regulation of turnover rates has helped understand adrenergic mechanisms in terms of their regulation and function. It is believed that the regulation of catecholamine turnover is coupled to nerve activity, and plays a role in maintaining constancy of transmitter concentrations in the face of the changing rates of nerve activity (Montanari, Costa, Beavan, and Brodie, 1963; Oliverio and Stjärne, 1965; Alousi and Weiner, 1966; Gordon, Reid, Sjoerdsma, and Udenfriend, 1966; Neff and Costa, 1966; Sedvall and Kopin, 1967). An awareness of this regulatory process has served to uncover the mode of action of many drugs which exert an effect on adrenergic nerve terminals, but which do not change the steady-state concentrations of the transmitter.

From studies of adrenergic neurons in the periphery and in the central nervous system of various animal species, a tenet has emerged which states that nerve activity controls the steady state of catecholamine transmitters by changing catecholamine turnover rate (see reviews by Costa, 1970, and Costa and Neff, 1970). The measurement of catecholamine steady-state concentrations is thus relatively uninformative in relating adrenergic nerve participation to adaptation to environmental changes, e.g., cold exposure (Oliverio and Stjärne, 1965), and in defining the site of action of drugs on adrenergic nerves (Costa and Neff, 1970).

The availability of catecholamines for release by nerve impulses appears to be regulated by three major mechanisms: (1) change of the rate of DOPA formation through feedback control by end product inhibition (Costa and Neff, 1966; Alousi and Weiner, 1966; Spector, Gordon, Sjoerdsma, and Udenfriend, 1967); (2) reuptake of released transmitter operating within a wide range of changes in neuronal activity as a first-order process (Folkow, Häggendal, and Lisander, 1967); and (3) regulation of synthesis of tyrosine 3-hydroxylase, the rate-limiting enzyme for catecholamine biosynthesis (Axelrod, Mueller, and Thoenen, 1970). While the change listed in (3) has value in slow adaptative modifications of neuronal activity, the other two mechanisms function in maintaining optimal levels of transmitters during rapid shifts of neuronal activity.

Circadian rhythms have been described in adrenergic and cholinergic neurons (Albrecht, Visscher, Bittner, and Halberg, 1956; Quay, 1965; Wurtman and Axelrod, 1966; Wurtman, Chou, and Rose, 1967; Reis, Weinbren, and Corvelli, 1968; Scheving, Harrison, Gordon, and Pauly, 1968;

Friedman and Walker, 1969*a, b;* Hanin, Massarelli, and Costa, 1970*a*). These diurnal variations do not negate but actually delineate tolerance limits in steady-state variation within normal oscillations of neuronal function. In the case of adrenergic neurons, circadian changes might well be linked to the functioning of a feedback control by end product inhibition (Costa and Neff, 1966; Alousi and Weiner, 1966; Spector et al., 1967). However, because we lack a complete understanding of the regulatory mechanisms in the cholinergic system, any suggestions about the cause of circadian rhythmicity of acetylcholine concentrations in brain must be speculative.

Studies of the *in vivo* regulation of cholinergic function have followed two main methodological approaches: (1) measurements of acetylcholine concentrations and specific activity in tissues superfused and/or perfused with fluids containing high concentrations of cholinesterase inhibitors, or (2) measurements of acetylcholine specific-activity changes with time after injections of radioactive choline.

The former approach has undergone several modifications to suit particular tissues. Generally, it has required the presence of considerable concentrations of a cholinesterase inhibitor (most frequently neostigmine or physostigmine in concentrations of 2.5×10^{-4} to 1.25×10^{-3} M) to block acetylcholine degradation completely (Mitchell, 1963; Szerb, 1964; Pepeu, Bartolini, and Deffenu, 1970). Therefore, before any conclusion is reached, the action of these inhibitors on acetylcholine turnover rate should be objectively evaluated. Since a reuptake of choline formed during the degradation of released acetylcholine is one of the main control mechanisms of cholinergic functions (Perry, 1953; Collier and MacIntosh, 1969), it follows that the presence of cholinesterase inhibitors may disrupt one of the main control processes of acetylcholine steady state. One should, consequently, consider the probability that cholinesterase inhibitors used at these high concentrations do not affect the system solely by inhibiting cholinesterase.

Initial steady-state concentrations of plasma choline have not been maintained when brain acetylcholine has been labeled by intravenously administered pulse injections of radioactive choline (Schuberth, Sparf, and Sundwall, 1969, 1970). Since brain choline acetyltransferase is not saturated by normal endogenous concentrations of choline (Potter and Glover, 1970), the question must be raised concerning the physiological significance of turnover rate calculations based upon such an experimental approach. Furthermore, such experiments exhibit a biphasic decline in brain choline specific radioactivity (Schuberth et al., 1969). This adds an uncertainty to the problem by imposing the necessity, in these calculations, to account for various compartments of choline in the brain.

Such considerations suggest that other labeling procedures should be developed to circumvent the problems created by the discrepancies inherent in the above-mentioned approaches.

CHOICE OF PRECURSOR FOR ESTIMATING TURNOVER RATE OF ACETYLCHOLINE

Results of *in vitro* studies have disclosed that there are several compounds which may function as physiological precursors of acetyl coenzyme A (CoA), the immediate precursor of the acetyl moiety of acetylcholine: pyruvate (see review by Quastel, 1955; also, Browning and Schulman, 1968; Nakamura and Cheng, 1969), acetate (Nakamura and Cheng, 1969), glucose (Browning and Schulman, 1968), and citrate (see reviews by Quastel, 1955, and Sörbo, 1970) fulfill some of the requirements for being acetylcholine precursors but none of these compounds can be singled out as an ideal candidate to be used to attain an efficient labeling of acetylcholine. Despite this necessarily conservative approach, Cheney, Gubler, and Jaussi (1969) and Tuček and Cheng (1970) have concluded from their *in vivo* studies in mammals that pyruvate is the most important precursor of the acetyl moiety of brain acetylcholine, while Fitzgerald and Cooper (1967) have maintained that acetate is the precursor of choice for the biosynthesis of acetylcholine in the corneal epithelium of the rabbit.

Choline has been used more extensively as the precursor for acetylcholine synthesis in mammalian brain and peripheral tissues (Birks and MacIntosh, 1961; Hebb, Ling, McGeer, McGeer, and Perkins, 1964; Friesen, Kemp, and Woodbury, 1964; Saelens and Stoll, 1965; Wallach, Goldberg, and Shideman, 1967; Chakrin and Shideman, 1968; Browning and Schulman, 1968; Collier and Lang, 1969; Schuberth et al., 1969; Potter, 1970; Diamond, 1971, and others). The reason for favoring choline is a practical one: this compound is an immediate precursor of acetylcholine in the cytoplasm of peripheral and central neurons. The nervous system is incapable of synthesizing choline (Bremer and Greenberg, 1961). Consequently, this quaternary compound has to be supplied to the brain from the periphery across the lipoid membranes of the blood-brain barrier by some specialized carrier. Whether choline is first converted into a lipid soluble form and then transported across the blood brain barrier (Ansell and Spanner, 1968, 1970, 1971) or transported from blood to brain without any metabolic alteration by a saturable carrier-mediated process (Diamond, 1971) has yet to be resolved. Nevertheless, passage of labeled choline from periphery into brain has been shown following either its intravenous injection (Groth, Bain, and Pfeiffer, 1958; Ansell and Spanner, 1968; Schuberth et al., 1969; Diamond, 1971) or its parenteral administration (Potter, Glover, and Saelens, 1968). In some of these experiments, however, steady state of plasma choline following injection of the radiolabeled choline was not maintained.

Carrier-mediated transport of choline has also been demonstrated *in vitro* in erythrocytes (Askari, 1966; Martin, 1968), in kidney slices (Sung and Johnstone, 1965), in brain slices (Schuberth, Sundwall, and Sörbo, 1967), and in isolated synaptic nerve endings and vesicles (Marchbanks, 1968; Potter, 1968; Diamond and Kennedy, 1969; Bosmann and Hemsworth, 1970), implying that uptake of choline across a lipoid barrier is a common occurrence in various mammalian cells and is not restricted to neurons.

Figure 1 lists in schematic form all possible immediate precursors involved in the biosynthesis of acetylcholine, with the intention of indicating possible ways of labeling tissue acetylcholine. An additional necessary condition not portrayed in Fig. 1 concerns the identification of the rate-

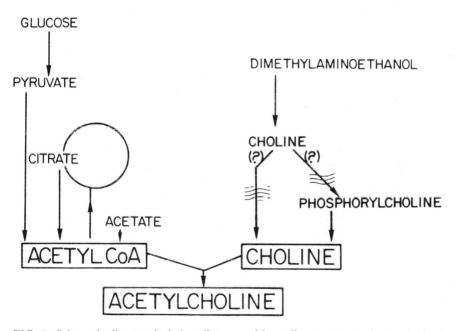

FIG. 1. Schematic diagram depicting all proposed immediate precursors for synthesis of acetylcholine in tissue extracts. Pathways which have not been definitely substantiated are identified by question marks. Three wavy lines indicate blood-brain barrier.

limiting process for acetylcholine biosynthesis. Available evidence does not suggest that the choline acetyltransferase step is rate-limiting for acetylcholine biosynthesis (Potter and Glover, 1970). Formation of acetyl CoA (Smallman, 1958), its rate of transfer from the mitochondria, or alternately the rate of choline reuptake may be investigated as rate limiting processes for acetylcholine biosynthesis.

In view of these uncertainties on this central issue of the control of cholinergic mechanisms, the *in vivo* rate of acetylcholine synthesis should be estimated concurrently by two methods: labeling both the choline moiety and the acetate moiety of acetyl CoA, each method being complementary to the other.

In these studies we have used phosphoryl (Me-^{14}C) choline as the precursor of the choline moiety for intracellular synthesis of radiolabeled acetylcholine. This approach was prompted by the suggestion of Ansell and Spanner (1970, 1971) that free choline is supplied to the central nervous system in the lipid-bound form, the source being, presumably, phosphatidylcholine or its lyso-derivative. The first and very rapid step in the conversion of choline to phosphatidycholine is the phosphorylation of choline by choline kinase to phosphorylcholine (Ansell and Spanner, 1968). Thus, phosphorylcholine might be a necessary intermediate in the transport of choline across a membrane barrier.

Our rationale in using this compound as a precursor was to see if we could achieve an efficient labeling of intracellular choline with relatively low concentrations of labeled phosphorylcholine. In this manner we would not affect steady-state levels of the neurotransmitter, which is one of the prime preconditions for turnover studies *in vivo*.

CHOICE OF TISSUE FOR STUDYING ACETYLCHOLINE TURNOVER *IN VIVO*

The submaxillary and sublingual salivary glands were chosen as a model for turnover rate measurements of acetylcholine *in vivo* because of their anatomical simplicity in comparison with the brain and other organs. These glands are parasympathetically innervated by fibers which originate in the superior salivatory nucleus, and pass via the chorda tympani (seventh cranial nerve) and submaxillary ganglion. Sensory fibers from these glands traverse the lingual nerve and connect with the trigeminal nerve (fifth cranial nerve). They are also innervated by sympathetic nerves originating from the superior cervical ganglion. Both innervations are easily accessible in the rat, and one set of glands from each pair can serve as a control for the set decentralized by unilateral surgery. It appeared to us that the salivary glands are ideal as a simple model for studying cholinergic function *in vivo*. For example, the effect of sympathetic denervation (superior cervical ganglionectomy), parasympathetic decentralization (chorda tympani section), and receptor atrophy (salivary duct ligation) on turnover rates can be studied with the contralateral glands serving as a normal control. In this model we can also study changes of turnover rates elicited by drugs affecting acetylcholine degradation or blocking muscarinic and nicotinic receptor sites. These surgical and pharmacological perturbations could yield important information on the mechanisms that control turnover of transmitter in cholinergic nerves.

The advantage of using a simple model to study cholinergic events at the level of the nerve ending is evident from the amount of information obtained using the phrenic nerve diaphragm and isolated superior cervical ganglion preparations (Brown and Feldberg, 1936; Friesen, Kemp, and Woodbury, 1965; Collier and MacIntosh, 1969; Potter, 1970).

SIMULTANEOUS GAS CHROMATOGRAPHIC MEASUREMENTS OF CHOLINE AND ACETYLCHOLINE SPECIFIC RADIOACTIVITY

The gas chromatographic procedure for estimating acetylcholine (Hanin and Jenden, 1968) and choline in tissue extracts (Hanin, Massarelli, and Costa, 1970*b*) was utilized and adapted to the *in vivo* measurements of acetylcholine and choline specific radioactivity (Hanin, Massarelli, and Costa, 1972). With this procedure we could estimate the change of choline and acetylcholine specific radioactivity with time, following injection of a radioactive precursor. We refer, for general information on this procedure, to the above-mentioned publications (Hanin and Jenden, 1968; Hanin et al., 1970*b*, 1972). Here we shall briefly review the methodology employed in these studies.

Preliminaries to Gas Chromatography

Choline and its analogs were extracted from the salivary glands into 0.4 N perchloric acid, precipitated as the Reinecke salts, and converted to the chlorides using Biorex 9 resin (Hanin and Jenden, 1968). They were next treated with hexanoyl chloride in methyl ethyl ketone, in order to esterify choline and any endogenous alcohols from the tissue extracts to their corresponding hexanoyl esters (Fig. 2) (Hanin et al., 1970*b*). Excess methyl ethyl ketone and unreacted hexanoyl chloride were evaporated, and the remaining products were washed with trimethylamine in pentane (0.1 M).

This last step quantitatively eliminates any tertiary amines present in the medium (Jenden, *personal communication*), and is very important for the following reasons: (1) dimethylaminoethanol, which might be the precursor for endogenous synthesis of choline, is present in various tissues (Bremer and Greenberg, 1959; Honneger and Honneger, 1959); and (2) Biorex 9, which is used in this procedure, has been found to yield an unidentified contaminant which is eluted from the gas chromatographic column with a retention time identical to that of choline. If the endogenous dimethylaminoethanol and the Biorex contaminant are not eliminated before analyzing the tissues for choline by gas chromatography, the compounds will give a false value of the concentration of choline in the tissue extract. In this regard, the trimethylamine wash is important because it quantitatively eliminates all traces of these two interfering compounds.

The samples were then demethylated with sodium benzenethiolate in methyl ethyl ketone (Fig. 3), and the volatile tertiary amines formed were concentrated and extracted into 5 μl of chloroform; an aliquot of this was injected into the gas chromatograph. The sensitivity of this procedure is of the order of 50 pmoles for acetylcholine and 100 pmoles for choline.

The chemical identity of tissue acetylcholine and choline has been obtained by gas chromatography–mass spectrometry (Hammar, Hanin, Holmstedt, Kitz, Jenden, and Karlén, 1968, and Hanin et al., 1972, respectively) using this gas chromatographic approach.

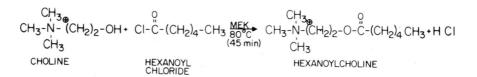

FIG. 2. Conversion of choline to its hexanoyl ester using hexanoyl chloride.

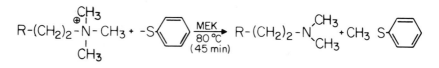

(R= OH, CH₃COO⁻, CH₃CH₂COO⁻, etc.)

FIG. 3. Demethylation reaction for quaternary ammonium compounds using sodium benzenethiolate.

Radio-Gas Chromatographic Assay

Estimation of the radioactivity as well as the total concentrations of each compound injected into the gas chromatographic column was made possible by using the Barber Colman 5000 Gas Chromatograph-Radioactivity Monitoring System. With this unit we have simultaneously assayed the concentration and the radioactivity of the labeled compounds and have expressed their specific activities in terms of cpm/nanomole. A typical radio gas chromatogram is shown in Figure 4.

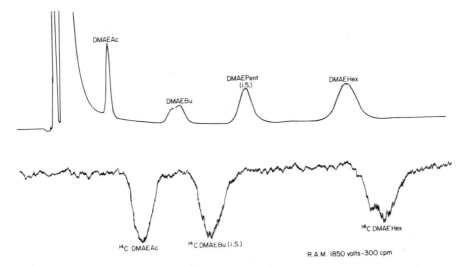

FIG. 4. Radio gas chromatogram of demethylated esters of choline. *Top record:* Flame ionization detector response. *Lower record:* Radioactive detector response. DMAEAc = dimethylaminoethyl acetate, 10 nmoles; DMAEPent (I.S.) = dimethylaminoethyl pentanoate, 20 nmoles, (internal standard); DMAEHex = dimethylaminoethyl hexanoate, 40 nmoles; ^{14}C DMAEAc, ^{14}C DMAEBu (I.S.), and ^{14}C DMAEHex = ^{14}C-labeled dimethylaminoethyl acetate (3,137 cpm), dimethylaminoethyl butyrate (9,377 cpm) (internal standard), and dimethylaminoethyl hexanoate (6,565 cpm), respectively. (DMAEBu is partially obscured by an impurity peak on the flame ionization detector record.) This factor will not interfere with calculations of the quantity of radioactive component in the sample).

Gas flow rates: argon (carrier), 15 ml/min (70 psi); air, 200 ml/min (20 psi); hydrogen, 40 ml/min (14 psi); propane (quench gas), 1.5 ml/min (20 psi). *Temperatures:* column oven, 185°C; front detector bath, 250°C; injection port, 220°C. *Column:* 6-ft. long, U-shaped, 2.5 mm i.d., glass, silanized. Two different column packings were used interchangeably in this study: (a) 1% PDEAS (Analabs, Inc.) on PAR 1 (80–120 mesh) (HP); and (b) 28% Pennwalt 223 plus 4% KOH on Gas Chrom R (80–100 mesh) (Applied Science Laboratories).

CHANGES WITH TIME OF CHOLINE AND ACETYL-CHOLINE SPECIFIC RADIOACTIVITY IN SALIVARY GLANDS OF RATS RECEIVING PHOSPHORYL (Me-^{14}C) CHOLINE

Choline and acetylcholine specific activities were determined at various times after the intravenous injection of phosphoryl (Me-^{14}C) choline (New England Nuclear, NEC 544) into Sprague-Dawley male rats (25 μC/kg; 23.2 mC/mmole). Both submaxillary and sublingual glands were assayed for choline and acetylcholine specific radioactivity. Data obtained are summarized in Table 1. Steady-state levels of choline and acetylcholine per gram of tissue were not affected by the administration of phosphorylcholine. This is to be expected since the total amount of phosphorylcholine injected was 179 nmoles per rat (200 g body weight) and, assuming uniform distribution of this phosphorylcholine in various tissues, the highest concentrations reached would be less than 0.9 nmoles/g. Available data suggest that the phosphorylcholine concentration in rat brain approximates 400 nmoles/g fresh tissue (Dawson, 1955; Porcellati, 1958; Ansell and Spanner, 1968) or more than 400 times the concentration of the label injected, assuming uniform distribution.

The changes with time of both choline and acetylcholine specific radioactivity were different. Acetylcholine specific activity reached a maximum within 10 min from injection, followed by a gradual decrease to a value which was still measurable at 80 min. Choline specific activity, on the other hand, declined rapidly and reached a level which was not detectable by the sensitivity of the method within 20 to 40 min. The two curves crossed over between 5 and 7 min.

TABLE 1. *Specific activity of choline and acetylcholine in salivary glands of rats receiving 25 μC/kg intravenously of phosphoryl (Me-^{14}C) choline*

Time after injection (min)	Specific activity (cpm/nmole $\pm$ SE) $\times 10^2$	
	Acetylcholine	Choline
2	0.53 $\pm$ 0.14	0.91 $\pm$ 0.43
10	1.05 $\pm$ 0.44	0.32 $\pm$ 0.15
20	0.84 $\pm$ 0.25	0.13 $\pm$ 0.08
40	0.87 $\pm$ 0.10	< 0.03
80	0.46 $\pm$ 0.06	< 0.03

Each value represents mean $\pm$ SE of three values. Control levels of acetylcholine and choline expressed in terms of mean $\pm$ SE were 13.5 $\pm$ 1.2 and 141.2 $\pm$ 5.9 nmoles/g wet weight, respectively (n = 17 in both cases).

EFFECT OF DECENTRALIZATION ON CHOLINE AND ACETYLCHOLINE SPECIFIC RADIOACTIVITY IN SALIVARY GLANDS OF RATS RECEIVING PHOSPHORYL (Me-¹⁴C) CHOLINE

Having established this pattern of changes in specific activities of acetylcholine and its precursors in normal glands, the next experiment was designed to determine if this pattern is controlled by impulses origi-

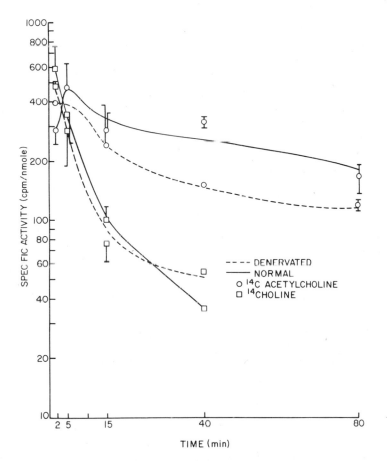

FIG. 5. Effect of unilateral decentralization of submaxillary and sublingual glands (chorda tympani section; 2 weeks after surgery) on turnover of choline and acetylcholine. Specific activities of choline and acetylcholine are plotted on the ordinate; time course comprises the abscissa. Rats were injected with phosphoryl (Me-¹⁴C) choline (25 μC/kg i.v.). Each point is the average ± SE of three sets of glands.

nating from the central nervous system. The right chorda tympani was sectioned at the level of the tympanic membrane and levels of acetylcholine and choline were first determined in these glands and compared with their contralateral normal controls 2 weeks after surgery. There was no statistically significant difference in these levels. We did observe, however, a weight loss of approximately 30% in the decentralized glands 2 weeks following surgery. This condition was still present 6 weeks after surgery.

Specific activities of choline and acetylcholine were next determined in decentralized glands and in their contralateral normal controls 2 weeks following surgery, after injection of phosphoryl (Me-^{14}C) choline as described in the previous experiment. Choline and acetylcholine steady-state concentrations were not altered by the injection of phosphorylcholine in either the normal or the decentralized glands. Choline specific radioactivities showed essentially the same trend in normal and decentralized glands over an 80-min time period. There was, however, a significant difference in acetylcholine specific activities between the normal and the decentralized glands (Fig. 5).

We are currently measuring the concentration of choline acetyl transferase in deafferented and normal glands to clarify if decentralization is associated with cholinergic neuron degeneration.

EFFECT OF PHARMACOLOGICAL AGENTS ON SPECIFIC RADIOACTIVITIES OF CHOLINE AND ACETYLCHOLINE IN NORMAL GLANDS OF RATS INJECTED WITH PHOSPHORYL (Me-^{14}C) CHOLINE

The glands of rats receiving atropine methylnitrate (45 mg/kg i.p.) behaved similarly to the decentralized glands when the animals had received the pulse labeling with phosphoryl (Me-^{14}C) choline 30 and 60 min earlier (Table 2). In contrast, although pilocarpine (100 mg/kg i.v.) stimulated copious parasympathetic salivary secretion lasting for 60 min or longer, it failed to change the form and sequence of change with time of choline and acetylcholine specific radioactivity. The experimental design followed in this experiment is schematized in Fig. 6. Phosphoryl (Me-^{14}C) choline (50 μC/kg) was administered at zero time, and 20 min later rats were divided into three separate groups of six animals. Each group was injected with saline, methylatropine, or pilocarpine at the doses and in the manner described. Thirty and 60 min later, three animals of each pretreated group were sacrificed and specific activities of choline and acetylcholine were determined in the usual way.

TABLE 2. *Effect of methylatropine (45 mg/kg: i.p.) on specific activities of choline and acetylcholine in salivary glands of rats injected with phosphoryl* (Me-^{14}C) *choline (25 μC/kg: i.v.) 20 min prior to drug administration*

Time after injection (min)	Effector used	Specific activity (cpm/nmole $\pm$ SE) $\times 10^2$	
		Acetylcholine	Choline
30	Saline	3.9 ± 1.25	0.28 ± 0.05
	Me-Atropine	1.2 ± 0.42	0.35 ± 0.13
60	Saline	1.8 ± 0.05	< 0.03
	Me-Atropine	< 0.3	< 0.03

Each value represents mean $\pm$ SE of three animals. Control levels of acetylcholine and choline expressed in terms of mean $\pm$ SE were 7.4 ± 0.6 and 112.9 ± 13.2 nmoles/g wet weight, respectively (n = 15 in both cases).

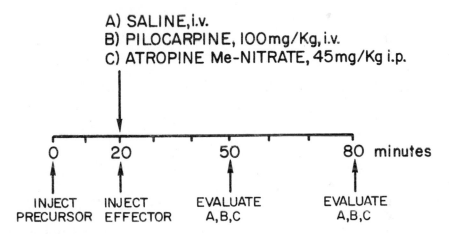

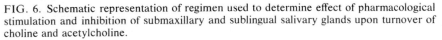

FIG. 6. Schematic representation of regimen used to determine effect of pharmacological stimulation and inhibition of submaxillary and sublingual salivary glands upon turnover of choline and acetylcholine.

DISCUSSION

The results obtained in this study have enabled us to construct a partial picture of the mechanism regulating cholinergic neurotransmitter metabolism in the rat submaxillary and sublingual glands.

The present understanding of the metabolic machinery functioning in the cholinergic nerve ending can be briefly summarized as follows. Choline is the immediate precursor for acetylcholine synthesis. It is transported across nerve membranes (Schuberth et al., 1967; Potter, 1968; Diamond and Kennedy, 1969), and synthesis of acetylcholine occurs in the cytoplasm of the nerve ending (Birks and MacIntosh, 1957; Angeles, Schueller, Lim, and Sotto, 1964). This synthesis is catalyzed by the enzyme choline acetyltransferase which is localized either in the cytoplasm (Fonnum, 1970) or in close vicinity of the vesicular membrane (McCaman, de Lores Arnaiz, and de Robertis, 1965; Saelens and Potter, 1966). Choline reacts with acetyl CoA in the presence of choline acetyltransferase to form acetylcholine. The mode of synthesis and source of acetyl CoA for synthesis of acetylcholine is presently a subject of deliberation.

The three compounds that may function as immediate precursors for this acetyl group in the mammalian system are now believed to be pyruvate, acetate, and/or citrate (see references earlier in the text). The newly formed acetylcholine in the cytoplasm is reported to redistribute itself into more than one pool: the "synaptosomal cytoplasmic" pool (Chakrin and Whittaker, 1969) and the "vesicular" pool (Marchbanks, 1968). The latter might be more resistant to release by nerve impulses whereas the former might be preferentially released. These inferences cannot be readily reconciled with the observation that nerve impulses increase the possibility that vesicles interact with nerve-ending membranes and release their content extraneuronally (Katz, 1971). The acetylcholine released from presynaptic nerve endings diffuses across the narrow synaptic cleft and reacts with receptors at the postsynaptic membrane (see review by Hebb, 1963) to induce a specific response. This action of acetylcholine is terminated partially by its enzymatic hydrolysis into choline and acetic acid. The choline might be either metabolized or taken up again by the nerve ending. This reuptake apparently contributes significantly to the turnover rate of neuronal choline (Perry, 1953; Collier and MacIntosh, 1969; Potter, 1970). It must be ascertained if the acetylcholine which has not been hydrolyzed is taken up to a minor extent by endings as suggested by Kramer, Seifter, and Bhagat (1968), Guth (1969), Liang and Quastel (1969), Polak (1969), Heilbronn (1970), Adamič (1970), and Schuberth et al. (1970). No physiological significance has yet been attached to this uptake.

The precursor product relationships for choline and acetylcholine (Table 1, Fig. 5) are thus predictable on the basis of this scheme. We have shown that, after administration of labeled phosphoryl (Me-^{14}C) choline in rats, there is a rapid incorporation of radioactivity into choline and an increase of acetylcholine specific radioactivity. The latter proceeds as long as the specific activity of choline is greater than that of acetylcholine. After the crossover point, the acetylcholine specific activity maintains a plateau and then declines at a rate slower than that of choline (as shown by the solid lines in Fig. 5). This sequence suggests, but does not prove, a precursor-product relationship (Zilversmit, 1960).

Twenty to 40 min after the pulse injection of radiolabeled phosphoryl choline, the specific activity of choline is not measureable. Since the specific activity of acetylcholine persists despite the low level of radioactive choline in the salivary glands, radioactive acetylcholine must be continuously formed from the labeled choline by processes with rate constants k_1' and k_1'' (Fig. 7). Several lines of evidence suggest that acetylcholine in

CHOLINERGIC NERVE ENDING

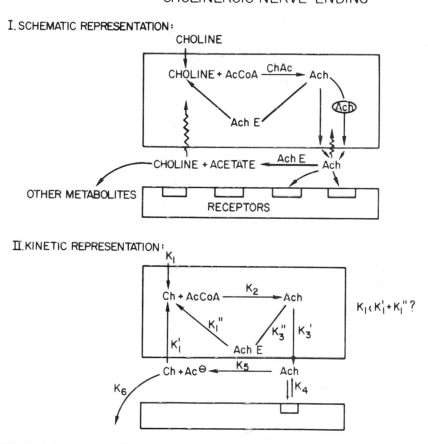

FIG. 7. Schematic and kinetic representation of the currently accepted biochemical regulatory mechanisms at the cholinergic nerve ending.

the synaptic cleft, after its extraneuronal release, is hydrolyzed by cholinesterase to form choline (Giacobini, 1959; Koelle, 1963; Augustinsson, 1963; Brzin, Tennyson, and Duffy, 1966) which is then reincorporated for the biosynthesis of acetylcholine in nerve terminals (Perry, 1953; Collier and MacIntosh, 1969). Hence, the origin of choline participating in synthesis of acetylcholine is contributed by a number of processes indicated in Fig. 7 by k_1, k_1', and k_1'', and these processes must have a key role in maintaining the acetylcholine at constant level.

When we reduce the nerve traffic by ablation of the chorda tympani, the acetylcholine level drops to a new steady state (same amount per gram of tissue despite the reduction in gland weight). Thus it can be postulated that synthesis relates to function. Moreover, the faster initial decline of acetylcholine specific activity to the right of the crossover point between the two specific activities (choline and acetylcholine) suggests that the processes with rate constant k_1' and k_1'' are important in causing the acetylcholine specific activity to endure, and that when nerve impulses are reduced the contribution by k_1' and k_1'' are proportionally reduced.

If reuptake of choline is the main mechanism operating in the homeostasis of cholinergic nerves, great importance should be given to this process in the study of cholinergic function. Hence, one wonders about the value of experiments where cholinesterase is blocked and acetylcholine efflux is measured with the intention to correlate cholinergic function with acetylcholine synthesis. Pharmacological stimulation or inhibition of the submaxillary ganglion innervating the glands would give us further insight into the contribution of neuronal input making synaptic connections at this site on the turnover of acetylcholine. Such studies are currently in progress.

Because of the high doses of methylatropine used in this study, the present data cannot rule out the possibility that methylatropine is interfering with the active reuptake of choline by process k_1' (Hemsworth, Darmer, and Bosmann, 1971)—a factor which would also contribute to a faster decrease in the specific activity of neuronal acetylcholine. The significant decrease in acetylcholine specific activity following methylatropine administration would, however, be consistent with the observation that atropine interacts extraneuronally with process k_3', increasing release of acetylcholine. This suggestion is in agreement with MacIntosh and Oborin (1953), Mitchell (1963), Giarman and Pepeu (1964), Szerb (1964), Celesia and Jasper (1966), and Polak and Meeuws (1966). This suggestion is further strengthened by observations of Pauling and Petcher (1970) which indicate from studies of the crystal structure of atropine that both atropine and acetylcholine interact with the muscarinic receptor in similar ways and at the same site. If hydrolysis of acetylcholine released by nerve impulses is maximal at this receptor site, atropine could, by occupying some of the receptors, be retarding the hydrolysis of acetylcholine in a competitive manner, thus decreasing reutilization of radioactive choline for the synthesis of acetylcholine.

The model which we have presented here is admittedly highly simplified in depicting cholinergic function, but it allows an initial kinetic approach to the study of *in vivo* turnover of acetylcholine. It is also flexible enough to incorporate changes and adaptations. Thus, with a further insight into the mechanisms involved in cholinergic nerve function, we will be able, if necessary, to modify this kinetic model in order to incorporate new information emerging from our work and the work of other investigators.

SUMMARY

An approach has been developed to study turnover of choline and acetylcholine on a simple model system *in vivo*. Phosphoryl (Me-^{14}C) choline (25 μC/kg) has been used as precursor for radioactive choline and acetylcholine formed *in situ*. Specific activities have been estimated by means of a gas chromatographic procedure for estimating tissue choline and acetylcholine, which has been adapted for use on a gas chromatograph–radioactivity monitoring system. Specific activities of choline and acetylcholine have been determined in rat submaxillary and sublingual glands as a function of time, to establish basal steady-state precursor-product conditions. Unilateral decentralization (chorda tympani section) in these salivary glands, when compared with the contralateral normal glands, appears to accelerate efflux of radioactive acetylcholine. Changes in steady-state conditions and in specific activities have been measured in normal glands following injections of a parasympathetic agonist (pilocarpine, 100 mg/kg i.v.) and antagonist (methylatropine, 45 mg/kg i.p.). Methylatropine increases acetylcholine efflux from the gland. A tentative model has been constructed to incorporate existing known factors functioning in the dynamics of the cholinergic nerve terminal. Our findings described in this manuscript have been interpreted on the basis of this model.

REFERENCES

Adamič, S. (1970): Accumulation of acetylcholine by the rat diaphragm. *Biochemical Pharmacology*, 19:2445–2451.

Albrecht, P., Visscher, M. B., Bittner, J. J., and Halberg, F. (1956): Daily changes in 5-hydroxytryptamine concentration in mouse brain. *Proceedings of the Society for Experimental Biology and Medicine*, 92:703–706.

Alousi, A., and Weiner, N. (1966): The regulation of norepinephrine synthesis in sympathetic nerves: Effects of nerve stimulation, cocaine, and catecholamine-releasing agents. *Proceedings of the National Academy of Sciences*, 56:1491–1496.

Angeles, L., Schueller, F., Lim, P., and Sotto, A. (1964): Effect of choline deficiency on HC-3 action. *Archives Internationales de Pharmacodynamie et de Therapie*, 152:253–256.

Ansell, G. B., and Spanner, S. (1968): The metabolism of [Me-¹⁴C] choline in the brain of the rat *in vivo*. *Biochemical Journal*, 110:201–206.

Ansell, G. B., and Spanner, S. (1970): The origin and turnover of choline in the brain. In: *Drugs and Cholinergic Mechanisms in the CNS*, edited by E. Heilbronn and A. Winter. Research Institute of National Defense, Stockholm, Sweden, pp. 143–159.

Ansell, G. B., and Spanner, S. (1971): Studies on the origin of choline in the brain of the rat. *Biochemical Journal*, 122:741–750.

Askari, A. (1966): Uptake of some quaternary ammonium ions by human erythrocytes. *Journal of General Physiology*, 49:1147–1160.

Augustinsson, K.-B. (1963): Classification and comparative enzymology of the cholinesterases and methods for their determination. In: *Handbuch der Experimentellen Pharmakologie*, *XV*, edited by G. B. Koelle. Springer-Verlag, Berlin, pp. 89–128.

Axelrod, J., Mueller, R. A., and Thoenen, H. (1970): Neuronal and hormonal control of tyrosine hydroxylase and phenylethanolamine N-methyl-transferase activity. In: *Bayer Symposium II*, edited by H. H. Schümann and G. Kroneberg. Springer-Verlag, Berlin, pp. 212–219.

Birks, R., and MacIntosh, F. C. (1957): Acetylcholine metabolism at nerve endings. *British Medical Bulletin*, 13:157–161.

Birks, R., and MacIntosh, F. C. (1961): Acetylcholine metabolism of a sympathetic ganglion. *Canadian Journal of Biochemistry and Physiology*, 39:787–827.

Bosmann, H. B., and Hemsworth, B. A. (1970): Synaptic vesicles: Incorporation of choline by isolated synaptosomes and synaptic vesicles. *Biochemical Pharmacology*, 19:133–141.

Bremer, J., and Greenberg, D. M. (1959): Mono- and dimethylethanolamine isolated from rat liver phospholipids. *Biochimica et Biophysica Acta*, 35:287–288.

Bremer, J., and Greenberg, D. M. (1961): Methyl transferring enzyme system of microsomes in the biosynthesis of lecithin (phosphatidylcholine). *Biochimica et Biophysica Acta*, 46:205–216.

Brown, G. L., and Feldberg, W. (1936): The acetylcholine metabolism of a sympathetic ganglion. *Journal of Physiology*, 88:265–283.

Browning, E. T., and Schulman, M. P. (1968): [¹⁴C]-Acetylcholine synthesis by cortex slices of rat brain. *Journal of Neurochemistry*, 15:1391–1405.

Brzin, M., Tennyson, V., and Duffy, P. (1966): Combined cytochemical-electron microscopic localization of cholinesterases in the nervous system. In: *Biochemistry and Pharmacology of the Basal Ganglia*, edited by E. Costa, L. J. Côté, and M. D. Yahr. Raven Press, New York, pp. 65–87.

Campbell, L. B., and Jenden, D. J. (1970): Gas chromatographic evaluation of the influence of oxotremorine upon the regional distribution of acetylcholine in rat brain. *Journal of Neurochemistry*, 17:1697–1699.

Celesia, G. G., and Jasper, H. H. (1966): Acetylcholine released from cerebral cortex in relation to state of activation. *Neurology*, 16:1053–1064.

Chakrin, L. W., and Shideman, F. E. (1968): Synthesis of acetylcholine from labeled choline by brain. *International Journal of Neuropharmacology*, 7:337–349.

Chakrin, L. W., and Whittaker, V. P. (1969): The subcellular distribution of [N-Me-³H] acetylcholine synthesized by brain *in vivo*. *Biochemical Journal*, 113:97–107.

Cheney, D. L., Gubler, C. J., and Jaussi, A. W. (1969): Production of acetylcholine in rat brain following thiamine deprivation and treatment with thiamine antagonists. *Journal of Neurochemistry*, 16:1283–1291.

Collier, B., and Lang, C. (1969): The metabolism of choline by a sympathetic ganglion. *Canadian Journal of Physiology and Pharmacology*, 47:119–126.

Collier, B., and MacIntosh, F. C. (1969): The source of choline for acetylcholine synthesis in a sympathetic ganglion. *Canadian Journal of Physiology and Pharmacology*, 47:127–135.

Costa, E. (1970): Simple neuronal models to estimate turnover rate of noradrenergic transmitters *in vivo*. In: *Biochemistry of Simple Neuronal Models*, edited by E. Costa and E. Giacobini. Raven Press, New York, pp. 169–204.

Costa, E., and Neff, N. H. (1966): Isotopic and non-isotopic measurements of the rate of catecholamine biosynthesis. In: *Biochemistry and Pharmacology of the Basal Ganglia*, edited by E. Costa, L. J. Côté, and M. D. Yahr. Raven Press, New York, pp. 141–155.

Costa, E., and Neff, N. H. (1970): Estimation of turnover rates to study the metabolic regulation of the steady-state level of neuronal monoamines. In: *Handbook of Neurochemistry*, Vol. 4, edited by A. Lajtha. Plenum Press, New York, pp. 45–90.

Crossland, J., and Merrick, A. J. (1954): The effect of anaesthesia on the acetylcholine content of brain. *Journal of Physiology*, 125:56–66.

Dawson, R. M. C. (1955): Phosphorylcholine in rat tissues. *Biochemical Journal*, 60:325–328.

Diamond, I. (1971): Choline metabolism in brain. *Archives of Neurology*, 24:333–339.

Diamond, I., and Kennedy, E. P. (1969): Carrier mediated transport of choline into synaptic nerve endings. *Journal of Biological Chemistry*, 244:3258–3263.

Fitzgerald, G. G., and Cooper, J. R. (1967): Studies on acetylcholine in the corneal epithelium. *Federation Proceedings*, 26:651.

Folkow, B., Häggendal, J., and Lisander, B. (1967): Extent of release and elimination of noradrenaline at peripheral adrenergic nerve terminals. *Acta Physiologica Scandinavica, Suppl.* 307.

Fonnum, F. (1970): Subcellular localization of choline acetyltransferase in brain. In: *Drugs and Cholinergic Mechanisms in the CNS*, edited by E. Heilbronn and A. Winter. Research Institute of National Defense, Stockholm, Sweden, pp. 83–95.

Friedman, A. H., and Walker, C. A. (1969a): Rat brain amines, blood histamine and glucose levels in relationship to circadian changes in sleep induced by pentobarbitone sodium. *Journal of Physiology*, 202:133–146.

Friedman, A. H., and Walker, C. A. (1969b): Circadian rhythms in central acetylcholine and the toxicity of cholinergic drugs. *Federation Proceedings*, 28:251.

Friesen, A. J. D., Kemp, J. W., and Woodbury, D. M. (1964): Identification of acetylcholine in sympathetic ganglia by chemical and physical methods. *Science*, 145:157–159.

Friesen, A. J. D., Kemp, J. W., and Woodbury, D. W. (1965): The chemical and physical identification of acetylcholine from sympathetic ganglia. *Journal of Pharmacology and Experimental Therapeutics*, 148:312–319.

Giacobini, E. (1959): The distribution and localization of cholinesterases in nerve cells. *Acta Physiologica Scandinavica* 45, *Suppl.* 156: pp. 1–45.

Giarman, N. J., and Pepeu, G. C. (1964): The influence of centrally acting cholinolytic drugs on brain acetylcholine levels. *British Journal of Pharmacology and Chemotherapy*, 23:123–130.

Gordon, R., Reid, J. V. O., Sjoerdsma, A., and Udenfriend, S. (1966): Increased synthesis of norepinephrine in the rat heart on electrical stimulation of the stellate ganglion. *Molecular Pharmacology*, 2:606–613.

Groth, D. P., Bain, J. A. and Pfeiffer, C. C. (1958): The comparative distribution of C^{14}-labeled 2-dimethylamine ethanol and choline in the mouse. *Journal of Pharmacology and Experimental Therapeutics*, 124:290–295.

Guth, P. S. (1969): Acetylcholine binding by isolated synaptic vesicles *in vitro*. *Nature*, 224:384–385.

Hammar, C.-G., Hanin, I., Holmstedt, B., Kitz, R. J., Jenden, D. J., and Karlén, B. (1968): Identification of acetylcholine in fresh rat brain by combined gas chromatography-mass spectrometry. *Nature*, 220:915–917.

Hanin, I., and Jenden, D. J. (1968): Estimation of choline esters in brain by a new gas chromatographic procedure. *Biochemical Pharmacology*, 18:837–845.

Hanin, I., Massarelli, R., and Costa, E. (1970a): Acetylcholine concentrations in rat brain: Diurnal oscillation. *Science,* 170:341–342.

Hanin, I., Massarelli, R., and Costa, E. (1970b): Environmental and technical preconditions influencing choline and acetylcholine concentrations in rat brain. In: *Drugs and Cholinergic Mechanisms in the CNS,* edited by E. Heilbronn and A. Winter. Research Institute of National Defense, Stockholm, Sweden, pp. 33–54.

Hanin, I., Massarelli, R., and Costa, E. (1972): An approach to the *in vivo* study of acetylcholine turnover in rat salivary glands by radio gas chromatography. *Journal of Pharmacology and Experimental Therapeutics,* 181:10–18.

Hebb, C. (1963): Formation, storage, and liberation of acetylcholine. In: *Handbuch der Experimentellen Pharmakologie,* Erg. XV, edited by G. B. Koelle. Springer-Verlag, Berlin, pp. 55–88.

Hebb, C., Ling, G., McGeer, E., McGeer, P., and Perkins, D. (1964): Effect of locally applied hemicholinium on acetylcholine content of the caudate nucleus. *Nature,* 204:1309–1311.

Heilbronn, E. (1970): Further experiments on the uptake of acetylcholine and atropine and the release of acetylcholine from mouse brain cortex slices after treatment with phospholipases. *Journal of Neurochemistry,* 17:381–389.

Hemsworth, B. A., Darmer, K. I., Jr., and Bosmann, H. B. (1971): The incorporation of choline into isolated synaptosomal and synaptic vesicle fractions in the presence of quaternary ammonium compounds. *Neuropharmacology,* 10:109–120.

Honneger, C. G., and Honneger, R. (1959): Occurrence and quantitative determination of 2-dimethylaminoethanol in animal tissue extracts. *Nature,* 184:550–552.

Katz, B. (1971): Quantal mechanism of neural transmitter release. *Science,* 173:123–126.

Koelle, G. B. (1963): Cytological distributions and physiological functions of cholinesterases. In: *Cholinesterases and Anticholinesterase Agents. Handbuch der Experimentellen Pharmakologie,* Erg. XV, edited by G. B. Koelle. Springer-Verlag, Berlin, pp. 187–298.

Kramer, S. Z., Seifter, J., and Bhagat, B. (1968): Regional distribution of tritiated acetylcholine in rat brain. *Nature,* 217:184–185.

Liang, C. C., and Quastel, J. H. (1969): Uptake of acetylcholine in rat brain cortex slices. *Biochemical Pharmacology,* 18:1169–1185.

MacIntosh, F. C. (1941): The distribution of acetylcholine in the peripheral and the central nervous system. *Journal of Physiology,* 99:436–442.

MacIntosh, F. C., and Oborin, P. E. (1953): Release of acetylcholine from intact cerebral cortex. *Abstract XIX International Physiology Congress:* 580–581.

Marchbanks, R. M. (1968): The uptake of [^{14}C]-choline into synaptosomes *in vitro. Biochemical Journal,* 110:533–541.

Martin, K. (1968): Concentrative accumulation of choline by human erythrocytes. *Journal of General Physiology,* 51:497–516.

McCaman, R. E., Arnaiz, G. R. de L., and DeRobertis, E. (1965): Species differences in subcellular distribution of choline acetylase in the CNS. A study of choline acetylase, acetylcholinesterase, 5-hydroxytryptophan decarboxylase and monoamine oxidase in four species. *Journal of Neurochemistry,* 12:927–935.

Mitchell, J. F. (1963): The spontaneous and evoked release of acetylcholine from the cerebral cortex. *Journal of Physiology,* 165:98–116.

Montanari, R., Costa, E., Beaven, M. A., and Brodie, B. B. (1963): Turnover rates of norepinephrine in hearts of intact mice, rats, and guinea pigs using tritiated norepinephrine. *Life Sciences,* 4:232–240.

Nakamura, R., and Cheng, S.-C. (1969): Evidence for the metabolic compartmentalization of acetyl coenzyme A in rat brain slices and its relation to the synthesis of acetylcholine and glutamate. *Life Sciences,* 8:657–662.

Neff, N. H., and Costa, E. (1966): Effect of tricyclic antidepressants and chlorpromazine on brain catecholamine synthesis. *Proceedings of the First International Symposium on Antidepressant Drugs,* 122:23–34.

Oliverio, A., and Stjärne, L. (1965): Acceleration of norepinephrine turnover in mouse heart by cold exposure. *Life Sciences,* 4:2339–2343.

Pauling, P. J., and Petcher, T. J. (1970): Interaction of atropine with the muscarinic receptor. *Nature*, 228:673–674.

Pepeu, G. C., Bartolini, A., and Deffenu, G. (1970): Investigations into the increase of acetylcholine output from the cerebral cortex of the cat caused by amphetamine. In: *Drugs and Cholinergic Mechanisms in the CNS*, edited by E. Heilbronn and A. Winter. Research Institute of National Defense, Stockholm, Sweden, pp. 387–410.

Perry, W. L. M. (1953): Acetylcholine release in the cat's superior cervical ganglion. *Journal of Physiology*, 119:439–454.

Polak, R. L. (1969): The influence of drugs on the uptake of acetylcholine by slices of rat cerebral cortex. *British Journal of Pharmacology*, 36:144–152.

Polak, R. L., and Meeuws, M. M. (1966): The influence of atropine on the release and uptake of acetylcholine by the isolated cerebral cortex of the cat. *Biochemical Pharmacology*, 15: 989–992.

Porcellati, G. (1958): The levels of some free nitrogen-containing phosphate esters in nervous tissue. *Journal of Neurochemistry*, 2:128–137.

Potter, L. T. (1968): Uptake of choline by nerve endings isolated from the rat cerebral cortex. In: *The Interaction of Drugs and Subcellular Components on Animal Cells*, edited by P. N. Campbell. J. & A. Churchill Ltd., London, p. 293.

Potter, L. T. (1970): Synthesis, storage, and release of [^{14}C] acetylcholine in isolated rat diaphragm muscles. *Journal of Physiology*, 206:145–166.

Potter, L. T., and Glover, V. A. S. (1970): Choline acetyltransferase from mammalian brains. In: *Drugs and Cholinergic Mechanisms in the CNS*, edited by E. Heilbronn and A. Winter. Research Institute of National Defense, Stockholm, Sweden, pp. 75–81.

Potter, L. T., Glover, V. A. S., and Saelens, J. K. (1968): Choline acetyltransferase from rat brain. *Journal of Biological Chemistry*, 243:3864–3870.

Quastel, J. H. (1955): Acetylcholine synthesis in the central nervous system. In: *Neurochemistry*, edited by K. A. C. Elliott, I. H. Page, and J. H. Quastel. C. A. Thomas, Springfield, Ill., pp. 153–172.

Quay, W. B. (1964): Circadian and estrous rhythms in pineal melatonin and 5-hydroxyindole-3-acetic acid. *Proceedings of the Society for Experimental Biology and Medicine*, 115: 710–713.

Reis, D. J., Weinbren, M., and Corvelli, A. (1968): A circadian rhythm of norepinephrine regionally in cat brain: Its relationship to environmental lighting and to regional diurnal variations in brain serotonin. *Journal of Pharmacology and Experimental Therapeutics*, 164:135–145.

Saelens, J. K., and Potter, L. T. (1966): Subcellular localization of choline acetyltransferase in rat brain cortex. *Federation Proceedings*, 25:451.

Saelens, J. K., and Stoll, W. R. (1965): Radiochemical determination of choline and acetylcholine flux from isolated tissue. *Journal of Pharmacology and Experimental Therapeutics*, 147:336–342.

Scheving, L. E., Harrison, W. H., Gordon, P., and Pauly, J. E. (1968): Daily fluctuations (circadian and ultradian) in biogenic amines of the rat brain. *American Journal of Physiology*, 214:166–173.

Schuberth, J., Sundwall, A., and Sörbo, B. (1967): Relation between Na$^+$-K$^+$ transport and the uptake of choline by brain slices. *Life Sciences*, 6:293–295.

Schuberth, J., Sparf, B. and Sundwall, A. (1969): A technique for the study of acetylcholine turnover in mouse brain *in vivo*. *Journal of Neurochemistry*, 16:695–700.

Schuberth, J., Sparf, B., and Sundwall, A. (1970): On the turnover of acetylcholine in the brain. In: *Drugs and Cholinergic Mechanisms in the CNS*, edited by E. Heilbronn and A. Winters. Research Institute of National Defense, Stockholm, Sweden, pp. 177–186.

Sedvall, G. C., and Kopin, I. J. (1967): Acceleration of norepinephrine synthesis in the rat submaxillary gland *in vivo* during sympathetic nerve stimulation. *Life Sciences*, 6:45–51.

Smallman, B. N. (1958): The choline acetylase activity of rabbit brain. *Journal of Neurochemistry*, 2:119–127.

Sörbo, B. (1970): On the origin of the acetyl group of acetylcholine. In: *Drugs and Cholinergic*

Mechanisms in the CNS, edited by E. Heilbronn and A. Winter. Research Institute of National Defense, Stockholm, Sweden, pp. 133–139.

Spector, S., Gordon, R., Sjoerdsma, A., and Udenfriend, S. (1967): End product inhibition of tyrosine hydroxylase as a possible mechanism for regulating norepinephrine synthesis. *Molecular Pharmacology*, 3:549–555.

Sung, C.-P., and Johnstone, R. M. (1965): Evidence for active transport of choline in rat kidney cortex slices. *Canadian Journal of Biochemistry*, 43:1111–1118.

Szerb, J. C. (1964): The effect of tertiary and quaternary atropine on cortical acetylcholine output and on the electroencephalogram in cats. *Canadian Journal of Physiology and Pharmacology*, 42:303–314.

Takahashi, R., and Aprison, M. H. (1964): Acetylcholine content of discrete areas of the brain obtained by a near-freezing method. *Journal of Neurochemistry*, 11:887–898.

Tuček, S., and Cheng, S.-C. (1970): Precursors of acetyl groups in acetylcholine in the brain *in vivo*. *Biochimica et Biophysica Acta*, 208:538–540.

Wallach, M., Goldberg, A., and Shideman, F. (1967): The synthesis of labeled acetylcholine by the isolated cat heart and its release by vagal stimulation. *International Journal of Neuropharmacology*, 6:317–323.

Wurtman, R. J., and Axelrod, J. (1966): A 24-hour rhythm in the content of norepinephrine in the pineal and salivary glands of the rat. *Life Sciences*, 5:665–669.

Wurtman, R. J., Chou, C., and Rose, C. M. (1967): Daily rhythm in tyrosine concentration in human plasma: Persistence on low-protein diets. *Science*, 158:660–662.

Zilversmit, D. B. (1960): The design and analysis of isotope experiments. *American Journal of Medicine*, 29:832–848.

Advances in Biochemical Psychopharmacology, Vol. 6
Raven Press, New York © 1972

Biochemical Effects of Psychotomimetic Anticholinergic Drugs

John J. O'Neill, Trudy Termini, and Joanne G. Walker

*Department of Pharmacology, Ohio State University College of Medicine,
Columbus, Ohio 43210*

Atropine and scopolamine at high concentrations (5 to 10 mg) produce in man a peripheral muscarinic blockade of smooth muscle and, frequently, marked central nervous system stimulation. Glycolate esters are atropine-like in action, possessing marked antimuscarinic actions peripherally.

Ditran® (JB-329) and other anticholinergic drugs of this class are known to produce bizarre behavioral changes in animals and in normal human subjects (Abood and Biel, 1962). In efforts to understand the relationship between psychotomimetic properties and chemical structures, a large number of derivatives have been synthesized by Abood (1970). In Fig. 1, a few representative compounds of this class are shown. Much of our present study is concerned with the biochemical effects of JB-840 (phenyl-cyclopentyl) glycolic acid ester of 1-N-methyl-3-hydroxy piperidinol and JB-329 or Ditran (a 30 to 70% mixture of the phenyl cyclopentyl glycolic acid esters of 3-hydroxy-1-ethyl piperidinol and 3-hydroxymethyl-1-ethyl pyrollidinol).

In 1963 we (O'Neill, Simon, and Cummins) reported the inhibitory action of glycolate esters (Fig. 1) on stimulated respiration in rat brain cortex slices. In Table 1 are the results of similar studies. Attention should be directed to the compounds labeled JB-840 and JB-329. You will note that while these drugs have little effect on unstimulated respiration, potassium ion stimulation (105 mM) is inhibited by more than 60%.

Similarly, JB-329 or Ditran has a comparable (60%) inhibitory effect on stimulated respiration. Even the compound Daricon®, a potent spasmolytic in man which is devoid of central effects, inhibited stimulation by about 50%.

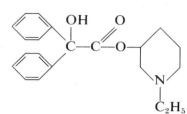

JB-318

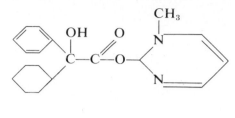

oxyphencyclimine
(Daricon)

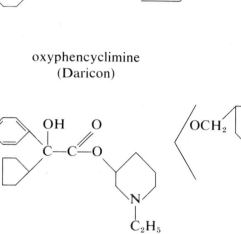

JB-336

30%

Ditran (JB-329)

70%

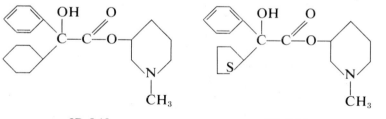

JB-840   JB-344

FIG. 1. Glycolic acid derivatives.

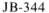

In like manner, JB-840 and Ditran caused selective inhibition of electrically stimulated respiration in guinea pig cortex slices (Table 2). A more detailed study of the action of JB-840 is presented in Table 3. It is to be noted that in unstimulated tissue the amounts of glucose utilized and lactate produced are not affected by the presence of JB-840 over a considerable concentration range. With stimulation however, the drug blocks the antici-

TABLE 1. *Inhibitory effect of cholinolytics on potassium ion-stimulated cerebral cortex respiration*[a]

Drug	Concn. (M)	Potassium ion (105 mM) stimulation		
		Unstimulated[b]	Stimulated[b]	Inhibition[c] (%)
Control		73	122	
JB-840	5×10^{-4}	68	87	62
	1×10^{-4}	73	135	0
Control		60	117	
JB-336	5×10^{-4}	59	91	44
	1×10^{-4}	59	108	13
	5×10^{-5}	59	103	23
Control		60	117	
JB-318	5×10^{-4}	56	76	64
	2.5×10^{-4}	58	94	37
	1×10^{-4}	54	100	18
	5×10^{-5}	57	115	0
Control		72	122	
JB-329	5×10^{-4}	72	91	61
	1×10^{-4}	62	109	4
Control		60	117	
JB-344	5×10^{-4}	56	100	26
	1×10^{-4}	53	103	14
Control		76	122	
		54	98	
Daricon	5×10^{-4}	77	98	52
	1×10^{-4}	54	85	31
	1×10^{-5}	56	94	15

[a] Rat brain.
[b] Rates are expressed as μmoles O_2/g fresh weight per hr.
[c] Inhibition (%) = $\dfrac{\text{control (stim} - \text{unstim)} - \text{drug (stim} - \text{unstim)}}{\text{control (stim} - \text{unstim)}}$ × 100. Recalculated from dry weight data previously published (O'Neill, Simon, and Cummins, 1963). Dry weight: wet weight ratio = 0.147; fresh weight:wet weight ratio = 0.70.

pated increase in glycolysis. Respiration, glucose consumption, and lactate production (Table 3) look very similar to unstimulated tissue. In Table 4 attention should again be given to the first two entries. Stimulated respiration is quite effectively blocked as are changes in glucose utilized and lactate formed.

Glycolysis alone may satisfy the energy demands of unstimulated brain slices which do not appear to be affected by the presence of drug. The energy demands at the excitable membrane level of stimulated tissue, however, can best be met through oxidative metabolism coupled through the respiratory chain. This increase in oxidative metabolism is undoubtedly

TABLE 2. *Inhibitory effect of cholinolytics on electrically stimulated cerebral cortex respiration*[a]

Drug	Concn. (M)	Electrical stimulation		
		Unstimulated[b]	Stimulated[b]	Inhibition (%)
Control		42	89	
JB-840	5×10^{-4}	54	59	87
	5×10^{-5}	54	72	56
Control		60	108	
JB-336	5×10^{-4}	51	68	64
	1×10^{-4}	52	75	51
Control		60	108	
JB-318	5×10^{-4}	51	58	84
	1×10^{-4}	56	72	65
Control		47	74	
JB-329	5×10^{-4}	49	49	100
	1×10^{-4}	45	62	36
Control		47	79	
JB-344	5×10^{-4}	50	64	56
	1×10^{-4}	46	64	51
Control		47	79	
Daricon	5×10^{-4}	56	65	70
	1×10^{-4}	48	68	40

[a] Guinea pig brain.
[b] Rates are expressed as μmoles O_2/g fresh weight per hr. Recalculated from dry weight data previously published (O'Neill, Simon, and Cummins, 1963). Dry weight:wet weight ratio = 0.147; fresh weight:wet weight ratio = 0.70.

TABLE 3. *Influence of JB-840 on cerebral cortex respiration and glycolysis*

Drug concn. (M)	Unstimulated			K+ (105 mM) Stimulation		
	Oxygen uptake	Lactate formed	Glucose utilized	Oxygen uptake	Lactate formed	Glucose utilized
Control	51 ± 5	27 ± 5	22 ± 2	104 ± 5	67 ± 4	46 ± 3
5×10^{-4}	56 ± 6	29 ± 9	23 ± 2	59 ± 6	34 ± 7	27 ± 6
10^{-4}	47	30 ± 4	24	86 ± 7	46 ± 4	25 ± 7
10^{-5}	57		25	99 ± 8	66 ± 3	43 ± 7
10^{-6}	49	30	24	90 ± 3	69 ± 6	41 ± 6
10^{-7}	49		22	99 ± 6	71 ± 2	43 ± 6
	50 ± 5	29 ± 6	23 ± 3			

Rates expressed as μmoles/wet g per hr, mean ± standard deviation; male guinea pig cortex. Glucose and lactate measurements are estimated from tissue content plus medium.

TABLE 4. *Influence of JB-840 on cerebral cortex respiration and glycolysis*

Drug concn. (M)	Unstimulated			Electrical (12 V) Stimulation		
	Oxygen uptake	Lactate formed	Glucose utilized	Oxygen uptake	Lactate formed	Glucose utilized
Control	51 ± 5	27 ± 5	22 ± 2	98 ± 11	50 ± 6	44 ± 8
5×10^{-4}	56 ± 6	29 ± 9	23 ± 2	56 ± 11	38 ± 8	23 ± 7
10^{-4}	47	30 ± 4	24	69 ± 14	33 ± 5	22 ± 8
10^{-5}	57		25	93 ± 10	41 ± 6	29 ± 5
10^{-6}	49	30	24	92 ± 9	43 ± 5	31 ± 5
10^{-7}	49		22	96 ± 13	51 ± 4	40 ± 7
	50 ± 5	29 ± 6	23 ± 2			

Rates expressed as μmoles/wet g per hr, mean $\pm$ standard deviation; male guinea pig cortex.

TABLE 5. *Influence of phosphate ion concentration on Ditran inhibition of K^+ stimulation*

	Glucose	Lactate	Pyruvate	G6P
5 mM P_i control	38	$8,140 \pm 560$	$1,540 \pm 255$	105 ± 30
+ Ditran (5×10^{-4} M)	30	$5,400 \pm 200$	$1,127 \pm 129$	81 ± 20
10 mM P_i control	67	$8,750 \pm 500$	$1,624 \pm 21$	94 ± 9
+ Ditran (5×10^{-4} M)	21	$4,970 \pm 300$	$1,015 \pm 22$	78 ± 6
15 mM P_i control	35	$10,140 \pm 1,090$	$1,135 \pm 125$	129 ± 47
+ Ditran (5×10^{-4} M)	17	$7,250 \pm 780$	794 ± 128	106 ± 20
20 mM P_i control	72	$7,010 \pm 300$	$1,616 \pm 146$	110 ± 25
+ Ditran (5×10^{-4} M)	12	$5,440 \pm 700$	$1,268 \pm 94$	81 ± 31
Zero time control	–	$3,340 \pm 400$	297 ± 76	64 ± 15

[+] 105 mM K^+ concentration.

Glucose in μmoles/fresh g per hr. All other results are μmoles/kg fresh weight (tissue plus medium).

accompanied by the rapid turnover of ATP and ADP plus P_i. This change in steady state brings about a secondary increase in glycolysis; Ditran blocks both.

The role of phosphate ion in glycolysis has been emphasized in the studies on phosphofructokinase by Passonneau and Lowry (1962) and on hexokinase and glyceraldehyde-3-phosphate dehydrogenase by Racker (1965).

Table 5 shows changes in glycolytic intermediates in the presence of Ditran. With increasing P_i concentration there appears to be an increase in the glucose consumption of stimulated controls, an effect not seen with Ditran; indeed, Ditran inhibition appears to increase with increasing phosphate concentration. Since all values represent tissue content plus medium, a pyruvate "leak" similar to the lactate "leak" may account for high pyruvate values, which normally would be in the range of 100 to 200 μmoles/kg.

At high P_i (15 mM), changes in pyruvate (Table 6) range from 600 to 700 μmoles/kg per hr in unstimulated tissue to 1,100 μmoles/kg per hr in stimulated controls, but to less than 800 μmoles at high Ditran concentrations.

Potassium ions cause a depolarization of nerve endings and increase respiratory activity; both would lead to an accelerated conversion of pyruvate to acetyl-coenzyme A. The changes may be linked directly to the stimulation of acetylcholine metabolism. Ditran appears to have an inhibitory effect at this step.

In Table 7 data are presented for some important glycolytic intermediates and the amino acids, glutamate, and aspartate. Glucose-6-phosphate does not change significantly with stimulation (entries 1 and 3) and actually

TABLE 6. *Influence of Ditran on brain metabolites at high (15 mM) phosphate*

Treatment	Glucose	Lactate	Pyruvate
Control (unstimulated)	15	6,520 ± 560	712 ± 43
Ditran (5 × 10⁻⁴ M) (unstimulated)	12	6,400 ± 810	605 ± 49
Control (stimulated)	35	10,140 ± 1,090	1,135 ± 125
Ditran (5 × 10⁻⁴ M) (stimulated)	17	7,250 ± 780	794 ± 178
5 × 10⁻⁵ M	31	8,190 ± 610	946 ± 86
5 × 10⁻⁶ M	41	9,750 ± 220	1,064 ± 154
Zero time control	–	3,300 ± 450	96 ± 13

For units of concentration, see Table 5.

TABLE 7. *Influence of Ditran on some brain metabolites at high (15 mM) phosphate*[a]

Treatment	Glucose-6-P	Fructose 1,6-diP	Triose P	α-GOP
Control (unstimulated)	159 ± 32	22 ± 6	81 ± 8	104 ± 32
Ditran (5 × 10⁻⁴ M) (unstimulated)	127 ± 15	43 ± 6	87 ± 22	74 ± 23
Control (stimulated)	129 ± 47	32 ± 28	126 ± 26	95 ± 13
Ditran (5 × 10⁻⁴ M) (stimulated)	106 ± 20	95 ± 25	110 ± 4	82 ± 10
Zero time control	46 ± 5	13 ± 2	149 ± 11	124 ± 58

[a] μmoles/kg fresh weight ± SEM.

falls in the presence of Ditran. Fructose diphosphate is an excellent indicator for adequacy of tissue oxygenation. Even under conditions of stimulation, the four-fold increase in fructose-diphosphate levels is consistent with the change in glycolytic flux. Levels of 200 to 300 μmoles/kg would be expected if tissues become hypoxic.

Heilbronn (1970) has described very provocative studies on phospholipid changes caused by glycolate esters. With potassium stimulation in the presence of Ditran, she observed an increase in ^{32}P-incorporation into phospholipids of brain slices. This suggested to her that glycolate esters may have caused an increase in tissue glycerol phosphate concentration. In our experiments, in the presence of Ditran, alpha-glycerol-phosphate (α-GOP) always appears to be lower than in the control tissues (Table 7). Since alpha-glycerolphosphate level is directly controlled by the redox and phosphorylation potential of the tissue, the change in tissue content in the presence of drug is understandable.

The changes in glucose-6-phosphate levels in the presence of Ditran (Table 7) suggest a decreased availability of ATP. The influence of Ditran on high-energy compounds is shown in Table 8. In unstimulated tissue there is some decrease in "total" high-energy phosphates but little difference in adenine nucleotide content. With stimulation, control tissues show the expected fall in ATP, phosphocreatine, and total high-energy content. It is surprising to observe the fall in these intermediates with Ditran present since other indices of stimulation, i.e., respiration and glycolysis, did not respond to stimulation by high potassium.

It has been suggested by Abood (1970) that Ditran behaves like calcium in brain tissue, probably acting at the excitable membrane level. Much earlier Adams and Quastel (1956) had shown that a number of organic bases can replace calcium ion to support anaerobic glycolytic fluxes.

TABLE 8. *Influence of Ditran on high-energy compounds at high (15 mM) phosphate*[a]

Treatment	ATP	ADP	5'-AMP	PC
Control (unstimulated)	$1,093 \pm 265$	$260 + 10$	$64 + 8$	$3,700 \pm 130$
Ditran (5×10^{-4} M) (unstimulated)	$1,035 \pm 55$	256 ± 65	45 ± 32	$1,750 \pm 560$
Control (stimulated)	353 ± 194	249 ± 61	166 ± 9	792 ± 50
Ditran (5×10^{-4} M) (stimulated)	747 ± 151	265 ± 62	68 ± 7	$1,645 \pm 195$
Zero time control	$1,323 \pm 90$	436 ± 46	182 ± 34	$1,550 \pm 257$

[a] μmoles/kg fresh weight $\pm$ SEM.
$Ca^{++} = 2.9$ mM.

In Table 9 data from preliminary experiments on the effect of Ditran at no or low (0.75 mM) calcium ion concentration are presented. All tissues were stimulated with 105 mM potassium ions, and, in the presence or absence of calcium, there was increased glycolysis. Ditran profoundly blocked glucose utilization, especially when calcium was omitted from the medium. Presence of low calcium did not appear to produce a significant change, except in the case of pyruvate, which appeared to be elevated. Data from these same experiments on levels of high-energy phosphates are shown in Table 10. At low calcium (0.75 mM) and low phosphate (1.4 mM), the levels of ATP and phosphocreatine were not influenced by the presence of Ditran during incubation with K^+. When slices were stimulated with K^+ at 2.9 mM calcium and 15 mM phosphate, the ATP and phosphocreatine levels did not decrease to the same extent as when Ditran was present (Table 8), and were similar to the levels found during K^+ stimulation at low calcium and low phosphate. The fall in ATP and phosphocreatine (PC) with stimula-

TABLE 9. *Effect of Ditran on intermediary metabolites during K^+-stimulated respiration at low calcium concentration*

Treatment	Glucose	Lactate	Pyruvate
Minus Ca⁺⁺			
Control + EGTA (3 mM)	51	$9,290 \pm 760$	882 ± 153
+ Ditran (5×10^{-4} M)	11	$5,610 \pm 200$	860 ± 52
Plus Ca⁺⁺ (0.75 mM)			
Control	48	$8,300 \pm 1,430$	802 ± 150
+ Ditran (5×10^{-4} M)	15	$6,210 \pm 563$	$1,010 \pm 62$

$[K^+] = 105$ mM; $[PO_4^=] = 1.4$ mM.
For units of concentration, see Table 5.

TABLE 10. *Effect of Ditran on high-energy compounds during K^+-stimulated respiration at low calcium concentration*

Treatment	ATP	ADP	5'-AMP	PC
Minus Ca⁺⁺				
Control + EGTA (3 mM)	555 ± 15	111 ± 139	77 ± 19	$1,530 \pm 160$
+ Ditran (5×10^{-4} M)	745 ± 15	131 ± 48	38 ± 7	$1,246 \pm 293$
Plus Ca⁺⁺ (0.75 mM)				
Control	673 ± 74	154 ± 60	19 ± 3	$1,570 \pm 49$
+ Ditran (5×10^{-4} M)	700 ± 29	859 ± 216	49 ± 3	$1,698 \pm 500$
Zero time control	650 ± 42	262 ± 42	63 ± 10	$1,027 \pm 594$

$[K^+] = 105$ mM; $[PO_4^=] = 1.4$ mM.
μmoles/kg fresh weight $\pm$ SEM.

tion can be prevented by Ditran or by lowering calcium and/or phosphate in the medium. These changes may be related to differences in the lactate: pyruvate ratio. Very high PC:ATP ratios may be obtained depending on the oxidation-reduction state of the tissue (Siesjo and Messeter, 1971). Since ATP-creatine transphosphorylase requires Mg^{++}, calcium ion antagonism may play a role in maintaining the usual PC:ATP ratio of 3:2, an effect lost when calcium is omitted. In any event, these changes are not consistent with those normally observed with stimulation; further work is needed to clarify this point. The role of calcium in Ditran action does not appear to be at a metabolic level, but perhaps it is more closely related to its actions on acetylcholine metabolism, which was not examined in the present studies.

In the presence of Ditran, it was consistently observed that high-energy phosphate content always fell with stimulation, although there was no change in glycolytic flux. It occurred to us that the primary effect might be an interference with some step in oxidative phosphorylation in mitochondria of nerve endings. This would be expected to occur with increased conversion of ATP to ADP and P_i during the depolarization-repolarization cycle which accompanies stimulation.

In the present studies we have examined this possibility directly. Mitochondria were isolated from homogenates of guinea pig cerebral cortex in Tris-buffered isotonic sucrose containing 1 mM EGTA. The crude pellet was gently resuspended in the same medium. Oxygen consumption was measured with a Clark-type electrode at 21°C. A 1- or 2-ml system containing approximately 1 mg of mitochondrial protein was used. Ditran was added during a preincubation period while air was bubbled through the system.

Not all Krebs cycle intermediates supported coupled respiration of brain mitochondria; this probably reflects the permeability characteristics of the mitochondira to exogenous substrates. Glutamate, succinate, and pyruvate (plus malate) supported coupled respiration, showing transition from state 4 to state 3 respiration upon addition of ADP, and a return to state 4 after the ADP had been depleted. Respiratory control ratios (RCR)— the ratio of the rate of oxygen consumption in state 3 to the subsequent rate in state 4—provided an index to the tightness of coupling. With additions of 1 to 300 nmoles of ADP, typical respiratory control ratios were obtained (for glutamate 5 to 6, for succinate 2 to 3, and for pyruvate 3 to 4).

Figure 2 shows the effect of Ditran on respiratory control with glutamate as substrate. Typical oxygen electrode records are shown for controls and preparations exposed to the indicated concentrations of Ditran. ADP additions were made at the points indicated. Rates of oxygen con-

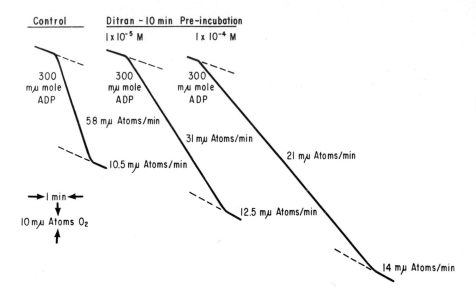

FIG. 2. Ditran effect on respiratory control of brain mitochondria; glutamate 10 mM as substrate.

sumption are shown to the right of the respective slopes. For the control, the respiratory control ratio is 58 (state 3) over 10.5 (state 4) or 5.5. In the presence of 10^{-5} M Ditran, the state 3 rate is half that of the control, the state 4 rate about the same. The respiratory control ratio is 2.5. At higher Ditran concentrations, the state 3 rate is further reduced (to 2.1), and the respiratory control ratio is 1.5. These concentrations of Ditran are in the range which blocked stimulated respiration of brain slices.

The experiments shown in Fig. 3 were identical to those presented in the previous figure, except that succinate was the substrate. The relatively high state 4 rate suggests that a substantial portion of succinate oxidation is not coupled to the production of ATP. ADP addition does stimulate respiration to state 3, and it returns to state 4, but the respiratory control ratio of succinate control is 2.5, half the value of the glutamate control. Ditran clearly does not affect respiratory control with succinate as substrate. The selectivity of Ditran for glutamate is emphasized in Fig. 4.

In these experiments, 10^{-4} M Ditran was present during a 10-min preincubation with glutamate as substrate. Challenge of the system with ADP shows that a block does exist for glutamate. The respiratory control ratio here is 1.5. Succinate is then added to a final concentration of 10 mM. The state 4 rate increases, and the respiratory control ratio after ADP addi-

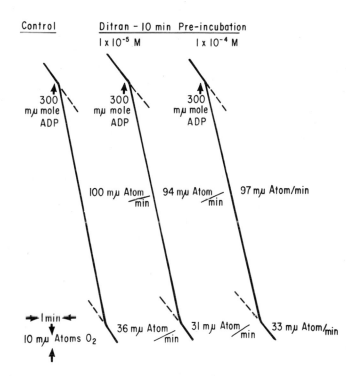

FIG. 3. Ditran effect on respiratory control of brain mitochondria; succinate 10 mM as substrate.

tion is typical of that for succinate controls. If succinate is added prior to ADP challenge, the trace looks like a typical succinate control with no evidence of a Ditran effect. Ditran has some effect on pyruvate control, but the concentrations required to reduce the respiratory control ratio with pyruvate by 25% are much greater than those which have a similar effect on glutamate control.

The time course of Ditran's effect on glutamate control is illustrated in Fig. 5. Respiratory control ratios are plotted as a function of the time between Ditran addition and the initial challenge with ADP. The most rapid change occurred within the first 10 min. Thereafter the ratio decreased more slowly.

Earlier results (Fig. 2) gave some indication that the effect of Ditran on glutamate is dose dependent. Of even greater interest is the finding that this dose-effect relationship is a function of the phosphate concentration of the medium. In Fig. 6, experiments carried out in media containing 1, 2, 10, or

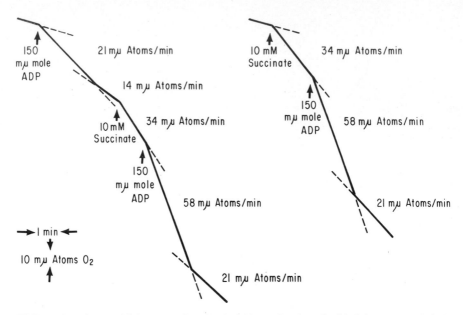

FIG. 4. Succinate addition to brain mitochondria preincubated with Ditran (1×10^{-4} M) and glutamate (10 mM).

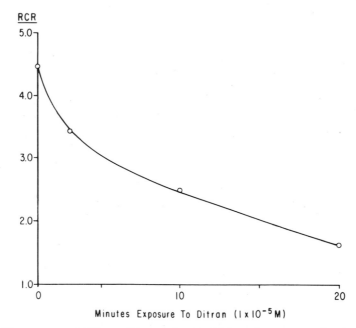

FIG. 5. Time course of Ditran effect on mitochondrial respiratory control ratios (RCR) with glutamate.

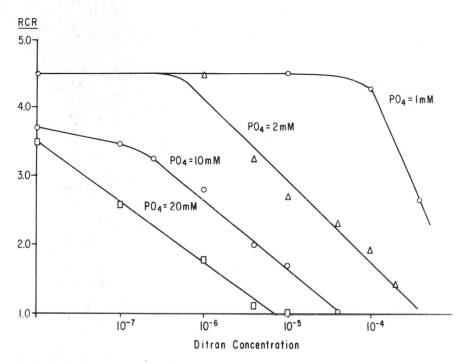

FIG. 6. Dose-effect relationship of Ditran on respiratory control ratios (RCR) of brain mitochondria utilizing glutamate.

20 mM phosphate are presented. Samples were preincubated with Ditran for 10 min. Ditran concentrations are plotted on the log scale of the ordinate. The higher the phosphate concentration of the medium, the more sensitive are the brain mitochondria to Ditran's effect on respiratory control in the presence of glutamate. In 2 mM phosphate, 5×10^{-5} M Ditran reduces the respiratory control ratio to 50% of the control value; in 20 mM phosphate, 1×10^{-7} M Ditran, 500 times less concentrated, has a comparable effect.

This preliminary evidence suggests that phosphate's effect is to facilitate the entry of drug into the mitochondria or to its site of action. Thus, the greater the phosphate concentration, the lower the concentration of Ditran required to produce an effective concentration at the critical site. A similar sort of effect was seen earlier with slice preparations.

The effect of Ditran at two levels of glutamate is seen in Table 11. Its effect on oxygen consumption appears to be the most marked. The amount of ADP consumed and the corresponding amount of ATP produced also drops significantly. You will note, however, that the total glutamate consumed with respect to the amount of aspartate formed does not appear to

TABLE 11. *Influence of Ditran on metabolic intermediates*

| | O_2 (μatoms) | (μM) Concentration changes[a] in state 3 | | | | |
		Glu[b]	Asp	AMP	ADP[b]	ATP
Control	$0.85 \pm <0.01$	$0.94 \pm .33$	0.42 ± 0.03	0.33 ± 0.03	2.61 ± 0.03	1.74 ± 0.04
	$0.83 \pm <0.01$	$0.59 \pm .20$	0.39 ± 0.01	0.32 ± 0.03	2.65 ± 0.05	1.72 ± 0.04
Ditran	0.24 ± 0.06	$0.45 \pm .14$	0.25 ± 0.03	0.55 ± 0.04	0.86 ± 0.10	0.60 ± 0.17
	0.35 ± 0.01	$0.74 \pm <.01$	0.30 ± 0.04	0.34 ± 0.08	1.22 ± 0.08	0.82 ± 0.08

[a] Mean $\pm$ SEM.
[b] Indicates disappearance.
Reaction mixture: 40 mM Tris, pH 7.1, mitochondria (0.1 ml = 2 mg), glutamate (12 or 6 mM), ADP (1.26 mM), P_i (5 mM), KCl (100 mM), and Ditran (0.1 mM) when added. Final volume = 2.3 ml.

be as significantly influenced. We interpret this to indicate that while the influence of Ditran on glutamate utilization may be linked to the decline in the production of oxaloacetate as the amino group acceptor, Ditran does not seem to be inhibiting glutamic-oxaloacetate transaminase directly. We are still in the process of defining precisely how Ditran affects glutamate control, but from the data already presented, it is possible to sharpen the focus on its possible sites of action.

The schematic diagram (Fig. 7) depicts that portion of the Krebs cycle relevant to this discussion, showing glutamate entry into the chain through α-ketoglutarate, and the respiratory chain coupling oxidation to phosphorylation. It seems unlikely that Ditran interferes with the coupling process directly, either by limiting the supply of ADP or by blocking access to the flow of electrons in the chain itself. If ADP were limiting, the coupling of all substrates should be affected equally. This is not the case. Ditran certainly does not block the flow of electrons into or from site II, since succinate control is unaffected by the drug. If Ditran blocked at site I, the drug should affect pyruvate control to the same extent that it impairs glutamate control, since pyruvate also feeds electrons into site I. Again, this is not the case.

It may be that Ditran interferes with the oxidation of glutamate by inhibiting glutamic dehydrogenase. It does not appear to interfere with transamination directly, since glutamate-aspartate ratio is maintained. Ditran may, by blocking the conversion of glutamate to α-ketoglutarate and ultimately oxaloacetate, indirectly interfere with transamination. The steady-state concentration of oxaloacetate is very low (4 μmoles/kg) and limiting in the glutamic-oxaloacetate transamination. An equally plausible explanation is that Ditran blocks the permeability of glutamate into the mitochondrial

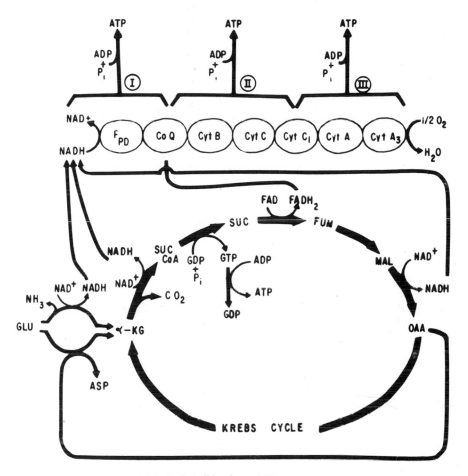

FIG. 7. Possible sites of Ditran action.

matrix just as it blocks the depolarizing action of potassium ions in the whole slice. It is well known that brain slices take up enormous amounts of L-glutamate by a specific pumping mechanism. It would appear that Ditran limits the entrance of glutamate into mitochondria as well as inducing an ATPase activity in the mitochondria, thereby accounting for the change in respiratory control ratios.

The question as to where Ditran acts cannot be answered on the basis of oxygen electrode studies alone. We are currently engaged in studies using isotopically labeled substrates which we hope will provide a more definitive answer to the question.

Regardless of how it acts, Ditran does interfere with the ability of brain mitochondria to utilize glutamate for the production of ATP. To what extent this may impinge upon the neuron's capacity to meet energy requirements of stimulation is uncertain. It is well known, however, that the concentration of glutamate in brain is extremely high *in vivo* (10 to 12 mM), making it a potentially important substrate in this tissue.

In addition to the possibility that Ditran may interfere with the bioenergetics of neurons by blocking glutamate control, there is also the question of how the Ditran block may affect intracellular glutamate concentrations and how this, in turn, may affect neuronal function. Recently, a number of studies have suggested that glutamate may play an important role in excitable tissues.

Abood and Biel (1962) have pointed out that the antagonism of acetylcholine at some membrane receptor site is probably of secondary importance in explaining the action of anticholinergic compounds on the central nervous system. Bertels-Meeuws and Polak (1968) have suggested a blocking of a feedback mechanism on presynaptic membranes in order to explain the increases in acetylcholine turnover. Our study provides evidence that glycolates have direct effects on energy production at the organelle level. It is conceivable that these effects may provide insights as to the primary mechanism of action of these compounds on central cholinergic mechanisms.

REFERENCES

Abood, L. I. (1970): Stereochemical and membrane studies with the psychotomimetic glycolate esters. In: *Psychotomimetic Drugs*, edited by D. Efron. Raven Press, New York.

Abood, L. I., and Biel, J. N. (1962): Anticholinergic psychotomimetic agents. *International Review of Neurobiology*, 4:218–273.

Adams, D. H., and Quastel, J. H. (1956): Factors influencing the anaerobic glycolysis of brain and tumour. *Proceedings of the Royal Society*, B145:742–756.

Bertels-Meeuws, M. M., and Polak, R. L. (1968): Influence of antimuscarinic substances on in vitro synthesis of acetylcholine by rat cerebral cortex. *British Journal of Pharmacology*, 33:368–380. In: *Drugs and Cholinergic Mechanisms in the CNS*, edited by E. Heilbronn and A. Winter. Forsvarets Forskingsanstalt, Stockholm, Sweden.

Heilbronn, E. (1970): Further experiments on the uptake of acetylcholine and atropine and the release of acetylcholine from mouse brain cortex slices after treatment with phospholipases. *Journal of Neurochemistry*, 17:381–389. In: *Drugs and Cholinergic Mechanisms in the CNS*, edited by E. Heilbronn and A. Winter. Forsvarets Forskingsanstalt, Stockholm, Sweden.

O'Neill, J. J., Simon, S. H., and Cummins, J. T. (1963): Inhibition of stimulated cerebral cortex respiration and glycolysis by cholinolytic drugs. *Biochemical Pharmacology*, 12:809–820.

Passonneau, J. V., and Lowry, O. H. (1962): Phosphofructokinase and the Pasteur effect. *Biochemical and Biophysical Research Communications*, 7:10–15.

Racker, E. (1965): *Mechanisms of Bioenergetics*. Academic Press, New York.

Siesjo, B. K., and Messeter, K. (1971): The effect of intracellular acidosis upon the energy metabolism of the brain. *Third International Meeting of the International Society for Neurochemistry. Abstracts.*

Advances in Biochemical Psychopharmacology, Vol. 6
Raven Press, New York © 1972

Hypophysectomy and Rat Brain Metabolism: Effects of Synthetic ACTH Analogs

D. H. G. Versteeg, W. H. Gispen, P. Schotman, A. Witter, and D. de Wied

Rudolf Magnus Institute for Pharmacology and Department of Physiological Chemistry, Medical Faculty, University of Utrecht, Vondellaan 6, Utrecht, The Netherlands

INTRODUCTION

For several years our group has been interested in the role of the hormones of the pituitary-adrenal system in avoidance conditioning in the rat. In particular, the performance of the hypophysectomized rat has been investigated in some detail (for a review, see de Wied, 1969). It was found that hypophysectomy markedly impaired the acquisition of a conditioned avoidance response in a shuttle box.

Treatment of hypophysectomized rats with ACTH restored the deficient performance toward almost normal levels (de Wied, 1964). However, experiments with MSH, which hardly affects adrenocortical activity, and with the synthetic ACTH analogs $ACTH_{1-10}$ and $ACTH_{4-10}$, which lack endocrine and metabolic effects, also showed a similar facilitation of avoidance conditioning in hypophysectomized rats (de Wied, 1969). Treatment of control rats with the same peptides delayed the extinction of a conditioned avoidance response (de Wied, 1966; de Wied, Bohus, and Greven, 1968; van Wimersma Greidanus and de Wied, 1971). Moreover, $ACTH_{1-10}$ − 7-D-phe facilitated extinction under the same experimental conditions in normal rats, and failed to facilitate acquisition of a conditioned avoidance response in hypophysectomized rats (Bohus and de Wied, 1966; de Wied, 1969). These experiments were interpreted as indicating that the pituitary contains neuropeptides which may affect formation of new behavior patterns.

On the basis of these data, a program was started to investigate the effects of hypophysectomy on brain metabolism and the possible effects of synthetic ACTH analogs on central nervous system metabolism in hypophysectomized rats.

HYPOPHYSECTOMY AND BRAIN METABOLISM

Hypophysectomy leads to dramatic disorders in metabolic processes in endocrine organs and other peripheral organs and tissues. As a consequence of the disturbance of hormonal regulating mechanisms, atrophy occurs in endocrine organs which are normally under the control of pituitary hormones, and metabolic changes can be observed in organs such as liver and muscle. The extensive literature dealing with the effects of hypophysectomy on metabolic parameters in peripheral organs and tissues will not be reviewed here.

Relatively little is known about the effects of hypophysectomy on the metabolism of the central nervous system. Reiss (1961) found little change in oxygen consumption of the cortex following hypophysectomy, while anaerobic glycolysis increased by more than 100%. Libertun, Moguilevsky, Schiaffini, and Foglia (1969) and Moguilevsky, Libertun, and Foglia (1970) observed a significant increase in oxygen uptake in certain parts of the hypothalamus of hypophysectomized rats. Although the effect of hypophysectomy on macromolecular metabolism has not been extensively studied, some evidence has been obtained for alterations in such metabolism. Decreases have been observed in both phenylalanine incorporation in a brain cell-free system and in poly-U stimulated amino acid incorporation in a system prepared from brain tissue following hypophysectomy (Dunn and Korner, 1966). Takahashi, Penn, Lajtha, and Reiss (1970) reported that after hypophysectomy the incorporation of isotopically labeled phenylalanine into brain protein was diminished. Hypophysectomy was found to lead to a significant decrease in RNA/DNA ratio in the brainstem (DeVellis and Inglish, 1968). Significant decreases in weight of the cortex and in content of DNA, RNA, protein, and water were found in the brains of young rats 3 weeks after hypophysectomy (Cheek and Graystone, 1969).

Data concerning monoamine levels and turnover in brain or brain regions of hypophysectomized rats are controversial. DeMaio (1959) found an increase in the serotonin level in medulla oblongata and brainstem after hypophysectomy, but Yeh, Solomon, and Chow (1959) could not confirm these findings. Resnick and Gray (1961) were also unable to detect any changes in brain levels of serotonin in hypophysectomized rats. However, Hyyppä and Valavaara (1970) reported an increase in the noradrenaline and serotonin content of anterior and posterior hypothalamus, but not of the cortex, 3 months after hypophysectomy. An increase in noradrenaline content of hypothalamic regions of the brain of hypophysectomized rats was also described by Shchedrina (1970). These findings suggest an effect of removal of the pituitary on monoamine levels in circumscribed brain areas, while levels in other regions of the brain seem unaffected. Few data are available concerning monoamine turnover. Landsberg and Axelrod (1968) described an unchanged noradrenaline turnover in the brain of rats 62 days after hypophysectomy; Fuxe, Corrodi, Hökfelt, and Jonsson (1970) mentioned a reduction in noradrenaline turnover in central neurons of hypophysectomized rats.

In view of these data, we felt it would be desirable to extend these observations concerning macromolecular and monoamine metabolism in the brains of hypophysectomized rats. Since the data should have a direct bearing on the influence of hypophysectomy on conditioned avoidance behavior, the same time schedule was used as in the previous behavioral experiments.

HYPOPHYSECTOMY AND MACROMULECULAR AND MONOAMINE METABOLISM IN THE BRAIN

In all experiments, except those to study monoamine metabolism, male rats were used. Hypophysectomy was performed via the transauricular route under light ether anesthesia on rats weighing approximately 120 g. Two or 3 weeks after hypophysectomy or sham operation, the rats were sacrificed by decapitation. Brains were dissected out immediately after the decapitation and processed as described below. Decrease in body weight, adrenal atrophy, and macroscopical inspection of the sella turcica were used as parameters for the completeness of the removal of the pituitary.

Total RNA Content

To investigate the effect of hypophysectomy on RNA metabolism in the brain, first total RNA content was determined in different brain areas. The brains were dissected into brainstem, cortex, and cerebellum (see Gispen, Schotman, and de Kloet, *in press*). RNA content was determined by the method of Munro and Fleck (1966); DNA content was measured

TABLE 1. *Gross localization of the effect of hypophysectomy on RNA content in rat brain*

Location	RNA (mg/g fresh tissue)	DNA (mg/g fresh tissue)	Ratio RNA/DNA
Intact			
Cortex (5)	1.77 ± 0.04	1.03 ± 0.06	1.74 ± 0.07
Cerebellum (4)	2.07 ± 0.08	4.91 ± 0.29	0.43 ± 0.01
Brainstem (4)	1.46 ± 0.05	0.99 ± 0.04	1.47 ± 0.04[a]
Hypophysectomized			
Cortex (6)	1.55 ± 0.02	1.04 ± 0.04	1.51 ± 0.07
Cerebellum (5)	1.90 ± 0.04	4.83 ± 0.23	0.40 ± 0.01
Brainstem (5)	1.35 ± 0.03	1.13 ± 0.03	1.19 ± 0.04[a]

No. of animals in parentheses. Values are mean $\pm$ SEM.
[a] $p < 0.025$ (*t*-test).

following the method of Burton (1956), using calf thymus DNA as a standard.

From Table 1 it can be seen that there is no significant difference in the RNA/DNA ratio, which represents a measure of RNA content per cell, between sham-operated and intact control rats weighing 120 g on the day of analysis. A lower RNA/DNA ratio was found in the brainstem of hypophysectomized rats, but not in the cortex and cerebellum. These data are in good agreement with the findings of De Vellis and Inglish (1968), who suggested that the effect of hypophysectomy on brain RNA was located mainly in brainstem areas.

Further studies revealed that in the brainstem, where the largest decrease was found in RNA/DNA ratio, the diencephalon, the mesencephalon, and the medulla oblongata all showed a decrease in RNA content following hypophysectomy (Gispen et al., *in press*). For these reasons, the brainstem was chosen for further study.

Subcellular Localization: Polysomes

With the same techniques of analysis, an attempt was made to localize the effect of hypophysectomy on RNA content at a subcellular level. Brainstems of hypophysectomized and control rats were homogenized and fractionated as described previously (Gispen, de Wied, Schotman, and Jansz, 1970). RNA content of homogenate, cell nuclei, mitochondria plus synaptosomes, microsomes, and the postmicrosomal supernatant was determined. As can be seen from Table 2, the only significant difference in RNA content between fractions from hypophysectomized and control rats

TABLE 2. *Subcellular localization of the effect of hypophysectomy on brainstem RNA*

| Location | Brainstem RNA (mg/g fresh tissue) | | | |
	Intact rats	Hypophysectomized rats	$\%^a$	p^b
Homogenate	1.727 ± 0.002 (9)	1.425 ± 0.002 (11)	-17.5	<0.001
Purified nuclei	0.020 ± 0.002 (4)	0.018 ± 0.002 (4)	-10.0	n.s.
Crude mitochondria	0.156 ± 0.011 (7)	0.163 ± 0.010 (11)	$+ 4.5$	n.s.
Microsomes	0.352 ± 0.018 (7)	0.287 ± 0.009 (11)	-18.5	<0.01
Post-microsomal supernatant	0.379 ± 0.030 (7)	0.341 ± 0.014 (6)	-10.0	n.s.

Values are mean $\pm$ SEM. No. of animals in parentheses.
[a] Proportional difference between values obtained from intact and hypophysectomized rats setting the value of intact rats at 100%.
[b] *t*-test.

was found in the fractions containing the microsomes. This result indicates that hypophysectomy might alter macromolecule metabolism by a deficiency on the ribosomal or polysomal level, as suggested by Korner (1969) for liver tissue.

The main RNA components of the microsomal fraction are the ribosomal RNA's, and further *m*-RNA and *t*-RNA's in minor quantities. Thus, a decrease in the microsomal RNA content suggests a decrease in ribosomes and polysomal aggregates. To test this hypothesis, polysomes were isolated using a technique described by Adair, Wilson, and Glassman (1968). The polysomal fraction was separated into monosomes, disomes, trisomes, and others by centrifugation through linear sucrose gradients (Gispen et al., 1970). The amounts of monosomes, disomes, trisomes, and large polysomes were determined by computing the areas under the peaks, obtained by a continuous recording of the optical density of the gradients at 260 nm. In Fig. 1, the mean values of intact and hypophysectomized rats are compared. It can be seen that hypophysectomy affects mainly the content of polysomes, especially of large polysomes ($\geq$ trisomes), implying a reduced number of structures active in protein synthesis.

Uridine Incorporation into RNA

We next investigated whether the reduction in polysome content following hypophysectomy was due to a decreased RNA synthesis or to a decreased stability of the polysomal aggregates. For liver tissue, a decreased

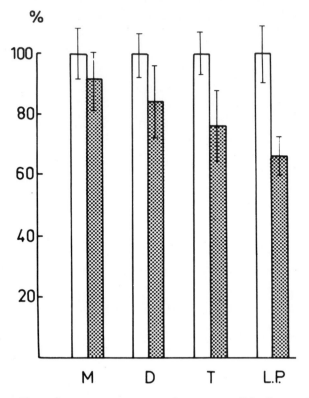

FIG. 1. Effect of hypophysectomy on content of monosomes (M), disomes (D), trisomes (T), and large polysomes (LP) in the rat brainstem. Values obtained for fractions from brainstems of hypophysectomized rats are expressed as percent of values for fractions from brainstems of intact rats. *Open columns:* intact rats; mean ± SEM; n = 15. *Stippled columns:* hypophysectomized rats; mean ± SEM; n = 11. For hypophysectomized trisomes, $p < 0.005$. For hypophysectomized large polysomes, $0.01 < p < 0.025$. (p values determined by t-test).

RNA synthesis, an increased RNAse activity, and a ribosomal deficit have been suggested to explain the changes in macromolecule metabolism in the hypophysectomized rat (Korner, 1970; Cardell, 1967; Brewer, Foster, and Sells, 1969; Foster and Sells, 1969). However, in brain tissue no ribosome deficit has been found (Dunn and Korner, 1966). Therefore, the turnover of RNA in the brainstem of hypophysectomized rats was studied. This was carried out by using radioactive labeled uridine as a precursor for RNA.

In order to study the *in vivo* incorporation of radioactive labeled uridine into different cell fractions, a double labeling method was used, in which (5-³H)- or (2-¹⁴C)-uridine was administered by injection into the diencephalon (Valzelli, 1964) either alternatively to control and hypophysectomized rats or to two control rats. The incorporation of the [3]H- and ^{14}C-label into several RNA fractions after 70 and 180 min of incorporation was measured and corrected for the relative [3]H- and ^{14}C-radioactivity of the precursor pool as described before (Gispen et al., 1970). Using two

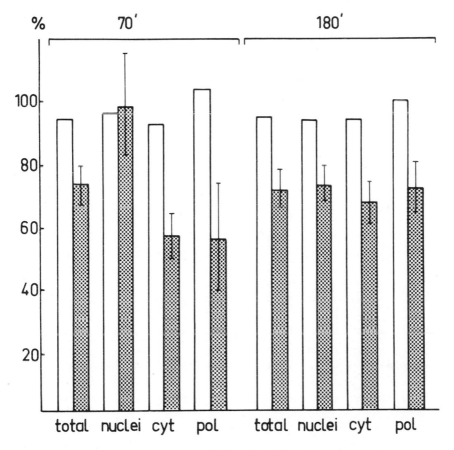

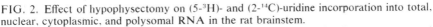

FIG. 2. Effect of hypophysectomy on (5-^{3}H)- and (2-^{14}C)-uridine incorporation into total, nuclear, cytoplasmic, and polysomal RNA in the rat brainstem.

The ratio of [3]H- and ^{14}C-label or [14]C- and ^{3}H-label in the RNA fractions was corrected for the ratio in the precursor pool. In the figure, the corrected ratios obtained for pairs consisting of one hypophysectomized and one intact rat are expressed as percent of the ratios obtained for pairs of two intact rats, which did not differ from unity.

Open columns: ratios of incorporation of label into RNA fractions from the brainstems of two intact rats. *Stippled columns:* ratios of incorporation of label into RNA fractions from the brainstems of a pair consisting of one hypophysectomized and one intact rat. Mean ± SEM; n = 3.

intact rats, one receiving ^{3}H- and the other ^{14}C-uridine, the corrected iso-tope ratio of the cell fractions differed by less than 7% from the theoretical value of one. However, using pairs of one hypophysectomized and one con-trol rat, the isotope ratio was 25 to 40% lower, indicating a decreased in-corporation of uridine into RNA in the brainstem of hypophysectomized rats (Fig. 2). The decrease was not limited to any particular cell fraction. Characterization of this rapidly labeled RNA indicated that after 70 min mainly m-RNA was labeled, whereas after 180 min of incorporation, pre-sumably all types of RNA had been labeled (Gispen et al., 1970; Schotman, in preparation). The reduced incorporation of uridine into RNA, presumably reflecting a decreased synthesis of m-RNA, accompanies and could account for the observed reduction in RNA content and polysomes.

Leucine Incorporation into Proteins

As a consequence of the reduction in the RNA metabolism, an altered protein synthesis in the brains of hypophysectomized rats can be expected. This led us to investigate the turnover of both proteins and polypeptides in the brain. The in vivo incorporation of (4,5-^{3}H)-leucine into proteins from various cell fractions was studied 5 min after the injection of the pre-cursor into the diencephalon. The brainstem was homogenized, and from the homogenate a fraction containing crude nuclei, mitochondria, the postmito-chondrial supernatant, and polysomes was isolated.

In all fractions, the ^{3}H-radioactivity incorporated into acid-insoluble proteinous material was determined. Samples of the supernatant after precipitation of the macromolecules were also assayed for radioactivity; these values were taken as precursor pool values. In order to compare the incorporation between different animals, the ratio of radioactivity of the acid-insoluble fractions over radioactivity of the acid-soluble precursor pool was determined in the various cell fractions. The values obtained for hypophysectomized and intact rats are shown in Fig. 3. As a result of hypo-physectomy, a decrease in leucine incorporation was observed, which was about equal in all cell fractions. Only a minor part of the labeled insoluble material appeared to consist of RNAse-sensitive material (probably labeled aminoacyl-t-RNA), whereas a large part could be degraded by incubation with pronase. The latter result indicates that the rapidly labeled material is of a protein nature (Schotman, in preparation). A short incorporation time was used, since it was found in pilot studies that 5 min after injection of ^{3}H-leucine into the brainstem, the radioactivity in the acid soluble pre-cursor pool was at a maximum.

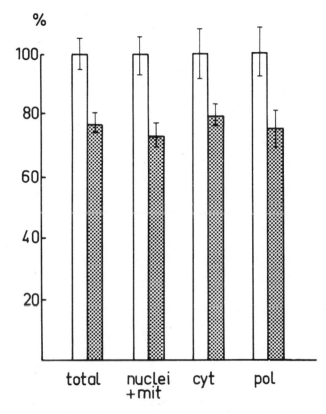

FIG. 3. Effect of hypophysectomy on incorporation of (4,5-³H)-leucine into rat brainstem proteins during an incorporation period of 5 min.

The acid-insoluble radioactivities of the isolated cell fractions were divided by the radioactivity of the acid-soluble precursor pool. Values obtained from hypophysectomized rats in this way were expressed as percent of the values obtained from intact rats.

Open columns: intact rats; mean ± SEM; n = 10. *Stippled columns:* hypophysectomized rats; mean ± SEM; n = 8. mit = mitochondrial fraction; cyt = postmitochondrial cytoplasmic fraction; pol = polysomes. *p* values (*t*-test) for hypophysectomized rats: *total*, $0.0005 < p < 0.001$; *nuclei + mit*, $0.001 < p < 0.005$; *cyt* and *pol*, $0.01 < p < 0.025$.

At later times, there appeared to be a net loss of radioactivity. This is in good agreement with the results of Lajtha and Toth (1961) who also reported a rapid loss of administered amino acids from the brain. Moreover, it was found that 5 min after (³H)-leucine injection, brainstem polysomes were labeled with high specific activity (dpm/µg protein), indicating an optimal labeling of growing peptide chains. Usually an incorporation period of 1 hr is used in order to obtain optimal labeling of overall cell protein *in vivo*.

Therefore, in another series of experiments, the effect of hypophysectomy on protein metabolism was studied using a 1-hr incorporation period.

Incorporation of a Mixture of ^{14}C-amino Acids into Insoluble Proteins and Soluble Polypeptides

A procedure was developed which allowed a differentiation between radioactivity incorporated into 0.1 N HCl-soluble polypeptides and into the insoluble protein residue. Rats were injected (Valzelli, 1964) with 5 μC U-^{14}C-amino acid mix. The animal was decapitated 1 hr later, and the brain-stem (440 $\pm$ 30 mg) was isolated and subjected to ultrasonic disintegration in 7.5 ml acetone for 1 min at 20 kcps and maximum power. The resulting homogenate was centrifuged (45 min, 4°C, 20,000 $\times g_{av}$), and the supernatant poured off, evaporated, dissolved in 1 ml Soluene-100, and counted. The precipitate was washed twice with acetone; total radioactivity in the acetone extracts is designated as AE. The final acetone-dried powder precipitate was extracted twice with 7.5 ml chloroform by stirring 1 hr and filtering the mixture by suction through a G-2 sintered glass filter. Total radioactivity in the chloroform extracts is designated as CE. The final chloroform-dried powder precipitate was extracted with 2.5 ml 0.1 N HCl by the aforementioned ultrasonic treatment and centrifuged. The residue was washed twice with 1 ml 0.1 N HCl, and the combined extracts were gel filtrated on Sephadex G 25 (see Fig. 4), yielding a polypeptide peak PEP and an amino acid peak AA, which were counted separately. The 0.1 N HCl-insoluble proteinous residue PR was dissolved in 2 ml Soluene-100 and counted. The yields of radioactivity in the various fractions are expressed as percentages of the total recovery $\pm$ SD. Radioactivity was measured in 10 ml of scintillation solution, consisting of toluene and Triton-X 100 (11:18, v/v) and containing 4 g 2,5-diphenyloxazole (PPO) per liter. Counting efficiencies were determined by the channels ratio method.

The combined radioactivity in AE, CE, and AA was regarded to represent the precursor pool; control experiments in which the amino acid mixture was added to the brainstem homogenate of non-injected animals as well as 0-hr incorporation experiments revealed that 98% of the total recovered radioactivity was present in these three fractions. The combined radioactivity in PEP and PR was used as a measure for incorporated radioactivity. For eight different incorporation periods, ranging from 0 to 17 hr, there was close agreement between data obtained by this method and values obtained by homogenization of the brainstem in 5% trichloroacetic acid (TCA) and counting the TCA-soluble respectively the TCA-insoluble frac-

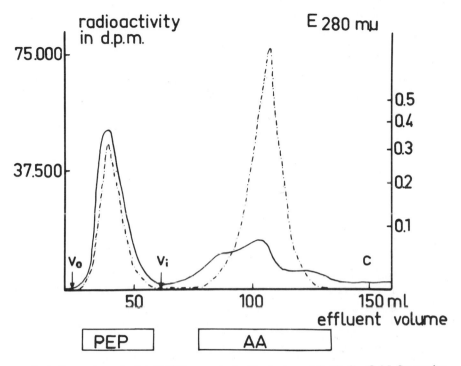

FIG. 4. Separation of a 0.1 N HCl extract of rat brainstem on Sephadex G 25. Separation was carried out on a 1.9 × 70 cm Sephadex G-25 column, equilibrated with 0.1 M acetic acid. Elution was performed with the same solvent at a rate of 12 ml/hr, and fractions of 1 ml were collected. V_o and V_i indicate the theoretical values for void and internal volume.

. . . . . – radioactivity, ——————— = extinction at 280 mμ.

tions. The former procedure has the advantage of discriminating between 0.1 N HCl-insoluble proteins, of which virtually all radioactivity is solubilized by incubation with pronase, and 0.1 N HCl-soluble polypeptides, which remain open for further investigation. When this procedure was applied to compare 1-hr incorporation of the ^{14}C-amino acids into proteins and polypeptides in the brains of intact rats and of rats hypophysectomized 3 weeks before, a significant difference was found in incorporation of radioactivity into both polypeptides and proteinous residue (Table 3). It is interesting to note that hypophysectomy leads to a decrease in incorporation which is particularly pronounced in the labeling of 0.1 N HCl-soluble polypeptides. The incorporation into this PEP-fraction is obviously more affected by hypophysectomy than by incorporation into the insoluble proteinous residue.

TABLE 3. *Effect of hypophysectomy and hypophysectomy + ACTH treatment on 1-hr in vivo incorporation of U-^{14}C-amino acids into 0.1 N HCl-soluble polypeptides and insoluble proteins in the rat brainstem*

Group	U-^{14}C-amino acid incorporation					Total incorporated
	AE	CE	AA	PEP	PR	
Intact	7.2 ± 0.4	7.2 ± 0.5	33.8 ± 1.9	14.1 ± 1.7	36.7 ± 3.2	51.3 ± 2.6
Hypophysectomy	7.9 ± 0.6	10.9 ± 1.4	40.7 ± 1.9[a]	7.9 ± 0.7[a]	31.4 ± 2.6[b]	39.8 ± 3.1[a]
Hypophysectomy +ACTH$_{4-10}$	7.2 ± 0.6	10.7 ± 0.8	39.1 ± 3.1	8.7 ± 1.6	33.0 ± 2.6	42.2 ± 4.0

Six animals in each group.
[a] $p < 0.0005$.
[b] $p < 0.02$ (*t*-test).

Monoamine Metabolism

In view of the finding that amino acid incorporation into proteins is decreased in the brains of hypophysectomized rats, suggesting a decrease in protein synthesis, one might expect that the activity of enzymes, which are the products of protein synthesis, will also show a decrease. A group of enzymes of considerable importance in the regulation of brain function are those involved in the synthesis of neurotransmitters. Therefore, the turnover of serotonin, noradrenaline, and dopamine was studied in the brains of hypophysectomized rats.

Serotonin turnover was studied by measuring the increase in brain levels of serotonin and the decrease in brain levels of 5-hydroxyindole acetic acid (5-HIAA) following monoamine oxidase inhibition by tranylcypromine (10 mg/kg, i.p.), according to Neff and Tozer (1968). Noradrenaline and dopamine turnover rates were determined by measuring the decrease in brain levels of these amines after inhibition of the enzyme tyrosine hydroxylase with α-methyltyrosine methylester (H44/68). Spectrofluorimetric techniques were used to determine serotonin and 5-HIAA (Bogdanski, Pletscher, Brodie, and Udenfriend, 1956), and also noradrenaline and dopamine (Taylor and Laverty, 1968).

The turnover rates of serotonin, noradrenaline, and dopamine were determined in the brain of female intact rats, weighing 140 to 150 g, and of hypophysectomized and sham-operated rats, operated when weighing 140 to 150 g. Turnover rates were measured 2 and 3 weeks following the operation. No significant differences were observed in the steady-state levels of the three amines and 5-HIAA in the various groups.

The turnover rates of the three amines in the brains of sham-operated rats, both 2 and 3 weeks after the operation, did not differ from those in the

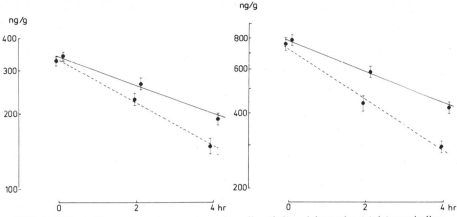

FIG. 5. Effect of hypophysectomy on noradrenaline (*left*) and dopamine (*right*) metabolism in the rat brain. The rate of depletion of noradrenaline and dopamine was determined in the brains of sham-operated and hypophysectomized rats, 3 weeks after the operation, after synthesis inhibition with α-methyltyrosine methylester (H44/68, 250 mg/kg i.p.). Each point represents mean $\pm$ SEM for at least six animals.

Left: Slope for hypophysectomized rats, -0.0703 ± 0.0080; for sham operated rats, -0.0939 ± 0.0081. ($0.025 < p < 0.05$.)

Right: Slope for hypophysectomized rats, -0.0728 ± 0.0073; for sham operated rats, -0.1024 ± 0.0084. ($0.01 < p < 0.02$.)

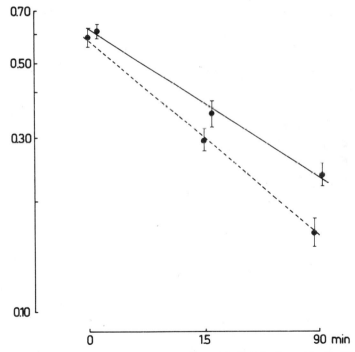

FIG. 6. Effect of hypophysectomy on serotonin metabolism in the rat brain. The rate of depletion of 5-HIAA was determined in the brains of sham-operated and hypophysectomized rats, 3 weeks after the operation, after inhibition of monoamine oxidase with tranylcypromine (10 mg/kg, i.p.). Each point represents the mean $\pm$ SEM for at least six animals. Slope for hypophysectomized rats, -0.0045 ± 0.0004; for sham operated rats, -0.0063 ± 0.0004. ($0.001 < p < 0.005$.)

brains of intact rats. Significant decreases, however, were found in the rates of turnover of serotonin, noradrenaline, and dopamine in the brains of hypophysectomized rats, 2 and 3 weeks after the operation, as compared with the turnover rates in the brains of rats which were sham-operated at the same time (Figs. 5 and 6).

Discussion

As a consequence of hypophysectomy, production and secretion of hormones by the target organs of the pituitary trophic hormones will decrease. These hormones and the hormones of the pituitary itself are known to act as regulators of metabolic processes in specific tissues, and participate as such in the homeostasis of the organism as a whole. Several of the pituitary hormones and the hormones in their target organs have been found to exert effects on metabolic processes in the central nervous system. Hormone actions on protein metabolism in the developing brain have received particular attention. The regulatory role of hormones capable of promoting growth and functional maturation (such as growth hormone, thyroid hormones, and steroids) on protein synthesis in the central nervous system is well established in this respect (for a review, see Geel and Timiras, 1970). However, evidence is accumulating that in the adult and near-adult brain, hormones may continue to have effects on brain metabolism. For instance, ACTH has been found to enhance protein synthesis in the adult brain (Jakoubek, Semiginovský, and Dědičová, 1971). The decreased tryptophan hydroxylase activity in the brains of adrenalectomized rats is partially restored by cortisone administration, possibly through a regulation of protein synthesis at a translational level (Azmitia and McEwen, 1968). Takahashi et al. (1970) mention that certain biochemical functions show no response in the normal animal, but are markedly affected after hypophysectomy. They found that after hypophysectomy the incorporation of isotopically labeled phenylalanine into brain protein is diminished, and that administration of growth hormone caused a significant stimulation to near-normal levels. Reiss (1961) found that the oxygen consumption in the brain of hypophysectomized rats cannot be significantly altered by the administration of growth hormone alone. Thyrotropic hormone or thyroxine could increase oxygen consumption and reduce the anaerobic glycolysis. Reiss and Rees (1961) found that treatment with ACTH can reduce the increased ^{32}P uptake by brain cortex following hypophysectomy.

The consequences of changes in the activity of the pituitary-adrenal system for noradrenaline and serotonin metabolism in the central nervous system have been reviewed by Fuxe et al. (1970). Treatment with gluco-corticoids did normalize both the increased noradrenaline turnover and the decreased serotonin metabolism in the brains of adrenalectomized rats. All these data indicate a hormonal control of brain metabolism, and it is, therefore, reasonable to ascribe the changes in RNA, protein, and mono-amine metabolism in the brain of hypophysectomized rats to the complete disturbance of hormonal balance. It could be that the primary effect of hypophysectomy might be an alteration at the transcriptional level, leading to a changed RNA synthesis and an altered protein synthesis, accounting for diminished enzyme activities. The turnover rates of all three monoamines investigated show a decrease, indicative of a lower rate of production of synthesizing enzymes. Adrenalectomy has been shown to lead to an increase in central noradrenaline metabolism and a decrease in that of serotonin (Fuxe et al., 1970). Hypophysectomy, however, brings about a decrease in the turnover rates of both amines. Therefore, it seems likely that the effect of hypophysectomy on monoamine metabolism is due to a direct ac-tion of one or more of the pituitary hormones on brain metabolism and not to a lower rate of secretion of glucocorticoids from the adrenal cortex. In this respect it is interesting to note that a decrease has been found in the activities of adrenal tyrosine hydroxylase (Mueller, Thoenen, and Axel-rod, 1970) and of dopamine-β-hydroxylase (Weinshilboum and Axelrod, 1970) following hypophysectomy, which could be prevented by ACTH administration.

It must be pointed out, however, that in our studies the effects of re-placement therapies on the various altered metabolic parameters have not yet been investigated. Therefore, a conclusion as to which of the hormones, alone or in concert, are involved in the control of brain metabolism is as yet not warranted.

ACTH ANALOGS AND BRAIN METABOLISM IN HYPOPHYSECTOMIZED RATS

The effects of the ACTH analogs $ACTH_{1-10}$ and $ACTH_{4-10}$ were studied because there is substantial evidence that these peptides affect conditioned avoidance behavior in hypophysectomized as well as in intact rats (see Introduction). These ACTH analogs have no appreciable endocrine or systemic effects (de Wied, 1969). It is more likely that they exhibit their behavioral effect via a direct action on brain structures. This hypothesis received extra support from experiments by van Wimersma Greidanus (1971), who showed that not only subcutaneous administration of the peptides, but also direct implantation into the brain resulted in resistance to extinction (van Wimersma Greidanus and de Wied, 1971). Localization studies revealed that in particular the centrum medianum in the diencephalon is sensitive to the behavioral influence of the peptides. The locus of action of the peptides in a circumscript area of the brain suggests the existence of a receptor site in this brain area for an amino acid sequence shared by ACTH and α- and β-MSH. This receptor site appears to be different from the receptor site for ACTH in the adrenal cortex. Hofmann, Wingender, and Finn (1970) found that although a particulate fraction from beef adrenal cortex tissue did bind isotopically labeled $ACTH_{1-20}$, it failed to bind radioactively labeled $ACTH_{1-10}$.

In the biochemical experiments reported here, similar amounts of the ACTH analogs were administered for the same period of time as used in the behavioral studies in order to determine a possible relation between behavioral and neurochemical phenomena. These peptides were administered as long-acting zinc phosphate preparations in a dose of 20 μg s.c. each 48 hr, generally during a 13-day period.

In previous experiments it had been found that treatment with $ACTH_{1-10}$, in combination with shuttle-box conditioning of hypophysectomized rats, increased the content of polysomes (Gispen, de Wied, Schotman, and Jansz, 1971). However, no effect of the peptide treatment *per se* on polysome patterns could be detected. From this and other experiments, it was concluded that this biochemical alteration in the brainstems of hypophysectomized rats, which acquired the response as a result of peptide treatment, was related to an interaction of the peptide treatment with the process of acquisition (Gispen et al., 1971).

The aim of the experiments reported in this chapter was to find a first cue with which to unravel the mechanism of action of $ACTH_{1-10}$ and $ACTH_{4-10}$ at a neurochemical level. Treatment with $ACTH_{1-10}$ or $ACTH_{4-10}$ failed to affect polysome patterns, uridine incorporation into various RNA fractions, and turnover of serotonin, noradrenaline, and dopamine in the brain of hypophysectomized rats. However, a significant increase in labeled leucine incorporation into rapidly labeled proteins was observed in the brainstems of hypophysectomized rats treated with $ACTH_{1-10}$. The *in vivo* incorporation of $4,5-{}^3H$-leucine into proteins 5 min after injection was measured as described above, the day after the last injection of the $ACTH_{1-10}$ preparation.

Brainstems of an $ACTH_{1-10}$-treated or a placebo-treated hypophysectomized rat were homogenized, and the homogenate was fractionated as described. The radioactivities in the acid-soluble precursor pool and in the acid-insoluble proteins were calculated as part of the total recovery. A

28% ($p < 0.01$) increase in the incorporation of leucine into the acid-insoluble fraction was found as a result of treatment with $ACTH_{1-10}$ (Fig. 7). Although there was a similar tendency in the 1-hr labeled amino acid incorporation into protein, no significant effect could be demonstrated in this respect. Pilot experiments suggest that ^{3}H-leucine incorporation into proteins 5 min after injection is diminished when $ACTH_{1-10}$-7-D-phenylalanine is administered.

Thus, it is obvious that $ACTH_{1-10}$ exhibits a specific effect on metabolism in the brain of the hypophysectomized rat, which runs parallel

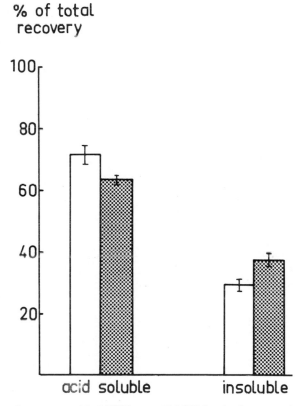

FIG. 7. Effect of treatment with $ACTH_{1-10}$ on (4,5-^{3}H)-leucine incorporation into proteins in the rat brainstem, during a 5-min incorporation period. From the brainstem homogenates, the total acid-insoluble and the total soluble fractions were isolated and assayed for the incorporated radioactivity as described in the text. Values obtained were expressed as percent of total recovered radioactivity in the homogenates

Open columns: placebo treatment (mean ± SEM, n = 6). *Stippled columns:* $ACTH_{1-10}$ treatment (mean ± SEM, n = 6); $0.005 < p < 0.01$.

with the behavioral effect. It appears that $ACTH_{1-10}$ exerts this influence on brain metabolism at a translational level. Other endocrine and metabolic disturbances seem to be unaffected. Jakoubek et al. (1971) reported an increased brain protein synthesis *in vivo* and *in vitro* as a result of ACTH administration. Our data with the ACTH analog $ACTH_{1-10}$ are in good agreement with this observation and might imply that ACTH exerts this effect via an extra-adrenal mechanism.

As stated before, it was concluded from implantation experiments that specific brain areas are sensitive to the behavioral effect of the synthetic ACTH analogs. At present we do not know which of the neurotransmitters are involved in this brain system. Influences on neurotransmitter metabolism may become evident when more defined brain regions are investigated.

It is not yet known how the ACTH analogs affect neuronal processes. There are very few data in the literature concerning the physiological effects of these peptides (for a review, see de Wied et al., *in press*). Summarizing this review, one might suggest that these peptides affect neurophysiological parameters via an interaction with neuronal membranes, possibly implying an involvement in the formation of new synaptic connections.

Further studies are in preparation to determine if membrane interactions are indeed involved in the observed biochemical and behavioral effects of $ACTH_{1-10}$ and $ACTH_{4-10}$.

SUMMARY

The effects of hypophysectomy on the metabolism of neuromolecules and monoamines in the rat brain were studied for up to 3 weeks after the operation. When compared with intact rats or sham-operated rats, hypophysectomized animals showed a decrease in RNA content in the brainstem; in polysome content, especially in large polysomes in the brainstem; in incorporation of ^3H- and ^{14}C-uridine into acid-precipitable material; in incorporation of ^3H- and ^{14}C-uridine into nuclear, cytoplasmic, and polysomal RNA; in incorporation of ^3H-leucine into acid-insoluble proteins; in incorporation of a ^{14}C-amino acid mixture into proteins and polypeptides; and in turnover rates of serotonin, noradrenaline, and dopamine. No differences were found in total protein content or steady-state levels of serotonin, 5-HIAA, noradrenaline, and dopamine.

Hypophysectomy reduces the rat's ability to acquire a shuttle-box avoidance response. This deficient behavior of hypophysectomized rats can be restored by treatment with ACTH analogs. To determine what relationship might exist between macromolecular metabolism in the brain and behavior, the influence of the ACTH analogs $ACTH_{1-10}$ and $ACTH_{4-10}$ on the respective biochemical parameters was investigated. No effects could be detected after chronic treatment of hypophysectomized rats with these peptides on polysome patterns, on ^3H- and ^{14}C-uridine incorporation into RNA, on incorporation of ^{14}C-amino acids into proteins and polypeptides, or on the turnover rates of serotonin, noradrenaline, and dopamine. However, a 28% increase was found in ^3H-leucine incorporation into rapidly labeled proteins in the brains of hypophysectomized rats after treatment with $ACTH_{4-10}$.

REFERENCES

Adair, L. B., Wilson, J. E., and Glassmann, E. (1968): Brain function and macromolecules. III. Uridine incorporation into polysomes of mouse brain during short-term avoidance conditioning. *Proceedings of the National Academy of Sciences*, 60:606–613.

Azmitia, E. C., Jr., and McEwen, B. S. (1968): Corticosterone regulation of tryptophan hydroxylase in midbrain of the rat. *Science*, 166:1274–1276.

Bogdanski, D. F., Pletscher, A., Brodie, B., and Udenfriend, S. (1956): Identification and assay of serotonin in brain. *Journal of Pharmacology and Experimental Therapeutics*, 117: 82–88.

Bohus, B., and de Wied, D. (1966): Inhibitory and facilitory effect of two related peptides on extinction of avoidance behavior. *Science*, 153:318–320.

Brewer, E. M., Foster, L. B., and Sells, B. H. (1969): A possible role for ribonuclease in the regulation of protein synthesis in normal and hypophysectomized rats. *Journal of Biological Chemistry*, 244:1389–1392.

Burton, K. (1956): A study of the conditions and mechanism of the diphenylamine reaction for the colorimetric estimation of deoxyribonucleic acid. *Biochemical Journal*, 62:315–323.

Cardell, R. R. (1967): Subcellular alterations in rat liver following hypophysectomy. *Biochimica et Biophysica Acta*, 148:539–552.

Cheek, D. B., and Graystone, J. E. (1969): Action of insulin, growth hormone and epinephrine on cell growth in liver, muscle and brain of the hypophysectomized rat. *Pediatric Research*, 3:77–88.

De Maio, D. (1959): Influence of adrenalectomy and hypophysectomy on cerebral serotonin. *Science*, 129:1678–1679.

DeVellis, J., and Inglish, D. (1968): Hormonal control of glycerol phosphate dehydrogenase in the rat brain. *Journal of Neurochemistry*, 15:1061–1070.

Dunn, A. I., and Korner, A. (1966): Hypophysectomy and amino acid incorporation in a rat brain cell-free system. *Biochemical Journal*, 100:76P.

Foster, L. B., and Sells, B. H. (1969): Functional capacity of intact and hybrid ribosomes from livers of normal and hypophysectomized rats. *Archives of Biochemistry and Biophysics*, 132:561–564.

Fuxe, K., Corrodi, H., Hökfelt, T., and Jonsson, G. (1970): Central monoamine neurons and pituitary-adrenal activity. *Progress in Brain Research*, 32:42–56.

Geel, S. E., and Timiras, P. S. (1970): The role of hormones in cerebral protein metabolism. In: *Protein Metabolism of the Nervous System*, edited by A. Lajtha. Plenum Press, New York, pp. 335–353.

Gispen, W. H., de Wied, D., Schotman, P., and Jansz, H. S. (1970): Effects of hypophysectomy on RNA metabolism in rat brainstem. *Journal of Neurochemistry*, 17:751–761.

Gispen, W. H., de Wied, D., Schotman, P., and Jansz, H. S. (1971): Brainstem polysomes and avoidance performance of hypophysectomized rats subjected to peptide treatment. *Brain Research*, 31:341–351.

Gispen, W. H., Schotman, P., and de Kloet, E. R.: Brain RNA and hypophysectomy: A topographical study. *Neuroendocrinology* (*in press*).

Hofmann, K., Wingender, W., and Finn, F. M. (1970): Correlation of adrenocorticotropic activity of ACTH analogs with degree of binding to an adrenal cortical particulate preparation. *Proceedings of the National Academy of Sciences*, 67:829–836.

Hyyppä, M., and Valavaara, M. (1970): Effect of castration and hypophysectomy on the content of noradrenaline and serotonin in the hypothalamus of the rat. *Experientia*, 26:193–194.

Jakoubek, B., Semiginovský, B, and Dědičová, A. (1971): The effect of ACTH on the synthesis of protein in spinal motoneurons as studied by autoradiography. *Brain Research*, 25:133–141.

Korner, A. (1964): Regulation of the rate of synthesis of messenger ribonucleic acid by growth hormone. *Biochemical Journal*, 92:449–456.

Korner, A. (1969): The hormonal control of protein synthesis. *Biochemical Journal*, 115:30P–31P.

Lajtha, A., and Töth, I. (1961): The brain barrier system II. Uptake and transport of amino acids by the brain. *Journal of Neurochemistry*, 8:216–225.

Landsberg, L., and Axelrod, J. (1968): Influence of pituitary, thyroid, and adrenal hormones on norepinephrine turnover and metabolism in the rat heart. *Circulation Research*, 22:559–571.

Laverty, R., and Taylor, K. M. (1968): The fluorometric assay of catecholamines and related compounds. *Analytical Biochemistry*, 22:269–279.

Libertun, C., Moguilevsky, J. A., Schiaffini, O., and Foglia, V. G. (1969): Effects of hypophysectomy on the oxidative and glycolytic metabolism of hypothalamus. *Experientia*, 25:196–197.

Moguilevsky, J. A., Libertun, C., and Foglia, V. G. (1970): Oxidative metabolism of the hypothalamus in hypophysectomized-castrated rats. *Experientia*, 26:421–422.

Mueller, R. A., Thoenen, H., and Axelrod, J. (1970): Effect of pituitary and ACTH on the maintenance of basal tyrosine hydroxylase activity in the rat adrenal gland. *Endocrinology*, 86:751–755.

Munro, H. N., and Fleck, A. (1966): The determination of nucleic acids. In: *Methods of Biochemical Analysis*, vol. XIV, edited by D. Glick. Interscience Publishers. New York, pp. 113–176.

Neff, N. H., and Tozer, T. N. (1968): In vivo measurement of brain serotonin turnover. *Advances in Pharmacology*, 6A:97–109.

Reiss, M. (1961): Hormones in mental disease. In: *Chemical Pathology of the Nervous System; Proceedings of the 3rd International Neurochemical Symposium* (Strasbourg, 1958), edited by J. Folch-Pi. Pergamon Press, New York, pp. 432–455.

Reiss, M., and Rees, D. S. (1947): Pituitary and carbohydrate metabolism of the brain. *Endocrinology*, 41:437–440.

Resnick, R. H., and Gray, S. J. (1961): Serotonin release by hydrochloric acid: Possibility of a feed-back mechanism. *American Journal of Physiology*, 201:1017–1019.

Shchedrina, R. N. (1970): Correlation of hypothalamic and adrenal catechol amines during hypophysectomy. *Doklady Akademiĭ Nauk SSSR*, 194:475–477.

Takahashi, S., Penn, M. W., Lajtha, A., and Reiss, M. (1970): Influence of growth hormone on phenylalanine incorporation into rat brain protein. In: *Protein Metabolism of the Nervous System*, edited by A. Lajtha. Plenum Press, New York, pp. 355–366.

Weinshilboum, R., and Axelrod, J. (1970): Dopamine-β-hydroxylase activity in the rat after hypophysectomy. *Endocrinology*, 87:894–899.

de Wied, D. (1964): Influence of anterior pituitary on avoidance learning and escape behaviour. *American Journal of Physiology*, 207:255–259.

de Wied, D. (1966): Inhibitory effect of ACTH and related peptides on extinction of conditioned avoidance behaviour in rats. *Proceedings of the Society for Experimental Biology and Medicine,* 122:28–32.

de Wied, D. (1969): Effects of peptide hormones on behaviour. In: *Frontiers in Neuroendocrinology,* edited by W. F. Ganong and L. Martini. Oxford University Press, London, pp. 97–140.

de Wied, D., Bohus, B., and Greven, H. M. (1968): Influence of pituitary and adrenocortical hormones on conditioned avoidance behaviour in rats. In: *Endocrinology and Human Behaviour,* edited by R. P. Michael. Oxford University Press, London, pp. 188–199.

de Wied, D., van Delft, A. M. L., Gispen, W. H., Weijnen, J. A. W. M., and van Wimersma Greidanus, Tj. B. (*in press*): The role of pituitary-adrenal system hormones in active avoidance conditioning. *Hormones and Behavior,* edited by S. Levine. Academic Press, New York (*in press*).

van Wimersma Greidanus, Tj. B., and de Wied, D. (1971): Effects of systemic and intracerebral administration of two opposite acting ACTH-related peptides on extinction of conditioned avoidance behaviour. *Neuroendocrinology,* 7:291–301.

Yeh, S. D., Solomon, J. D., and Chow, B. F. (1959): Influence of vitamin B_6 on tissue serotonin levels in rats. *Federation Proceedings,* 18:357.

Advances in Biochemical Psychopharmacology, Vol. 6
Raven Press, New York © 1972

Effect of L-DOPA on S-Adenosylmethionine Levels and Norepinephrine Metabolism in Rat Brain

R. J. Wurtman

Massachusetts Institute of Technology, Cambridge, Massachusetts 02139

It has generally been assumed that L-DOPA produces its therapeutic effect in Parkinson's disease by being converted to dopamine in the surviving neurons of the nigro-neostriatal tract. However, it has never been demonstrated that a major fraction of administered L-DOPA actually undergoes this fate. Endogenous L-DOPA is normally transformed to dopamine within the neurons and chromaffin cells that synthesize it from L-tyrosine. Little, if any, of the amino acid is released into the bloodstream or can be measured within the mammalian brain. Conversely, administered L-DOPA is carried by the circulation to every cell in the body. Moreover, because of its structural similarity to circulating L-phenylalanine and L-tyrosine, L-DOPA apparently is taken up by all cells and transformed within most of them by enzymes that are widely distributed in the body (e.g., catechol-O-methyl transferase, DOPA decarboxylase).[1]

We have examined the metabolic fate of administered L-DOPA in rats and mice and have observed that very little of the amino acid is converted to brain dopamine. Moreover, so much of the circulating amino acid is O-methylated that concentrations of the methyl donor S-adenosylmethionine (SAMe) in brain and other tissues are transiently depressed, causing an impairment in the methylation of other endogenous substrates (e.g., norepinephrine and dopamine).

---

[1] Skeletal muscle appears to differ from most other tissues in that it concentrates administered L-DOPA more effectively than any other tissue, but metabolizes very little of the amino acid by O-methylation or decarboxylation (Ordonez, Romero, and Wurtman, 1972). Muscle may thus function as a tissue reservoir for exogenous L-DOPA.

Isotopically labeled L-DOPA (10 to 100 mg/kg, administered intraperitoneally) was given to mice. The animals were killed after various intervals and their brains and the rest of the carcass assayed separately for unchanged ¹⁴C-DOPA, ¹⁴C-dopamine, and the major deaminated and O-methylated ¹⁴C-metabolites of these compounds (Wurtman, Chou, and Rose, 1970a). The administered L-DOPA was rapidly metabolized by O-methylation (Fig. 1); after 20 min, 59% had been transformed to such O-methylated catechols as 3-O-methyl-DOPA or to homovanillic acid (HVA) (Table 1). At no time was more than 0.02% of the injected dose of ¹⁴C-DOPA detectable in the brains as either ¹⁴C-dopamine or unchanged ¹⁴C-DOPA.

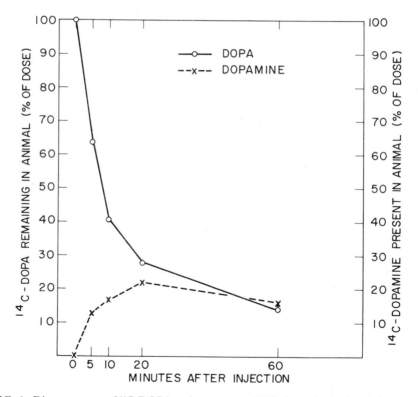

FIG. 1. Disappearance of ¹⁴C-DOPA and appearance of ¹⁴C-dopamine in the whole mouse. Animals were killed 5, 10, 20, or 60 min after receiving ¹⁴C-DOPA (0.5 μC, 0.5 mg/kg) intraperitoneally, and homogenized in nine volumes of 0.4 N perchloric acid. The ¹⁴C-DOPA and ¹⁴C-dopamine present in the supernatants after centrifugation at 10,000 × g were assayed by column chromatography. (Reprinted from Wurtman et al., 1970a.)

TABLE 1. *Identity of radioactive metabolites in whole mice 20 min after administration of ^{14}C-DOPA*

	Percentage of metabolite	
	Average	Range
Alumina eluate	41	32–47
DOPA	21	18–27
Catecholamines	19	15–21
Unidentified compounds	1	0–3
Alumina effluent	59	53–68
Homovanillic acid	20	18–26
3-O-methyl-DOPA	30	24–33
Unidentified compounds	9	6–15

Six mice received 5 μC (5 to 6 mg/kg) of ^{14}C-DOPA intraperitoneally. The homovanillic acid fraction might have contained small amounts of neutral O-methylated metabolites of ^{14}C-DOPA. (Data reprinted from Wurtman et al., 1970*a*.)

The extensive O-methylation of administered L-DOPA caused a marked decline (by 70 to 90%) in levels of the methyl donor SAMe (assayed by the method of Baldessarini and Kopin, 1966) in rat brain (Wurtman, Rose, Matthysse, Stephenson, and Baldessarini, 1970*b*) (Table 2). This decrease was maximal 45 to 60 min after L-DOPA injection, but persisted for less than 3 hr (Fig. 2) (i.e., only for the interval during which measurable quantities of L-DOPA were still detectable in the brain). Single doses of L-DOPA (10 mg/kg) also significantly depressed SAMe levels in the adrenal medulla; hepatic SAMe was not affected by single doses of the drug, but did decline by 20 to 25% 1 hr after the last of 10 daily doses (100 mg/kg).

TABLE 2. *Relation between dose of L-DOPA and extent of depletion of SAMe content in tissue*

	L-DOPA dose (mg/kg)			
Tissue	0	10	0.30	100
Brain	16.8 ± 0.6	16.0 ± 1.1	10.7 ± 0.3[a]	5.5 ± 0.4[a]
Adrenal	39.4 ± 1.8	19.4 ± 3.9[b]	15.1 ± 4.9[b]	14.1 ± 3.6[a]
Liver	56.8 ± 3.5	65.9 ± 2.0	71.2 + 5.3	61.4 ± 5.4

Groups of five rats received L-DOPA intraperitoneally and were killed 45 min later. Data are presented as mean concentration of SAMe (micrograms per gram of wet tissue) ± standard error of the mean.

[a] $P < 0.001$ differs from control group.

[b] $p < 0.01$ differs from control group. (Data reprinted from Wurtman et al., 1970*b*.)

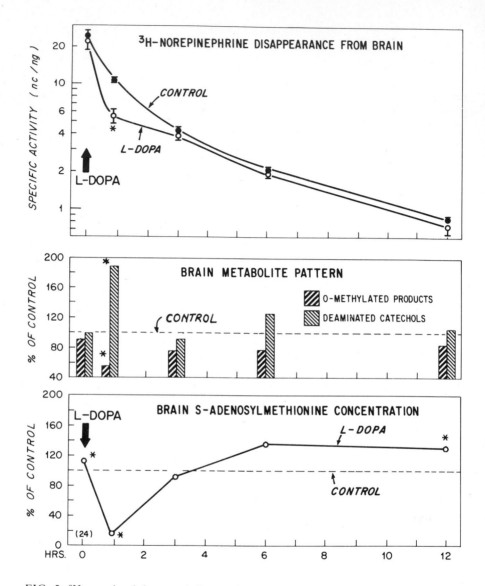

FIG. 2. ³H-norepinephrine metabolism and S-adenosylmethionine concentrations in rats given L-DOPA (100 mg/kg intraperitoneally) daily for 10 days, as described in Table 3. The "zero-time" animals had not received L-DOPA for 24 hr. Statistically significant changes calculated on the mean values are indicated by an asterisk. (Reprinted from Chalmers et al., 1971.)

To determine if the marked decrease in brain SAMe induced by L-DOPA was sufficient to interfere with the O-methylation of endogenous substrates, an isotopic label was introduced into brain norepinephrine stores by injecting tracer amounts of ^{3}H-norepinephrine intracisternally 5 min before rats received the last of 10 daily doses of L-DOPA (100 mg/kg, i.p.) (Chalmers, Baldessarini, and Wurtman, 1971). At intervals after L-DOPA administration when brain SAMe was depressed (i.e., 45 to 60 min), a profound reduction was also noted in the quantities of the methylated metabolites of ^{3}H-norepinephrine (primarily normetanephrine and VMA) present in the brain (Fig. 2). Concurrently, the concentration of unlabeled norepinephrine in the brain rose (by 15–40%), while the turnover and rate of disappearance of the ^{3}H-norepinephrine were markedly accelerated. Increases in norepinephrine content and decreases in the quantities of O-methylated ^{3}H-metabolites were detected in all brain regions examined (brain stem, cerebellum, telencephalon, hypothalamus-thalamus, and striatum) (Romero, Chalmers, Cottman, Lytle, and Wurtman, 1972).

Brain dopamine levels were also elevated by 15 to 40% after the administration of L-DOPA, both within the dopaminergic neurons of the basal ganglia and in nondopaminergic cells present in the rest of the brain. The increases in dopamine lasted for somewhat longer than those in brain norepinephrine. Three to 6 hr after the administration of L-DOPA, the turnover of brain ^{3}H-norepinephrine was markedly *slowed* in all of the brain regions mentioned except the hypothalamus (Table 3). This was the only effect of L-DOPA that we observed which occurred after L-DOPA molecules were no longer detectable in the brain. It may have resulted from a "pool effect," i.e., the L-DOPA may have caused the release of a "rapidly-turning-over" pool of ^{3}H-norepinephrine, leaving in the brain only molecules whose average rate of disappearance was slower than that of the ^{3}H-norepinephrine in brains of control animals (Hyyppa and Wurtman, *in press*).

These observations indicate that: (1) the metabolism of administered L-DOPA causes a sufficient reduction in brain SAMe to suppress the O-methylation of such endogenous substrates as norepinephrine; (2) the effects of L-DOPA on the brain are by no means restricted to the basal ganglia, to dopaminergic neurons, or even to the conversion of L-DOPA to catecholamines; and (3) the effects of L-DOPA on the SAMe and catecholamines in the brain are, for the most part, short-lived, persisting only so long as the L-DOPA itself is present in large quantities within the brain.

If the actions of L-DOPA on brain SAMe and norepinephrine participate in its therapeutic effects, it might be possible to attain similar benefit with other methyl acceptors which are not amino acids or monoamine precursors. Conversely, if these actions participate in the toxic effects of

TABLE 3. *Effects of* L-*DOPA on calculated rate of norepinephrine turnover in regions of rat brain*

Region	Interval after last L-DOPA dose (hr)		
	0–1	1–3	3–6
Striatum	185	35	30
Hypothalamus	100	140	140
Telencephalon	110	140	35
Cerebellum	150	280	45
Brain stem	145	130	70

Rats received daily intraperitoneal injections of L-DOPA (100 mg/kg) for 10 days. Twenty-four hours after the 10th injection, all rats received an intracisternal injection of ^{3}H-norepinephrine (17 μC). One group of animals was killed 5 min later to provide a zero-time point for the initial uptake of ^{3}H-norepinephrine that could be used to follow its disappearance from the brain. Three other groups of rats were given a last intraperitoneal injection of L-DOPA 5 min after the ^{3}H-norepinephrine injection and were killed 1, 3, or 6 hr later. Turnover was calculated as ng/g/hr by multiplying the average norepinephrine pool size by the rate of ^{3}H-norepinephrine disappearance. The rates for each region and time interval are given as the percent of control turnover. (Data reprinted from Romero et al., 1972).

L-DOPA, it might be possible to block their occurrence (and increase the effectiveness of the L-DOPA) by inhibiting the O-methylating enzyme catechol-O-methyl transferase.

REFERENCES

Baldessarini, R. J., and Kopin, I. J. (1966): S-adenosylmethionine in brain and other tissues. *Journal of Neurochemistry,* 13:769–777.
Chalmers, J. P., Baldessarini, R. J., and Wurtman, R. J. (1971): Effects of L-DOPA on brain norepinephrine metabolism. *Proceedings of the National Academy of Sciences,* 68:662–666.
Hyyppa, M., and Wurtman, R. J.: Different pools of norepinephrine in rat brain: Effects of treatment with L-DOPA. *Life Sciences. (in press).*
Ordonez, L. A., Romero, J. A., and Wurtman, R. J. (1972): Tissue distribution of L-DOPA: Evidence for a reservoir in skeletal muscle. *Fed. Proc.,* 31:589.
Romero, J. A., Chalmers, J. P., Cottman, K., Lytle, L. D., and Wurtman, R. J. (1972): Regional effects of L-dihydroxyphenylalanine (L-DOPA) on norepinephrine metabolism in rat brain. *Journal of Pharmacology and Experimental Therapeutics,* 180:277–285.
Wurtman, R. J., Chou, C., and Rose, C. (1970a): The fate of ^{14}C-dihydroxyphenylalanine (^{14}C-DOPA) in the whole mouse. *Journal of Pharmacology and Experimental Therapeutics,* 174:351–356.
Wurtman, R. J., Rose, C. M., Matthysse, S., Stephenson, J., and Baldessarini, R. J. (1970b): L-Dihydroxyphenylalanine: effect on S-adenosylmethionine in brain. *Science,* 169:395–397.

Index